Bipolar Disorder

Won-Myong Bahk • Moon-Doo Kim
Young Sup Woo • Young-Eun Jung
Editors

Bipolar Disorder

Bridging Clinical Practice and Evidence-Based Research

Springer

Editors
Won-Myong Bahk
Department of Psychiatry
College of Medicine,
The Catholic University of Korea
Seoul, Korea (Republic of)

Woo and Bahk Psychiatry Clinic
Seoul, Korea (Republic of)

Young Sup Woo
Woo and Bahk Psychiatry Clinic
Seoul, Korea (Republic of)

Moon-Doo Kim
Department of Psychiatry
Jeju National University Hospital,
School of Medicine,
Jeju National University
Jeju, Korea (Republic of)

Young-Eun Jung
Department of Psychiatry
Jeju National University Hospital,
School of Medicine,
Jeju National University
Jeju, Korea (Republic of)

ISBN 978-981-92-1322-1 ISBN 978-981-92-1323-8 (eBook)
https://doi.org/10.1007/978-981-92-1323-8

Translation from the Korean language edition: "Textbook of Bipolar Disorder, 4th edition" by Won-Myong Bahk et al., © KOONJA PUBLISHING INC. 2024. Published by KOONJA PUBLISHING INC.. All Rights Reserved.

This Springer imprint is published by the registered company Springer Nature Singapore Pte Ltd.
The registered company address is: 152 Beach Road, #21-01/04 Gateway East, Singapore 189721, Singapore

Preface: Questions Beyond the Textbook, Voices from the Clinical Frontline

Structure and Purpose: Why We Revisit Bipolar Disorder

For those of us in psychiatry, bipolar disorder remains both a source of intellectual fascination and a formidable clinical challenge. Despite the abundance of research findings and increasingly sophisticated treatment guidelines, the lived realities of the patients who enter our consultation rooms seldom conform neatly to textbook descriptions. While academic texts present a seemingly clear dichotomy of "alternating mania and depression," the individuals we encounter in daily practice often inhabit far more ambiguous terrain. They struggle within the blurred boundaries of mixed states, or they experience destabilizing mood episodes following antidepressant treatment initially prescribed for what appeared to be unipolar depression.

This volume was conceived from our shared recognition of the persistent gap between standardized academic frameworks and the complexities of real-world clinical care. We have intentionally moved away from the conventional model of compiling exhaustive theoretical knowledge. Instead, we have chosen to focus on the questions that continue to surface in the minds of clinicians—even those with years of experience. How can we meaningfully restore cognitive function in a patient whose mood symptoms have stabilized but whose executive abilities remain impaired? What guidance can we responsibly provide to a woman with bipolar disorder who wishes to become pregnant? How should we navigate treatment decisions when evidence-based recommendations intersect with deeply personal life circumstances?

These are not abstract inquiries. They are the daily questions of clinical practice.

Four Chapters Written in the Language of Clinical Reality

The architecture of this book reflects the natural progression of clinical reasoning. In Section I (Concepts and Diagnosis), we move beyond a simple recitation of diagnostic criteria. While established definitions are indispensable, they are often insufficient when confronted with the subtle distinctions between hypomania and normative temperament, or between bipolar depression and unipolar major depressive disorder. Accordingly, we present refined conceptual and practical tools intended to illuminate these gray zones and to support more confident diagnostic discernment.

In Sections II and III (Diverse Populations and Treatment), we explore the heterogeneity of bipolar disorder across the lifespan and across specific clinical contexts. We examine how the disorder manifests in women, in older adults, and in children and adolescents—populations in whom symptom expression and treatment response may diverge significantly from prototypical adult presentations. We also engage in a candid appraisal of antidepressant use in bipolar disorder, acknowledging both its potential benefits and its inherent risks. Importantly, we consider non-pharmacological interventions and multimodal strategies that extend beyond what guideline algorithms alone can resolve.

Perhaps the most distinctive dimension of this volume lies in Section IV (Miscellaneous). Traditional medical texts frequently confine themselves to symptomatology and pharmacotherapy. In contrast, we have deliberately widened the lens. We consider not only the disorder itself but also the person who lives with it—and the social and relational world that shapes their experience. What evidence-based reassurance can we offer to a parent overwhelmed by anxiety about the heritability of illness? How should we interpret the long-standing cultural association between "madness" and creativity in figures such as Van Gogh or Schumann? Are these merely romanticized narratives, or might they offer nuanced insights into the vulnerabilities and potentials present within our patients?

We do not regard such topics as peripheral. On the contrary, we believe that attention to these humanistic and societal dimensions is indispensable. To treat bipolar disorder effectively, we must see beyond diagnostic labels and engage with the whole person.

Responding to the Solitary Questions of the Clinic

This book does not aspire to function as a manual of definitive answers. Psychiatry, perhaps more than any other medical discipline, resists reduction to absolute certainty. Rather, this volume represents a gesture of solidarity toward fellow clinicians who persistently question, reflect, and strive to provide the best possible care amid uncertainty.

When the authority of textbooks reaches its limits, we hope that the practical reflections and multidimensional perspectives gathered here may serve as a modest but steady source of orientation within the consultation room. Our confidence does not lie in the illusion of complete understanding, but in the shared commitment to remain intellectually rigorous and emotionally present. As long as we continue to confront our patients' suffering with sincerity and perseverance, we believe that the intricate puzzle of bipolar disorder will gradually reveal a more coherent and meaningful picture.

As we brought this work to completion, we found ourselves reflecting on the countless conversations that have unfolded across our desks over the years. The moments that tested us most profoundly were not those in which we lacked familiarity with the latest data or clinical trials. Rather, they were the moments when neither evidence-based guidelines nor statistical probabilities could provide the singular, reassuring answer sought by the patient sitting before us in tears.

Patients ask questions that pierce beyond epidemiology:
"Why did this happen to me?"
"Will my child inherit this suffering?"
"Is there truly no alternative to this medication?"

Such questions inhabit the intersection of medicine and existential reflection. They demand more than numerical risk estimates; they call for thoughtful, humane engagement. We believe that to avoid these questions would be to abdicate a fundamental responsibility of care. For this reason, topics that might traditionally be relegated to a "Miscellaneous" section have, in this book, been granted structural and conceptual prominence. Addressing the distress of a patient's child, acknowledging the burdens entwined with creativity, and recognizing the silent grief carried by families are not tangential concerns—they may, in fact, lie at the heart of therapeutic work.

The process of compiling this volume has also reminded us that we are not solitary in our uncertainties. Within the contributions of colleagues from diverse subspecialties, we encountered reflections shaped by long nights of deliberation and shared clinical dilemmas. We are fellow travelers on a road without final answers, striving together to place clearer markers along its course.

As clinicians and as human beings, it is our collective hope that this book conveys to you, the reader, a simple but essential reassurance: you are not alone in confronting these complexities. If this volume provides even a small measure of clarity—or a renewed sense of courage as you begin tomorrow's consultations—then our efforts will have been worthwhile.

Seoul, Republic of Korea — Won-Myong Bahk
Jeju, Republic of Korea — Moon-Doo Kim
Seoul, Republic of Korea — Young Sup Woo
Jeju, Republic of Korea — Young-Eun Jung

Contents

Part I Concepts and Diagnosis

1 **Understanding and Applying Useful Instruments to Evaluate Bipolar Spectrum Disorder** 3
Sung-Yong Park and Bo-Hyun Yoon

2 **Distinguishing Bipolar Depression from Unipolar Depression and Its Clinical Significance** 13
Saeheon Jang and Duk-In Jon

3 **Mixed Features: Challenges in Diagnosis and Treatment** 29
In Hee Shim and Jong-Hyun Jeong

4 **Cognitive Dysfunction in Bipolar Disorder: A Comprehensive Review of Clinical Evidence and Implications** 41
Kang Soo Lee and Young-Min Park

5 **Normal, Hypomanic, and Manic States: Key Differences and Their Implications** 53
Jeongwan Hong and Moon-Doo Kim

Part II Bipolar Disorder in Diverse Populations and Clinical Contexts

6 **The Significance of Bipolar Disorder in Women** 63
Hangoeunbi Kang, Jyeheon Song, and Beomwoo Nam

7 **Characteristics and Treatment of Bipolar Disorder in the Elderly** 77
Eunsoo Moon and Jung goo Lee

8 **Child and Adolescent Bipolar Disorder** 89
MoonSoo Lee and Se Hoon Shim

9 **Bipolar Disorder and Attention-Deficit/Hyperactivity Disorder (ADHD): Importance and Differential Diagnosis** 101
Hyun-Ju Yang and Young-Eun Jung

10 **Obesity and Metabolic Syndrome in Bipolar Disorder** 109
Sung Hoon Yoon and Young Sup Woo

11 **Bipolar Disorder and Addiction** ... 123
Eunsung Lim and Inki Sohn

12 **Suicide in Bipolar Disorder** ... 133
Won-Seok Choi and Kyung Joon Min

Part III Treatment

13 **Pros and Cons: The Usefulness of Antidepressants in Bipolar Depressive Episodes** ... 145
Jeong Seok Seo and Kwanghun Lee

14 **Comparative Analysis of Bipolar Disorder Treatment Guidelines** ... 161
Chan-Mo Yang and Won-Myong Bahk

15 **Biological Non-pharmacological Treatments for Bipolar Disorder** ... 177
Min-Kyu Song and Jonghun Lee

Part IV Miscellaneous

16 **The Impact of Parental Bipolar Disorder on Children** ... 187
Chan-Mo Yang and Hyung-Mo Sung

17 **Historical Figures and Bipolar Disorder** ... 199
Jee Hyun Ha and Sang-Yeol Lee

18 **Bipolar Disorder and Creativity** ... 205
Won Kim and Young Joon Kwon

Part I

Concepts and Diagnosis

Understanding and Applying Useful Instruments to Evaluate Bipolar Spectrum Disorder

1

Sung-Yong Park and Bo-Hyun Yoon

The Importance of Early Detection and Assessment Tools in Bipolar Disorder

Bipolar disorder is one of the most common psychiatric conditions associated with significant disability. It is frequently comorbid with other disorders and is linked to high rates of suicide and unemployment, thereby imposing a considerable burden on individuals and society [1, 2]. Delayed diagnosis often exacerbates this burden, highlighting the importance of early detection. In this context, clinical assessment tools can serve as valuable resources for timely identification.

In cases of bipolar II disorder, bipolar disorder not otherwise specified (NOS), and subthreshold mania, patients often fail to recognize their own hypomanic or manic symptoms. As a result, they are less likely to seek clinical help. Even when patients do visit mental health services, they typically present during depressive episodes and may not report past hypomanic symptoms, making accurate diagnosis difficult [3].

In contrast, bipolar I disorder presents with distinct clinical features that meet the DSM-V (*Diagnostic and Statistical Manual of Mental Disorders, Fifth Edition*) criteria for manic episodes, making diagnosis more straightforward. In such cases, assessment tools are used not only to aid in diagnosis but also to objectively evaluate symptom severity and treatment response.

Therefore, regardless of a clinician's experience, standardized assessment tools are essential for increasing diagnostic accuracy and objectively measuring the severity of symptoms. They play a critical role in improving the detection and management of bipolar disorder.

Although structured diagnostic tools such as the Structured Clinical Interview for DSM-V (SCID-5) can be used to ensure diagnostic accuracy, they are often time-consuming and thus difficult to implement in routine clinical practice. In contrast, screening tools with high sensitivity and specificity are generally brief, easy to administer, and can be used even by evaluators without extensive professional training, making them highly practical in real-world settings.

However, concerns have recently been raised regarding the validity of screening tools used to identify bipolarity. One major criticism is that, from a methodological standpoint, these tools often demonstrate low diagnostic accuracy, particularly in the form of high false-positive rates [4].

Currently, several assessment tools are widely utilized for the evaluation of bipolar spectrum disorders. These include the Young Mania Rating Scale (YMRS) [5], the Bipolar Depression Rating Scale (BDRS) [6], the Mood Disorder Questionnaire (MDQ) [7], the Bipolar Spectrum

S.-Y. Park (✉)
Department of Psychiatry, Keyo Hospital,
Uiwang, Republic of Korea

B.-H. Yoon
Department of Psychiatry, Naju National Hospital,
Naju, Republic of Korea

W.-M. Bahk et al. (eds.), *Bipolar Disorder*, https://doi.org/10.1007/978-981-92-1323-8_1

Diagnostic Scale (BSDS) [8], and the Hypomania Checklist-32 (HCL-32) [9]. This chapter aims to provide a detailed overview of the key features of these instruments, as well as to discuss their limitations and clinical implications.

Young Mania Rating Scale (YMRS)

The Young Mania Rating Scale (YMRS) has long been one of the most widely used instruments for assessing manic symptoms. Young et al. introduced an 11-item clinician-administered Mania Rating Scale (MRS) and validated its reliability, validity, and sensitivity [5]. The results showed significant correlations between each of the 11 symptom items and the total YMRS score (Spearman's $rs = 0.41–0.85$), demonstrating the scale's internal homogeneity. In addition, strong agreement was found for both the total score and individual item ratings ($r = 0.93$ and $r = 0.66–0.95$, respectively; $p < 0.001$).

The YMRS is a clinician-rated tool designed to objectively assess manic symptoms. It consists of 11 items that evaluate the following core domains of mania:

1. Elevated mood (0~4 points)
2. Increased motor activity–energy (0~4 points)
3. Sexual interest (0~4 points)
4. Sleep (0~4 points)
5. Irritability (0~8 points)
6. Speech (rate and amount) (0~8 points)
7. Language–thought disorder (0~4 points)
8. Content (0~8 points)
9. Disruptive–aggressive behavior (0~8 points)
10. Appearance (0~4 points)
11. Insight (0~4 points)

Each item is scored on a 5-point scale (0–4), but for patients with more severe symptoms—particularly those who are uncooperative or provide insufficient information—four items (irritability, speech, content, and disruptive–aggressive behavior) are weighted double to compensate for limited self-reporting.

The scale is administered through a 15- to 30-minute structured clinical interview conducted by a trained clinician, evaluating the patient's behavior and subjective symptoms over the past 48 hours. Higher total scores indicate more severe manic symptoms. A total score of 20 or higher is typically considered clinically significant. According to the global severity ratings defined by Young et al. [5], the score ranges are interpreted as follows:

- 13–19: Minimal symptoms
- 20–25: Mild mania
- 26–37: Moderate mania
- 38–60: Severe mania

It is important to note that the YMRS is not appropriate for use in patients without manic symptoms.

Bipolar Depression Rating Scale (BDRS)

The Bipolar Depression Rating Scale (BDRS) was developed to assess the severity of depressive symptoms in individuals with bipolar disorder, including those presenting with mixed features and atypical symptom patterns [6]. Conventional depression rating scales commonly used in clinical settings—such as the Hamilton Depression Rating Scale (HAM-D) and the Montgomery–Åsberg Depression Rating Scale (MADRS)—were designed and validated primarily for major depressive disorder and focus on its core symptoms. As such, they often fail to capture the unique clinical features of bipolar depression.

Bipolar depression differs from unipolar depression in several significant ways. It tends to occur equally in men and women, has an earlier age of onset, and is characterized by more abrupt mood episode onset and remission. Patients are more likely to experience psychotic features, substance abuse, a family history of bipolar disorder, frequent recurrences, and atypical depressive symptoms such as hypersomnia and fatigue. Despite their limitations, general depression scales like HAM-D and MADRS have still been widely used in patients with bipolar disorder.

The BDRS specifically aims to evaluate both current and recent depressive and mixed symptoms. It comprises 20 items:

- Items 1–15 assess core depressive symptoms. Among these, items 2 and 3 specifically measure changes in sleep and appetite, which are commonly altered in bipolar depression.
- Items 16–20 evaluate mixed features often observed in bipolar depression.

Each item is scored on a 4-point Likert scale (0–3). Items may be assessed subjectively (based on patient self-report), objectively (based on the clinician's observation), or through a combined evaluation. In cases where subjective and objective ratings differ, greater weight should be given to the objective evaluation. If the clinician finds that a symptom's severity falls between two scores and additional questioning does not clarify the rating, the higher (more severe) score should be assigned.

Mood Disorder Questionnaire (MDQ)

The Mood Disorder Questionnaire (MDQ) is a self-report screening tool and is currently one of the most widely used instruments for identifying bipolar disorder [7]. It has been translated into numerous languages and has demonstrated global utility and reliability as a screening tool for bipolarity [10–12].

The MDQ consists of three sections:

- Section 1 contains 13 yes/no items that assess the lifetime presence of manic or hypomanic symptoms.
- Section 2 asks whether two or more symptoms occurred during the same time period.
- Section 3 assesses the degree of functional impairment caused by these symptoms.

Its brevity and ease of administration make the MDQ suitable for use in various clinical and community settings.

The original developers of the MDQ proposed that a positive screen for bipolar disorder is indicated when the respondent (1) endorses seven or more symptoms in Section 1, (2) confirms that several of these symptoms occurred simultaneously (Section 2), and (3) reports that these symptoms caused moderate or severe functional impairment (Section 3). In clinical validation studies, this criterion yielded a sensitivity of 73% and specificity of 90%, making it a reasonably effective screening tool [10].

However, when applied to the general population, the sensitivity dropped dramatically to 28%, indicating significant limitations in non-clinical samples [11]. In one Korean study by Bae et al. [13] involving university students, more than half of the participants scored above the threshold in Section 1, highlighting the difficulty of using the MDQ to screen for bipolar spectrum disorders in general populations.

To improve the MDQ's sensitivity, several researchers have proposed modifying or eliminating Section 3, as requiring moderate to severe impairment can reduce sensitivity excessively [14–18]. Some studies have reported optimal sensitivity and specificity when using only the 13 symptom items from Section 1 [19].

While the MDQ demonstrates adequate sensitivity and specificity in many clinical contexts, it consistently shows limitations in detecting bipolar II disorder and bipolar spectrum conditions, which often involve subtler symptoms [23, 24]. In response to this, some researchers have argued for excluding Section 3 to improve sensitivity in detecting these milder presentations [14–23].

Hypomania Checklist-32 (HCL-32)

The Hypomania Checklist-32 (HCL-32) was developed by Angst et al. to identify hypomanic symptoms in the general population and in individuals with major depressive disorder [24]. The tool consists of 32 self-report yes/no items assessing symptoms of mania or hypomania. In addition to these core symptom items, the checklist also includes questions assessing symptom severity, duration, and the positive or negative subjective experiences resulting from these symptoms across various functional domains. Compared to the MDQ, the HCL-32 requires more time to complete due to its broader scope. A revised version of the tool, the HCL-32-R2, which includes the original 32 items plus 2 additional items (e.g., *"I gamble more," "I eat more"*), has recently been developed and utilized.

In an initial validation study, a cutoff score of 14 on the HCL-32 yielded a sensitivity of 80% and a specificity of 51% for detecting bipolar spectrum disorders [24]. Although its specificity was lower than that of the MDQ in clinical samples, the HCL-32's higher sensitivity offers an advantage in identifying at-risk individuals, which is a critical function of screening tools. The positive predictive value (PPV) was 73%, and the negative predictive value (NPV) was 63%, suggesting adequate discriminatory power even when applied to general populations, where the base rate of bipolar spectrum disorders is relatively low. Cross-validation studies comparing the MDQ and HCL-32 have reported that the HCL-32 generally performs better in identifying bipolar spectrum disorders [25–27].

While most studies have used a cutoff of 14 [24, 26, 27], more recent research has reported improved performance at different thresholds (e.g., sensitivity 85%, specificity 78%) [28]. In a study conducted in China, a cutoff of 14 distinguished bipolar disorder from major depressive disorder, while a cutoff of 12 differentiated bipolar II disorder from major depression with sensitivity 86% and specificity 69%. However, neither cutoff was effective in distinguishing bipolar I from bipolar II disorder [29]. Conversely, Wu et al. reported that a cutoff of 21 could distinguish bipolar I from bipolar II with sensitivity 64% and specificity 73%, though these findings require further replication [27].

The HCL-32-R2, which incorporates two additional behavioral items (e.g., increased gambling and eating), shows similar psychometric properties to the original HCL-32, with a sensitivity of 82% and specificity of 57% [30].

In a recent Korean study, Yoon et al. examined the validity of the Korean version of the HCL-32-R2 [31] and found that:

- At a cutoff score of 16, the tool distinguished major depressive disorder from bipolar I disorder with sensitivity 73% and specificity 70%.
- At a cutoff of 15, it differentiated major depressive disorder from bipolar II disorder with sensitivity 67% and specificity 67%.

However, similar to previous findings, the HCL-32-R2 could not reliably distinguish between bipolar I and bipolar II disorders. The tool's positive predictive value (76%) and negative predictive value (63%) suggest it is a useful screening instrument for identifying bipolarity in clinical settings.

Hypomanic Personality Scale (HPS)

Among screening tools for bipolar spectrum disorders, instruments such as the Mood Disorder Questionnaire (MDQ) and the Hypomania Checklist-32 (HCL-32) have shown good validity when used with clinical populations. However, their validity in the general population remains limited [32, 33]. This limitation highlights the need for tools that can detect subtle hypomanic or manic-like symptoms in individuals who have limited insight into psychiatric symptoms and do not experience significant functional impairment—characteristics common in community samples [34].

The Hypomanic Personality Scale (HPS) was developed specifically to measure hypomanic traits in non-clinical populations. It is one of the most widely used tools for assessing vulnerability to bipolar spectrum disorders. The HPS is easy to interpret, quick to administer, and consists of true/false (yes/no) items, which contributes to its brevity and user-friendliness [35, 36].

Recent years have seen active cross-cultural adaptation and validation of the HPS in various countries. It is commonly used to identify hypomanic or manic-like tendencies in research samples, thus aiding in the valid selection of experimental groups or in distinguishing between population subtypes [37]. Furthermore, the HPS has been employed to understand maladaptive personality traits and predict real-life dysfunction in ecological momentary assessment (EMA) studies [38–40]. These uses demonstrate the HPS's utility beyond screening—extending into personality research and studies on psychological resilience and stress response.

In sum, the HPS is useful not only for identifying individuals at high risk for bipolar disorder, but also for detecting bipolar-like subclinical symptoms, understanding personality profiles, and predicting functional adaptation and reactivity to stress.

Bipolar Spectrum Diagnostic Scale (BSDS)

The Bipolar Spectrum Diagnostic Scale (BSDS) was developed by Pies et al. as a screening tool intended to facilitate the early identification of individuals exhibiting relatively mild symptoms within the bipolar spectrum [8]. The BSDS was specifically designed to overcome the limitations of the Mood Disorder Questionnaire (MDQ), which, although highly sensitive in detecting bipolar I disorder, demonstrates relatively lower sensitivity in identifying bipolar II disorder and bipolar disorder not otherwise specified (NOS).

The BSDS consists of two main components. The first part includes a narrative passage incorporating 19 symptom items related to bipolar disorder. Respondents are instructed to read through the passage and mark each statement that accurately reflects their personal experience, with 1 point awarded for each marked item,

The second part asks respondents to evaluate how well the overall narrative applies to them. They are given four response options:

- "This story fits me very well, or almost perfectly"—6 points
- "This story fits me fairly well"—4 points
- "This story fits me to some degree, but not in most respects"—2 points
- "This story does not describe me at all"—0 points

The maximum total score is 25 points, with 19 points possible from the first section and 6 points from the second. Based on validation studies, Ghaemi et al. proposed a cutoff score of 13, which yielded a sensitivity of 76% and a specificity of 85%, indicating robust diagnostic utility for identifying bipolar spectrum disorders [8].

Other Assessment Tools

The General Behavior Inventory (GBI) was developed to comprehensively assess both depressive and manic symptoms associated with bipolar disorder. Multiple versions of the GBI exist, ranging from 52 to 73 items, allowing for flexible application depending on the purpose of the assessment [41].

Other instruments include the Mood Spectrum Self-Report (MOODS-SR) [42] and the Temperament Evaluation of Memphis, Pisa, Paris, and San Diego—Auto-questionnaire version (TEMPS-A) [43]. These tools are designed to evaluate mood spectrum characteristics and affective temperaments, respectively.

Limitations and Significance of Assessment Tools for Detecting Bipolarity

As mentioned in the introduction, recent criticisms have been raised regarding assessment tools used to detect bipolarity. Notably, many patients who do not meet the diagnostic criteria for bipolar disorder according to SCID still test positive on these tools. Furthermore, patients with conditions such as post-traumatic stress disorder, substance use disorders, eating disorders, and impulse control disorders also show positive results. For example, the MDQ often yields similar positive rates in patients with borderline personality disorder as in those with bipolar disorder [44].

However, these comorbid conditions showing false positives are closely related to bipolar disorder. Especially in anxiety disorders, eating disorders, and substance abuse disorders, reports indicate that 41.4% of such cases progress to bipolar disorder [45]. Other studies have reported similarities between MDQ-positive individuals and bipolar disorder patients in terms of risk factors such as gender and age, high psychological distress, low social functioning, comorbid anxiety, alcohol and eating disorders, low employment rates, high suicide rates, frequent use of mood stabilizers and antidepressants, and high recurrence rates of depressive episodes [46].

Although these factors do not constitute the psychopathology of bipolar disorder themselves, screening tools for bipolarity can identify subthreshold bipolar patients who do not currently meet diagnostic criteria. While structured interviews like SCID can improve sensitivity in diagnosing bipolar disorder, some reports suggest that these interviews may also increase false-positive rates [47].

In conclusion, the current diagnostic rate of bipolar disorder is lower than its actual prevalence compared to major depressive disorder. Considering the potential progression from major depressive disorder to bipolar disorder, screening tools for bipolarity that identify subthreshold patients hold significant clinical value [48].

Clinical Applications and Selection Considerations

Selecting the most appropriate assessment tool for bipolar spectrum disorders requires consideration of each instrument's target population, psychometric properties, and clinical purpose. While screening tools such as the Mood Disorder Questionnaire (MDQ) and the Hypomania Checklist-32 (HCL-32) share conceptual overlap, they differ significantly in applicability and diagnostic focus.

For screening bipolar II or subthreshold bipolarity, the HCL-32 is generally preferred due to its higher sensitivity for mild hypomanic symptoms and its broader coverage of behavioral and energy-related changes. In contrast, the MDQ demonstrates superior specificity and is more efficient in busy outpatient settings where the goal is to detect clear bipolar I presentations. However, the MDQ's lower sensitivity for bipolar II and its high false-negative rate in community samples suggest caution when used in general population screening.

For depressive or mixed presentations, the Bipolar Depression Rating Scale (BDRS) extends beyond assessing pure depressive symptoms. By incorporating mixed and atypical features—such as psychomotor agitation, irritability, and energy changes—it provides valuable guidance for treatment monitoring. Clinicians can use BDRS subscale trends to evaluate the transition between depressive and hypomanic phases, adjust medication strategies (e.g., mood stabilizers vs. antidepressants), and assess residual mood instability that predicts relapse risk.

In practice, clinicians should integrate multiple instruments: use the MDQ or HCL-32 for initial screening, the YMRS for acute mania severity, and the BDRS for ongoing mood stabilization tracking. The Bipolar Spectrum Diagnostic Scale (BSDS) and Hypomanic Personality Scale (HPS) may supplement this process in cases with unclear longitudinal histories or when personality factors and subthreshold bipolarity are suspected (Table 1.1).

Summary

The YMRS is useful for monitoring the severity of manic symptoms and treatment response but has limitations in cases involving depressive or mixed episodes. The BDRS is effective for evaluating mixed features and atypical presentations observed in bipolar depression. The MDQ is the most widely translated and used screening tool,

Table 1.1 Summary comparison of bipolar spectrum disorder assessment instruments

Instrument	Items	Type	Strengths	Limitations	Target population	Psychometric highlights
YMRS (Young Mania Rating Scale)	11	Clinician--rated	Sensitive to manic symptom change; gold standard for mania severity	Not suitable for depressive or mixed states	clinical; inpatient/ outpatient	$r = 0.93$ (inter-rater); strong internal validity
BDRS (Bipolar Depression Rating Scale)	20	Clinician--rated	Captures atypical and mixed depressive features; guides treatment	Requires trained clinician; moderate administration time	Bipolar depression; mixed states	Sensitivity 85%; good construct validity
MDQ (Mood Disorder Questionnaire)	13 (+2)	Self-report	Brief, easy, high specificity	Low sensitivity for bipolar II; false negatives in general population	clinical and community	Sensitivity 73%; specificity 90%
HCL-32 (Hypomania Checklist-32)	32	Self-report	High sensitivity for subthreshold mania; broader behavioral coverage	Lower specificity; longer completion time	Bipolar II; MDD; community samples	Sensitivity 80%; specificity 51–78%
BSDS (Bipolar Spectrum Diagnostic Scale)	25	Self-report (narrative)	Effective for bipolar II and NOS; user-friendly	Subjective interpretation of narrative	Outpatient and research	Sensitivity 76%; specificity 85%
HPS (Hypomanic Personality Scale)	48	Self-report	Measures trait vulnerability; useful for research	Not standardized, limited clinical data	Non-clinical; personality research	$\alpha =$ 0.84–0.87; predictive validity for bipolarity
GBI (General Behavior Inventory)	52–73	Self-report	Comprehensive; covers depressive and hypomanic dimensions	Lengthy; impractical for clinics	Community; research	Sensitivity 80%; specificity 75%

with 13 brief items making it easy to administer; however, its sensitivity is lower for detecting bipolar II disorder and other unspecified bipolar disorders. To address these limitations, tools such as the HCL-32 and BSDS have been used for screening milder bipolar spectrum symptoms, but they require more time to complete and their reliability is less satisfactory compared to the MDQ. The HPS can be useful for detecting bipolar traits in the general population, but it has not yet been standardized. The GBI has demonstrated high sensitivity and specificity in general population samples, but its length of 73 items and lack of standardization limit its practical use in clinical settings.

When interpreting diagnostic tools, sensitivity and specificity are commonly considered; however, these metrics are influenced by disease prevalence. Therefore, positive predictive value (PPV) and negative predictive value (NPV) are more helpful in accounting for differences in prevalence [49]. Since the prevalence of bipolar spectrum disorders is reported to range between 3.0 and 6.5% [50, 51], general population studies gradually lower prevalence estimates from 50% to approximately 5%, while sensitivity and specificity remain unchanged. In this context, PPV decreases while NPV increases, as shown in Korean studies on the MDQ and BSDS, where NPV

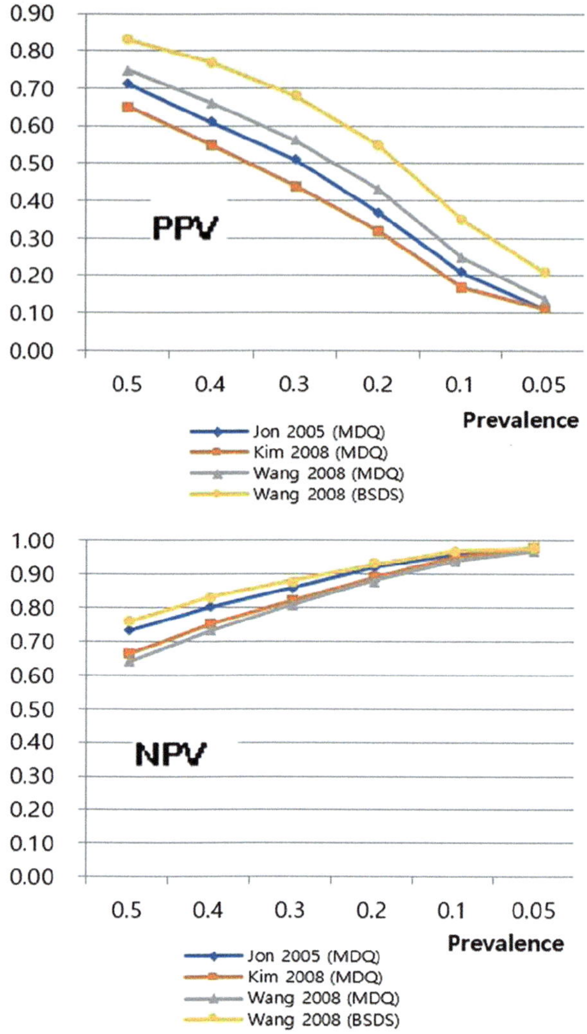

Fig. 1.1 Changes in positive predictive value (PPV) and negative predictive value (NPV) according to the prevalence of bipolar spectrum disorders. As prevalence decreases (e.g., from clinical samples to general populations), PPV markedly declines while NPV increases. This demonstrates that screening tools are more useful in clinical populations with higher base rates of bipolarity. (Adapted from [48, 49])

reached 0.97–0.98 at general population prevalence levels [2, 16, 28]. Thus, when screening the general population, a positive test result—due to low PPV—is insufficient to confirm bipolar spectrum disorder, whereas a negative result—due to high NPV—effectively excludes the disorder with approximately 97–98% certainty. However, in clinical settings where prevalence is higher, PPV also rises, making a positive screening result a stronger indicator of bipolar spectrum disorder. Therefore, bipolar spectrum screening tools are relatively more useful in clinical environments than for general population screening (Fig. 1.1).

Declarations

Competing Interests The author(s) has no competing interests to declare that are relevant to the content of this manuscript.

Ethics Approval The author(s) declares that this manuscript does not include primary research with human participants.

The author(s) declares that this manuscript does not include primary studies involving animals.

References

1. Angst J. Bipolar disorder–a seriously underestimated health burden. Eur Arch Psychiatry Clin Neurosci. 2004;254:59–60.
2. Fajutrao L, Locklear J, Priaulx J, Heyes A. A systematic review of the evidence of the burden of bipolar disorder in Europe. Clin Pract Epidemiol Ment Health. 2004;5:3. https://doi.org/10.1186/1745-0179-5-3.
3. Hantouche EG, Akiskal HS, Lancrenon S, Allilaire JF, Sechter D, Azorin JM, et al. Systematic clinical methodology for validating bipolar-II disorder: data in mid-stream from a French national multi-site study (EPIDEP). J Affect Disord. 1998;50:163–73.
4. Zimmerman M, Galione JN, Ruggero CJ, Chelminski I, Dalrymple K, Young D. Are screening scales for bipolar disorder good enough to be used in clinical practice? Compr Psychiatry. 2011;2011(52):600–6.
5. Young RC, Biggs T, Ziegler VE, Meyer DA. A rating scale for mania: reliability, validity, and sensitivity. Br J Psychiatry. 1978;133:429–35.
6. Michael B, Gin SM, Catherine C, Catherine C, Dusan HP, Mary TH, et al. The Bipolar Depression Rating Scale (BDRS): its development, validation and utility. Bipolar Disord. 2007;9(6):571–9. https://doi.org/10.1111/j.1399-5618.2007.00536.x.
7. Hirschfeld RMA. The mood disorder questionnaire: a simple, patient-rated screening instrument for bipolar disorder. Prim Care Companion J Clin Psychiatry. 2002;4(1):9–11. https://doi.org/10.4088/pcc.v04n0104.
8. Ghaemi SN, Miller CJ, Berv DA, Klugman J, Rosenquist KJ, Pies RW. Sensitivity and specificity of a new bipolar spectrum diagnostic scale. J Affect Disord. 2005;84(2–3):273–7. https://doi.org/10.1016/S0165-0327(03)00196-4.
9. Angst J, Adolfsson R, Benazzi F, Gamma A, Hantouche E, Meyer TD, et al. The HCL-32: towards a self-assessment tool for hypomanic symptoms in outpatients. J Affect Disord. 2005;88:217–33. https://doi.org/10.1016/j.jad.2005.05.011.
10. Hirschfeld RM, Williams JB, Spitzer RL, Calabrese JR, Flynn L, Keck PE Jr, et al. Development and validation of a screening instrument for bipolar spectrum disorder: the Mood Disorder Questionnaire. Am J Psychiatry. 2000;157:1873–5.
11. Hirschfeld RM, Calabrese JR, Weissman MM, Reed M, Davies MA, Frye MA, et al. Screening for bipolar disorder in the community. J Clin Psychiatry. 2003;64:53–9.
12. Hirschfeld RMA. The mood disorder questionnaire: A simple, patient-rated screening instrument for bipolar disorder. J Clin Psychiatry. 2002;4:9–11.
13. Bae SO, Kim MD, Lee JG, Seo JS, Won SH, Woo YS, et al. Prevalence of bipolar spectrum disorder in Korean college students according to the K-MDQ. Neuropsychiatr Dis Treat. 2013;9:869–74.
14. Miller CJ, Klugman J, Berv DA, Rosenquist KJ, Ghaemi SN. Sensitivity and specificity of the Mood Disorder Questionnaire for detecting bipolar disorder. J Affect Disord. 2004;81:167–71.
15. Weber Rouget B, Gervasoni N, Dubuis V, Gex-Fabry M, Bondolfi G, Aubry JM. Screening for bipolar disorders using a French version of the Mood Disorder Questionnaire (MDQ). J Affect Disord. 2005;88:103–8.
16. Chung KF, Tso KC, Cheung E, Wong M. Validation of the Chinese version of the Mood Disorder Questionnaire in a psychiatric population in Hong Kong. Psychiatry Clin Neurosci. 2008;62(4):464–71.
17. Twiss J, Jones S, Anderson I. Validation of the Mood Disorder Questionnaire for screening for bipolar disorder in a UK sample. J Affect Disord. 2008;110:180–4.
18. Graves RE, Alim TN, Aigbogun N, Chrishon K, Mellman TA, Charney DS, et al. Diagnosing bipolar disorder in trauma exposed primary care patients. Bipolar Disord. 2007;9:318–23.
19. Kim BS, Wang HR, Son JI, Kim CY, Joo YH. Bipolarity in depressive patients without histories of diagnosis of bipolar disorder and the use of the Mood Disorder Questionnaire for detecting bipolarity. Compr Psychiatry. 2008;49:469–75.
20. Zimmerman M, Posternak MA, Chelminski I, Solomon DA. Using questionnaires to screen for psychiatric disorders: a comment on a study of screening for bipolar disorder in the community. J Clin Psychiatry. 2004;65:605–10.
21. Bennazzi F. Improving the Mood Disorder Questionnaire to detect bipolar II disorder. Can J Psychiatr. 2003;48:770–1.
22. Mago R. Bipolar disorder questionnaire. Am J Psychiatry. 2001;158:1743–4.
23. Calabrese JR, Muzina DJ, Kemp DE, Sachs GS, Frye MA, Thompson TR, et al. Predictors of bipolar disorder risk among patients currently treated for major depression. Med Gen Med. 2006;8(3):38.
24. Angst J, Adolfsson R, Benazzi F, Gamma A, Hantouche E, Meyer TD, et al. The HCL-32: towards a self-assessment tool for hypomanic symptoms in outpatients. J Affect Disord. 2005;88:217–33.
25. Carta MG, Hardoy MC, Cadeddu M, Murru A, Campus A, Morosini PL, et al. The accuracy of the Italian version of the Hypomania Checklist (HCL-32) for the screening of bipolar disorders and comparison with the Mood Disorder Questionnaire (MDQ) in a clinical sample. Clin Pract Epidemiol Ment Health. 2006;2:2. https://doi.org/10.1186/1745-0179-2-2.
26. Vieta E, Sánchez-Moreno J, Bulbena A, Chamorro L, Ramos JL, Artal J, et al. Cross validation with the mood disorder questionnaire (MDQ) of an instrument for the detection of hypomania in Spanish: the 32 item hypomania symptom check list (HCL-32). J Affect Disord. 2007;101:43–55.
27. Wu YS, Angst J, Ou CS, Chen HC, Lu RB. Validation of the Chinese version of the hypomania checklist (HCL-32) as an instrument for detecting hypo(mania)

in patients with mood disorders. J Affect Disord. 2008;106:133–43.
28. Perugi G, Fornaro M, Maremmani I, Canonico PL, Carbonatto P, Mencacci C. Discriminative Hypomania Checklist-32 factors in unipolar and bipolar major depressive patients. Psychopathology. 2012;45:390–8.
29. Yang HC, Xiang YT, Liu TB, Han R, Wang G, Hu C, et al. Hypomanic symptoms assessed by the HCL-32 in patients with major depressive disorder: a multicenter trial across China. J Affect Disord. 2012;143:203–7.
30. Gamma A, Angst J, Azorin JM, Bowden CL, Perugi G, Vieta E, et al. Transcultural validity of the Hypomania Checklist-32 (HCL-32) in patients with major depressive episodes. Bipolar Disord. 2013;15:701–12.
31. Yoon BH, Angst J, Bahk WM, Wang HR, Bae SO, Kim MD, et al. Psychometric properties of the Hypomania Checklist-32 in Korean patients with mood disorders. Clin Psychopharmacol Neurosci. 2017;15:352–60.
32. Hirschfeld RM, Holzer C, Calabrese JR, Weissman M, Reed M, Davies M, et al. Validity of the mood disorder questionnaire: a general population study. Am J Psychiatry. 2003;160:178–80.
33. Bae SO, Kim MD, Lee JG, Seo JS, Won SH, Woo YS, et al. Is it useful to use the Korean version of the mood disorder questionnaire for assessing bipolar spectrum disorder among Korean college students? Asia Pac Psychiatry. 2014;6:170–8.
34. Chu H, Lin CJ, Chiang KJ, Chen CH, Lu RB, Chou KR. Psychometric properties of the Chinese version of the Bipolar Spectrum Diagnostic Scale. J Clin Nurs. 2010;19:2787–94.
35. Ratheesh A, Berk M, Davey CG, McGorry PD, Cotton SM. Instruments that prospectively predict bipolar disorder–a systematic review. J Affect Disord. 2015;179:65–73.
36. Sperry SH, Walsh MA, Kwapil TR. Measuring the validity and psychometric properties of a short form of the Hypomanic Personality Scale. Pers Individ Dif. 2015;82:52–7.
37. Preti A, Vellante M, Zucca G, Melis M, Marrone M, Masala C, et al. The validity and reliability of the Italian version of the Hypomanic Personality Scale (I-HPS). J Psychopathol. 2017;23:35–47.
38. Walsh MA, DeGeorge DP, Barrantes-Vidal N, Kwapil TR. A 3-year longitudinal study of risk for bipolar spectrum psychopathology. J Abnorm Psychol. 2015;124:486–97.
39. Sperry SH, Kwapil TR. What can daily life assessment tell us about the bipolar spectrum? Psychiatry Res. 2017;252:51–6.
40. Stanton K, Daly E, Stasik-O'Brien SM, Ellickson-Larew S, Clark LA, Watson D. An integrative analysis of the Narcissistic Personality Inventory and the Hypomanic Personality Scale: implications for construct validity. Assessment. 2017;24:695–711.
41. Depue RA, Krauss S, Spoont MR, Arbisi D. General Behavior Inventory identification of unipolar and bipolar conditions in a non-clinical university population. J Abnorm Psychol. 1989;98:117–26.
42. Dell'Osso L, Armani A, Rucci P, Frank E, Fagiolini A, Corretti G, et al. Measuring mood spectrum: comparison of interview (SCI-MOODS) and self-report (MOODS-SR) instruments. Compr Psychiatry. 2002;43:69–73.
43. Akiskal HS, Akiskal KK, Haykal RF, Manning JS, Connor PD. TEMPS-A: progress towards validation of a self-rated clinical version of the Temperament Evaluation of the Memphis, Pisa, Paris, and San Diego Autoquestionnaire. J Affect Disord. 2005;85(1–2):3–16. https://doi.org/10.1016/j.jad.2004.12.001.
44. Zimmerman M, Galione JN, Ruggero CJ, Chelminski I, Young D, Dalrymple K, et al. Screening for bipolar disorder and finding borderline personality disorder. J Clin Psychiatry. 2010;71:1212–7.
45. Serra G, Koukopoulos A, DeChiara L, Napoletano F, Koukopoulos AE, Curto M, et al. Features preceding diagnosis of bipolar versus major depressive disorders. J Affect Disord. 2015;173:134–42.
46. Carta MG, Zairo F, Saphino D, Sevilla-Dedieu C, Moro MF, Massidda D, et al. MDQ positive people's searching for effective and ineffective treatments for Bipolar Disorders: a screening study in France. J Affect Disord. 2013;149:84–92.
47. Kessler RC, Akiskal HS, Angst J, Guyer M, Hirschfeld RM, Merikangas KR, et al. Validity of the assessment of bipolar spectrum disorders in the WHO CIDI 3.0. J Affect Disord. 2006;96:259–69.
48. Carta MG, Angst J. Screening for bipolar disorders: A public health issue. J Affect Disord. 2016;15(205):139–43.
49. Phelps JR, Ghaemi SN. Improving the diagnosis of bipolar disorder: predictive value of screening tests. J Affect Disord. 2006;92(2-3):141–8.
50. Angst J, Gamma A, Lewinsohn P. The evolving epidemiology of bipolar disorder. World Psychiatry. 2002;1:146–8.
51. Benazzi F. Prevalence of bipolar II disorder in outpatient depression: a 203-case study in private practice. J Affect Disord. 1997;43:163–6.

Distinguishing Bipolar Depression from Unipolar Depression and Its Clinical Significance

2

Saeheon Jang and Duk-In Jon

Introduction

In the *Diagnostic and Statistical Manual of Mental Disorders, Fifth Edition, Text Revision* (DSM-V-TR) [1], bipolar disorder (BD) and major depressive disorder (MDD) are classified as distinct diagnostic entities, each with its own criteria. However, both share an identical definition of the major depressive episode, as the core depressive symptoms—such as low mood, anhedonia, and psychomotor changes—largely overlap. Consequently, differentiating bipolar depression from unipolar depression hinges primarily on the presence or absence of past (hypo) manic episode. This narrow diagnostic hinge is problematic, especially when patients present during depressive phases without a documented history of mania or hypomania.

This symptomatic overlap has led to frequent diagnostic misclassification. Studies suggest that up to 70% of individuals with BD are initially misdiagnosed with unipolar depression [2, 3], resulting in inappropriate treatment—most notably, antidepressant monotherapy without mood stabilization—which can precipitate manic switches, induce rapid cycling, or contribute to treatment resistance [4]. Among such misdiagnosed patients, 55% developed mania and 23% experienced rapid cycling following antidepressant exposure [2].

Beyond clinical destabilization, misdiagnosis carries broader healthcare implications. Patients with undetected BD experience significantly higher psychiatric service utilization, including nearly double the hospitalization rates and more than twice the emergency department visits compared to correctly diagnosed individuals [5, 6]. Misdiagnosed patients also incur higher treatment costs, with one analysis reporting a mean annual difference of over $3000 USD [6].

These findings underscore the need for more nuanced and multidimensional diagnostic strategies. While standard clinical assessment—including symptom chronology, family history, and comorbidities—remains essential, emerging tools may enhance diagnostic precision. Structured diagnostic interviews, biomarkers, neuroimaging profiles, and machine learning algorithms are increasingly being explored to improve differentiation between bipolar depression and unipolar depression, particularly during depressive phases.

This chapter integrates these complementary approaches into a unified diagnostic framework. It begins by tracing the historical evolution of the bipolar–unipolar distinction, followed by a comparative review of diagnostic systems (DSM-V-TR vs. ICD-11 [*International Classification of Diseases, 11th Revision*]) and clinical course

S. Jang (✉)
Department of Psychiatry, Bongseng Memorial Hospital, Busan, Republic of Korea

D.-I. Jon
Department of Psychiatry, Dong-A University Hospital, Busan, Republic of Korea

W.-M. Bahk et al. (eds.), *Bipolar Disorder*, https://doi.org/10.1007/978-981-92-1323-8_2

characteristics (e.g., age of onset, recurrence, episode duration); the final section examines how machine learning and multimodal data integration can support early and accurate identification. By weaving together historical, clinical, and data-driven perspectives, we aim to clarify the boundaries—and overlaps—between bipolar and unipolar depression, with the ultimate goal of improving diagnostic validity and treatment outcomes.

Historical Evolution of the Bipolar–Unipolar Distinction

The categorical separation between bipolar and unipolar depression is a relatively recent development in psychiatric nosology. Until the mid-twentieth century, all mood disorders were subsumed under the umbrella of manic-depressive illness, as proposed by Emil Kraepelin. The first formal distinction between unipolar and bipolar mood disorders was introduced by Karl Leonhard in 1957, and further elaborated upon in empirical studies by Angst, Perris, Winokur, and Clayton in the 1960s [7–9]. This binary framework was adopted into official classification systems with the publication of DSM-III in 1980 [10] and has been retained in subsequent revisions, including DSM-IV [11] and DSM-V-TR [1] (Fig. 2.1).

Despite the dominance of this categorical view, alternative models persist. Some scholars argue for a return to Kraepelin's dimensional perspective, wherein mood disorders lie along a continuum of affective instability, and the presence of manic episodes is merely one—albeit important—indicator of underlying bipolarity [12]. Others propose spectrum-based frameworks that accommodate overlapping features between bipolar depression and unipolar depression, while maintaining some diagnostic separation [13]. Still more conceptual models draw on premodern ideas, such as the classical "dual polarity" model rooted in the theory of the four humors, which posits mania and depression as fundamentally distinct illnesses sharing a depressive phenotype but differing in affective polarity [14].

Each of these models offers valuable insights into the nature of mood disorders, and they continue to influence modern classification systems and research directions. As diagnostic systems evolve (e.g., the shift toward dimensional specifiers in ICD-11), integrating historical perspectives with empirical data may help resolve ongoing ambiguities in mood disorder diagnosis.

Comparative Diagnostic Criteria for Bipolar and Unipolar Depression in DSM-V-TR and ICD-11 (Table 2.1)

The diagnostic frameworks for BD and unipolar depression differ in meaningful ways between the DSM-V-TR and the ICD-11 (*International Classification of Diseases, 11th Revision*) [15]. Although both systems define depressive episodes using largely overlapping core symptoms—such as depressed mood, anhedonia, and cognitive or somatic disturbances—their approaches to distinguishing bipolar from unipolar depression reflect different conceptual priorities.

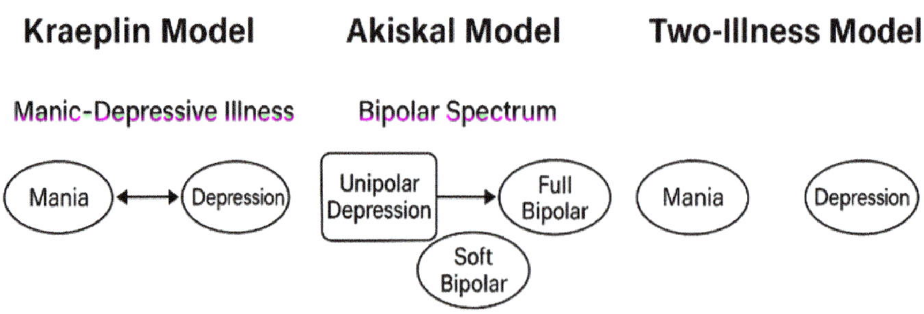

Fig. 2.1 Conceptual models of unipolar and bipolar depression: Kraepelin, Akiskal, and the Two-Illness frameworks

Table 2.1 Key differences between DSM-5-TR and ICD-11 in the diagnosis of bipolar and unipolar depression

Comparison aspect	DSM-5-TR	ICD-11
Diagnosis of bipolar depression	Requires at least one prior hypomanic (bipolar II) or manic (bipolar I) episode	Requires history of elevated or irritable mood; no strict episode count
Hypomania duration requirement	At least 4 consecutive days	No strict duration; diagnosis based on observable behavioral change
Diagnostic method	Checklist approach (symptom counting)	Narrative, descriptive guidelines emphasizing clinical judgment
Flexibility	Rigid, symptom-count based	Flexible, context-sensitive
Risk of misdiagnosis	Higher risk of misdiagnosing bipolar depression as unipolar depression	Lower risk due to broader clinical evaluation
Global applicability	Less adapted for diverse global settings	Designed for broader global applicability

A crucial point of divergence concerns the operationalization of hypomanic symptoms. DSM-V-TR adopts a categorical and threshold-based approach, requiring a documented hypomanic episode of at least four consecutive days for bipolar II disorder (BD II) or a manic episode for bipolar I disorder (BD I). While this duration criterion enhances diagnostic specificity and inter-rater reliability, it may fail to capture brief or subthreshold mood elevations that nonetheless carry prognostic significance. As a result, individuals presenting exclusively with depressive episodes may remain classified as having unipolar depression for prolonged periods.

ICD-11, by contrast, applies to a more flexible and descriptive framework. Although it similarly requires evidence of elevated or irritable mood for a bipolar diagnosis, it does not enforce a strict minimum duration for hypomania. Instead, greater emphasis is placed on observable changes in mood, behavior, and functioning, even when these changes are short-lived. This approach may increase sensitivity to bipolar features in patients who predominantly present with depression, particularly in early or ambiguous clinical stages.

The two systems also differ in diagnostic structure. DSM-V-TR relies on symptom counting and fixed time thresholds, prioritizing standardization and reproducibility. ICD-11, in contrast, uses narrative diagnostic guidelines that encourage clinicians to integrate symptom patterns with illness course, family history, and contextual factors. This descriptive style allows greater clinical discretion but also places higher demands on clinician expertise.

These nosological differences have important clinical implications. Under DSM-V-TR, patients with latent bipolarity who present with depression but lack clearly documented hypomania may be diagnosed with unipolar depression, potentially leading to treatment strategies—such as antidepressant monotherapy—that carry risks of mood destabilization. ICD-11's broader clinical framing may help mitigate this risk by allowing bipolarity to be considered earlier in the diagnostic process. However, this increased flexibility may also introduce variability in diagnostic practice, particularly across settings with differing levels of psychiatric training.

In summary, DSM-V-TR and ICD-11 represent complementary but distinct diagnostic philosophies. DSM-V-TR emphasizes categorical precision and reliability, whereas ICD-11 favors contextual sensitivity and clinical judgment. Understanding these differences is essential for interpreting epidemiological data, evaluating clinical courses, and integrating emerging biological and computational approaches discussed later in this chapter.

Epidemiology and Diagnostic Conversion Between Bipolar and Unipolar Depression (Table 2.2)

Large-scale epidemiological surveys consistently demonstrate that BD is less prevalent than MDD in the general population, yet the

Table 2.2 Epidemiological findings on the prevalence of and diagnostic transition in bipolar and unipolar depression.

Study	Disorder	Lifetime prevalence	12-month prevalence	Key findings
ECA Study (USA) [16]	BD I	0.8%	0.6%	
	BD II	0.5%	0.3%	
	MDD	4.9%	2.3%	
NCSR Study (USA) [17]	BD I	1.0%	0.6%	
	BD II	1.1%	0.8%	
	Bipolar spectrum	2.4%	1.4%	
	MDD	6.6%	16.2%	MDD 12-month prevalence higher
WHO WMH Survey [19]	BD I	0.6%	0.4%	
	BD II	0.4%	0.3%	
	Subthreshold bipolar	1.4%	0.8%	
Canadian Survey [20]	MDD	12.2%	4.8%	
Benazzi [21]	BD II	Up to 43.4%		Structured interviews
Akiskal et al. [22]	Bipolar spectrum	30–55%		Broader criteria reassessment
Angst et al. [23]	Expanded bipolar spectrum	23.6%		Close to depression spectrum (24.6%)
NIMH CDS [24]	MDD → BD II	8.6%		Over 11 years
	MDD → BD I	3.9%		Over 11 years
Ghaemi et al. [25]	MDD → Bipolar	40%		Mean 7.56 years to rediagnosis
Hantouche et al. [26]	BD II rise after evaluation	22% → 40%		Structured evaluation
Kim et al. [27]	Diagnostic stability	79% (MDD)		BD I: 89.3% retained
Sharma et al. [28]	MDD → Bipolar spectrum	52%		Within 1 year
Inoue et al. [29]	MDD → Bipolar	23.8%		Over 5.7 years

ECA, NCSR, NIMH CDS, WHO WMH

estimated prevalence varies substantially depending on diagnostic definitions and assessment methods. Community-based studies from the United States, the World Health Organization, and Canada show relatively stable prevalence estimates for BD I and II, while broader bipolar spectrum definitions markedly increase the proportion of individuals meeting criteria for bipolarity [16–20]. These findings underscore the strong influence of diagnostic thresholds and interview strategies on epidemiological estimates.

Importantly, studies employing structured and systematic assessments of hypomanic symptoms among patients presenting with major depressive episodes reveal a substantially higher rate of BD II than is typically identified in routine clinical practice [21]. When broader bipolar spectrum concepts are applied retrospectively, a sizeable proportion of individuals previously diagnosed with unipolar depression appear to fall within the bipolar spectrum [22, 23]. This highlights a fundamental limitation of cross-sectional diagnostic approaches that rely heavily on overt manic episodes.

Longitudinal data further reinforces the dynamic nature of mood disorder diagnoses. Follow-up studies demonstrate that a nontrivial proportion of patients initially diagnosed with unipolar depression are later reclassified as having BD over time, particularly bipolar II disorder [24–26]. At the same time, diagnostic stability remains relatively high for classic bipolar I disorder and for a majority of patients with MDD, suggesting that misdiagnosis is not universal but concentrated within specific subgroups [27].

Patients with treatment-resistant depression (TRD) appear to represent one such high-risk subgroup. Prospective studies indicate that a substantial fraction of individuals initially diagnosed with TRD later meet criteria for bipolar spectrum disorders, often within a relatively short time frame [28, 29]. Clinically, these findings suggest that apparent antidepressant nonresponse may, in some cases, reflect unrecognized bipolarity rather than true resistance to treatment.

Taken together, epidemiological and longitudinal evidence indicates that the distinction between bipolar and unipolar depression is not static but evolves over time. While population-level prevalence of BD is lower than that of MDD, diagnostic transition from unipolar to bipolar categories is common in selected clinical contexts, particularly when structured assessments, long-term follow-up, or treatment resistance are considered. These patterns emphasize the importance of longitudinal diagnostic vigilance and support the view that bipolarity exists along a spectrum rather than as a strictly categorical entity.

Differences in Clinical Course Between Bipolar and Unipolar Depression (Table 2.3)

Clinical differences between bipolar depression and unipolar depression are not defined by a single pathognomonic feature, but rather by a constellation of course-related characteristics that, when considered together, can enhance diagnostic accuracy. These include gender distribution patterns, age of onset, episode characteristics, recurrence patterns, and exposure to early life stressors.

Gender differences offer some diagnostic clues, although they are not definitive. While unipolar depression tends to be more prevalent in women, BD—particularly bipolar I disorder—does not show a consistent gender disparity [30]. Moreover, data from young adult populations suggest that male predominance may be more pronounced in bipolar depression than unipolar depression [31], although bipolar II disorder appears to mirror the gender ratio seen in unipolar depression [32]. These trends may help clinicians contextualize depressive presentations, particularly in women, where misdiagnosis of bipolar depression as unipolar depression is more common due to overlapping symptomatology and higher baseline rates of depression.

Table 2.3 Clinical feature comparison between bipolar depression (BD) and unipolar depression (UD)

Clinical feature	BD	UD	Controversial findings
Mood lability	More common [53–55]	Less common	No major controversy
Psychotic symptoms	More common [56]	Less common	No major controversy
Psychomotor retardation	Reported, but findings inconsistent [57–60]	Reported, but findings inconsistent	Conflicting findings across studies
Atypical features (hypersomnia, weight gain)	More common, but findings inconsistent [60–66]	Reported, but not distinguishing [69–72]	Conflicting findings across studies
Somatic symptoms (e.g., bodily pain)	Less common	More common [57, 67]	Generally accepted
Sleep disturbances	Less common	More common	Generally accepted
Emotional symptoms (anger, anxiety, agitation)	Less common	More common	Generally accepted
Weight loss	Less common	More common	Generally accepted
Anhedonia	Present	Present [68]	Generally accepted

Age of onset has emerged as a robust clinical indicator, with BD (especially type I) often beginning during adolescence or early adulthood, while unipolar depression typically presents later [30, 33, 34]. Several studies suggest that earlier onset of depressive symptoms—particularly in the teens or early twenties—should prompt a thorough assessment for underlying bipolarity [31, 35, 36]. This is especially relevant in cases marked by atypical features, psychomotor symptoms, or poor antidepressant response.

The temporal pattern of depressive episodes also differs meaningfully between the two disorders. BD tends to be characterized by shorter but more frequent depressive episodes, as well as briefer intervals between them [38–40]. In contrast, unipolar depression episodes may be more protracted and carry a greater risk of progressing to chronicity. These distinctions—though not absolute—can aid in longitudinal tracking and prognostication.

Recurrence patterns further differentiate between the two conditions. Long-term follow-up studies indicate that while both disorders are associated with high recurrence rates, BD patients often experience more total episodes and shorter cycle lengths than their unipolar depression counterparts [37–40]. Additionally, although some evidence suggests that recurrence intervals shorten over time in BD [41], this finding may not generalize beyond the earliest episodes [42]. Regardless, a high number of prior episodes—particularly within a relatively short timeframe—should alert clinicians to the possibility of bipolarity [33, 34].

Childhood trauma, especially emotional abuse, is another variable more commonly reported in individuals with bipolar depression than those with unipolar depression [31, 43]. Such early adverse experiences have been linked not only to increased risk for BD but also to more severe illness trajectories, including higher rates of recurrence and treatment resistance [44]. A thorough developmental and psychosocial history is therefore essential when evaluating recurrent or early-onset depression.

In summary, while individual features such as mood lability or psychomotor changes may be nonspecific, their co-occurrence—particularly in the context of early onset, high recurrence, and trauma exposure—can provide important diagnostic signals. Recognizing these patterns may reduce delays in appropriate diagnosis and treatment, ultimately improving clinical outcomes.

The Role of Heritability and Family History in Mood Disorders

Genetic factors play a pivotal role in differentiating BD from unipolar depression. BD exhibits markedly higher heritability estimates—up to 85%—compared to approximately 37% for unipolar depression, based on twin and meta-analytic studies [45, 46]. This contrast points to a stronger genetic contribution in BD.

Family studies offer additional evidence of this divergence. Meta-analytic findings show that relatives of individuals with BD are at elevated risk for both BD and unipolar depression, whereas relatives of those with unipolar depression show increased risk only for unipolar depression [47]. This pattern underscores a degree of genetic specificity in BD, suggesting that it carries a broader familial liability that spans both bipolar and depressive phenotypes, while unipolar depression demonstrates narrower heritability.

In clinical settings, family history of BD consistently emerges as one of the most reliable predictors of eventual bipolar diagnosis in patients presenting with depressive symptoms. Multiple studies have found that individuals later diagnosed with BD report a higher prevalence of BD among first-degree relatives than those with unipolar depression [31, 33, 48]. Moreover, family history is particularly valuable in identifying subthreshold or "soft" bipolarity, where overt manic symptoms may be absent but longitudinal patterns suggest bipolar diathesis [36].

Taken together, these findings highlight the importance of incorporating detailed family history assessments into diagnostic evaluations. Beyond aiding differential diagnosis, family history may also inform risk stratification, treatment selection, and psychoeducation, especially in cases of early-onset, recurrent, or atypical depression.

Clinical Symptomatology and Challenges in Differentiating Bipolar and Unipolar Depression

Although BD and unipolar depression share the full range of core depressive symptoms, numerous studies have sought to identify symptom-level differences that might assist in differential diagnosis. Historically, it was often assumed that the two disorders were clinically indistinguishable during depressive phases. However, accumulating evidence suggests that certain symptom patterns may diverge in clinically meaningful ways.

In broad terms, BD has been more frequently associated with greater mood lability, a higher incidence of psychotic features, and increased rates of atypical depressive symptoms such as hypersomnia and weight gain [49–62]. By contrast, unipolar depression tends to present more commonly with somatic complaints, sleep disturbances, anxious or agitated emotional states, and features such as weight loss or prominent anhedonia [53, 63, 64]. When interpreted within the broader longitudinal context of an individual patient, these contrasting symptom profiles may provide probabilistic, rather than definitive, diagnostic clues.

Nevertheless, symptom-based differentiation remains limited by substantial inconsistency across studies. Meta-analytic and comparative investigations have yielded conflicting results, particularly with respect to psychomotor features and atypical depressive symptoms. Psychomotor retardation, for example, has been reported as more pronounced in bipolar depression in some studies, more common in unipolar depression in others, or not significantly different between the two groups [50, 53, 55, 65, 66]. Similarly, atypical features such as hypersomnia or hyperphagia have not reliably distinguished bipolar II disorder from unipolar depression, with several studies finding no meaningful differences in their prevalence [65–68].

Given this variability, no single symptom or constellation of symptoms has demonstrated sufficient diagnostic accuracy to function as a stand-alone marker for differentiating bipolar depression from unipolar depression. Consequently, reliance on symptomatology alone is insufficient for diagnostic decision-making in routine clinical practice.

More accurate differentiation requires a multidimensional assessment that integrates the longitudinal course of illness, including episode duration and recurrence patterns, alongside family psychiatric history—particularly the presence of BD among first-degree relatives. Treatment response patterns, such as antidepressant-induced mood switching, as well as contextual factors including age of onset and psychiatric or medical comorbidities, also play an important role in diagnostic formulation.

Ultimately, while symptom patterns can guide clinical suspicion, diagnostic confirmation depends on careful longitudinal observation and contextual synthesis. A heightened index of suspicion is especially warranted in patients presenting with early-onset, recurrent, or treatment-resistant depressive episodes, where underlying bipolarity may only become evident over time.

The Importance of History-Taking and Screening Instruments in the Differential Diagnosis of Bipolar Depression

Patients who present during a depressive episode often do not spontaneously report hypomanic symptoms, making it difficult for clinicians—particularly those who are less experienced—to recognize underlying bipolarity [26]. Therefore, obtaining a thorough clinical history is essential for differentiating bipolar depression from unipolar depression. One of the most important steps in this process is identifying a family history of BD and inquiring, not only with the patient but also with close relatives or significant others, about any past episodes of (hypo)mania.

In addition to detailed history-taking, the use of screening tools with high sensitivity and specificity may support the diagnostic process. In clinical practice in South Korea, several standardized instruments are widely used for this purpose, including the Mood Disorder Questionnaire (MDQ) [69], the Bipolar Spectrum Diagnostic Scale (BSDS) [70], and the Hypomania Checklist-32 (HCL-32) [71].

Functional and Structural Neuroimaging Differences Between Bipolar and Unipolar Depression (Table 2.4)

Neuroimaging studies have made substantial contributions to elucidating both shared and distinct pathophysiological mechanisms underlying bipolar depression and unipolar depression. Although many abnormalities overlap between the two disorders, particularly within neural systems involved in emotion regulation, converging evidence indicates that differences in neural circuitry, functional connectivity, and structural integrity may offer insights relevant to differential diagnosis.

Table 2.4 Summary of key neuroimaging findings differentiating bipolar depression (BD) and unipolar depression (UD)

Study focus	Key researchers	Main findings
Functional imaging	Han et al. [76]	Comparison of functional and structural imaging in BD vs. UD
	Taylor et al. [77]	UD: impaired top-down regulation; BD: normal regulation
	Almeida et al. [78, 79]	BD: impaired vmPFC-amygdala connectivity; UD: heightened amygdala reactivity
	Grotegerd et al. [80]	UD: heightened amygdala excitability, differentiating with 80% accuracy
	Burger et al. [81]	UD: impaired bottom-up emotion processing
Structural imaging	Versace et al. [83]	BD: reduced FA in SLF; UD: reduced FA in ILF
	Silverstone et al. [84]	BD: increased deep white matter hyperintensities
	Savitz et al. [85]	BD: reduced habenular volume compared to UD and controls
	MacMaster et al. [86]	Both BD and UD: increased pituitary gland volume compared to controls

FA, ILF, SLF, vmPFC

Functional neuroimaging studies, primarily using functional magnetic resonance imaging (fMRI), consistently implicate frontolimbic network dysfunction in both BD and unipolar depression, albeit with distinct patterns of dysregulation. In unipolar depression, depressive states are more commonly associated with heightened bottom-up emotional reactivity, especially in response to negatively valanced stimuli, coupled with diminished regulatory engagement of prefrontal regions. Experimental paradigms such as reversal learning and subliminal emotional priming have demonstrated exaggerated amygdala responses alongside blunted activation in dorsomedial and ventrolateral prefrontal cortices in unipolar depression [72–76]. These findings are generally interpreted as reflecting impaired cognitive–emotional control and increased sensitivity to negative feedback.

In contrast, BD appears to be characterized by greater disruption of top-down modulation, particularly in the context of positive or reward-related stimuli. Reduced functional connectivity between the ventromedial prefrontal cortex and the amygdala has been reported in BD, a pattern that may underlie vulnerability to manic or hypomanic shifts [73, 74]. Moreover, emotional reactivity in BD tends to be more variable and context dependent than in unipolar depression, suggesting a distinct mode of affective regulation rather than a uniform amplification or attenuation of emotional responses.

Resting-state fMRI studies further extend these observations by examining intrinsic network organization. Both BD II and unipolar depression have been shown to exhibit inefficiencies within default mode and limbic networks. However, graph-theoretical analyses have identified disorder-specific alterations in local network hubs, indicating that network-level characteristics—rather than global dysfunction alone—may hold promise as differentiating features [77].

Structural neuroimaging provides complementary evidence for both shared and distinct neurobiological substrates. Diffusion tensor imaging (DTI) studies have identified differential patterns of white matter disruption, with reduced fractional anisotropy in the superior longitudinal fasciculus observed more prominently in BD, and similar alterations in the inferior longitudinal fasciculus reported in unipolar depression [78]. These findings suggest disorder-specific disturbances in long-range connectivity pathways involved in mood regulation, attention, and memory processing. In addition, BD has been associated with a higher burden of deep white matter hyperintensities, a finding that may reflect cumulative vascular or metabolic influences on illness course [79].

Subcortical structural differences have also been described. Notably, reduced habenular volume—a structure centrally involved in reward processing and aversive signaling—has been reported in BD but not in unipolar depression, pointing to altered midbrain neuromodulatory regulation in bipolar illness [80]. At the same time, not all structural findings distinguish the two disorders. Increased pituitary gland volume, for example, has been observed in both BD and unipolar depression, particularly among adolescents, suggesting a shared component of hypothalamic–pituitary–adrenal axis dysregulation across mood disorders [81].

Taken together, these neuroimaging findings indicate that BD and unipolar depression are characterized by partially overlapping yet distinguishable neural signatures. The most consistent distinctions appear to involve the directionality of emotional reactivity, differences in frontolimbic connectivity, and selective alterations in white matter integrity and subcortical structures. Although none of these markers are currently sufficient for standalone diagnostic use, their integration—particularly within multimodal neuroimaging frameworks or in combination with machine learning approaches—holds promise for improving diagnostic specificity and informing more personalized treatment strategies in the future.

Toward Biologically Informed Diagnosis of Bipolar and Unipolar Depression

Advances in neurobiology and data science have stimulated increasing interest in the use of biological markers to differentiate bipolar depression from unipolar depression. Although most candidate biomarkers remain at an investigational stage, they offer the potential to complement conventional clinical assessment and, in the longer term, to enhance diagnostic precision beyond symptom-based criteria alone.

Among peripheral biomarkers, Glycogen Synthase Kinase-3 (GSK3), particularly its β isoform, has been proposed as a candidate marker of bipolarity. Research examining peripheral blood mononuclear cells (PBMCs) has shown that GSK3β levels are significantly lower in patients with bipolar depression than in those with unipolar depression [82]. While GSK3α levels did not demonstrate significant group differences, the combined use of both isoforms in a serial classification model achieved very high sensitivity, approaching 100%, albeit at the cost of a substantial false-negative rate of approximately 26.7%. These findings suggest that GSK3β may represent a useful component of a future multi-marker panel, but they also underscore that its current applicability is confined to the research setting rather than routine clinical practice.

Beyond single-marker approaches, inflammatory cytokines and oxidative stress markers have been explored using machine learning techniques. In one study, support vector machine models identified interleukin-4, interleukin-10, and thiobarbituric acid reactive substances as key variables distinguishing bipolar depression from unipolar depression [83]. Distinct combinations of biomarkers were also found to differentiate each disorder from healthy controls. Although these classification results are encouraging, they require replication in larger and more clinically heterogeneous cohorts before any meaningful translation to clinical use can be considered.

Electrophysiological measures provide another line of biologically informed differentiation. Electroencephalographic (EEG) studies have reported state-independent differences between bipolar depression and unipolar depression, including distinct patterns of frontal EEG asymmetry and alterations in functional connectivity indices such as cordance and coherence in the theta and alpha frequency bands [84, 85]. In parallel, a meta-analysis of event-related potentials demonstrated that patients with bipolar depression consistently exhibit prolonged P300 latency compared with those with unipolar depression, both during acute depressive episodes and in euthymic states [86]. These observations suggest the presence of trait-like neural signatures, although their diagnostic specificity and robustness across clinical contexts remain to be fully established.

Neuroimaging combined with machine learning has further expanded the scope of biologically informed diagnostics. A multiple kernel learning framework integrating Tract-Based Spatial Statistics (TBSS) and Voxel-Based Morphometry (VBM) achieved a balanced accuracy of 73.65% in differentiating bipolar depression from unipolar depression [87]. Structural analyses revealed reduced gray matter volume in limbic and paralimbic regions, including the hippocampus, amygdala, and insula, in bipolar depression relative to unipolar depression, whereas TBSS analyses indicated more pronounced white matter microstructural abnormalities in unipolar depression. Despite their potential relevance, these findings are derived from relatively small samples and must therefore be interpreted cautiously.

Taken together, evidence from peripheral biomarkers, electrophysiological measures, and neuroimaging—particularly when integrated using advanced machine learning approaches—offers an increasingly detailed biological characterization of mood disorders. However, it is crucial to distinguish between promising research signals and clinically actionable tools. To date, most studies have been constrained by limited sample sizes, variable replication, and a lack of validation in real-world clinical settings.

Accordingly, while these multimodal approaches may eventually contribute to more refined and biologically informed diagnostic processes, especially in ambiguous or treatment-resistant cases, they are not yet suitable for routine clinical application. At present, they should be regarded as adjunctive research instruments that complement, rather than replace, comprehensive longitudinal clinical evaluation.

Differences in Treatment Response Between Bipolar and Unipolar Depression (Table 2.5)

Treatment response patterns in bipolar depression and unipolar depression diverge in ways that carry important implications for clinical management. Antidepressant monotherapy, while generally effective and widely used in unipolar depression, presents considerable risks in bipolar depression, particularly the induction of manic or mixed episodes—a phenomenon known as antidepressant-induced mood switching [88, 89]. As a result, such monotherapy is typically avoided in bipolar depression unless combined with mood stabilizers.

Mood stabilizers, particularly lithium, are a cornerstone of BD treatment, supported by strong evidence for reducing depressive symptoms and suicidal risk [90]. In contrast, they play a mini-

Table 2.5 Comparison of treatment response patterns in bipolar depression (BD) and unipolar depression (UD)

Treatment aspect	BD	UD
Antidepressant monotherapy	Risk of mood switching; prescribed only with mood stabilizers [94]	Standard treatment; often effective [93]
Mood stabilizers	Central to treatment; lithium reduces depression and suicide risk [90]	Rarely first-line; used only in augmentation for resistant cases
Use of antipsychotics	Quetiapine, lurasidone effective as primary treatments [91, 92]	Used mainly for augmentation in treatment-resistant depression
Treatment resistance	More frequent; related to cycling, comorbidity, and rapid switching [93, 94]	Also common; linked to chronicity and severity
Psychotherapy focus	Emphasizes mood stabilization, early symptom detection, and circadian rhythm maintenance	Targets cognitive distortions, behavioral activation

mal role in unipolar depression, where treatment strategies tend to focus on antidepressants, with augmentation reserved for resistant cases.

Atypical antipsychotics—such as quetiapine and lurasidone—have demonstrated efficacy as primary treatments for bipolar depression [91, 92], whereas in unipolar depression, their use is usually confined to augmentation in treatment-resistant depression. This distinction underscores the different pharmacodynamic targets and neurobiological profiles between the disorders.

Treatment resistance is a common challenge in both conditions, but it tends to manifest differently. In bipolar depression, resistance often correlates with comorbidities (e.g., anxiety, substance use), rapid cycling, or poor adherence, while in unipolar depression, chronicity and symptom severity are more predictive of poor outcomes [93, 94]. Recognizing these distinct pathways to resistance can guide more tailored treatment planning.

Psychotherapeutic approaches are effective in both disorders, but the therapeutic focus differs. In BD, interventions such as interpersonal and social rhythm therapy (IPSRT) emphasize mood stabilization, early symptom detection, and circadian rhythm regulation. In unipolar depression, cognitive-behavioral therapy (CBT) typically targets maladaptive cognitions and behavioral activation strategies.

In summary, while there is some overlap in available treatments, bipolar depression and unipolar depression differ meaningfully in their pharmacologic response profiles, risk of treatment-emergent mood destabilization, and psychological intervention targets. Understanding these differences is critical to optimizing individualized care strategies.

Conclusions

Accurately differentiating bipolar depression from unipolar depression remains a central challenge in clinical psychiatry. Misdiagnosis is not a trivial error; it can lead to inappropriate treatment strategies, illness destabilization, unnecessary exposure to medication-related risks, and increased long-term morbidity. Such diagnostic failures arise from multiple sources, including limited patient insight into past hypomanic symptoms, incomplete longitudinal assessment by clinicians, and the substantial phenomenological overlap between the two disorders during depressive episodes. Recognizing these structural vulnerabilities is a prerequisite for improving diagnostic accuracy and patient outcomes.

This chapter has traced the conceptual and empirical foundations of the bipolar–unipolar distinction, beginning with its historical evolution and continuing through its operationalization in contemporary diagnostic systems such as DSM-V-TR and ICD 11. Differences in epidemiology, sociodemographic patterns, age of onset, illness course, recurrence, family history, symptom expression, and treatment response were reviewed not as isolated findings, but as complementary dimensions that collectively shape diagnostic reasoning.

A key clinical implication emphasized throughout this chapter concerns treatment response. Antidepressant monotherapy, while effective and generally safe in unipolar depression, carries well-documented risks in bipolar depression, including mood switching, cycle acceleration, and treatment resistance. In contrast, mood stabilizers and certain atypical antipsychotics form the cornerstone of bipolar depression management, whereas antidepressants—often with augmentation strategies—remain first-line treatments for unipolar depression. These divergent response patterns underscore the practical importance of accurate diagnosis, particularly in early or ambiguous depressive presentations.

Screening instruments commonly used in clinical practice, such as the MDQ, BSDS, and HCL-32, may assist in identifying bipolar features among patients presenting with depression. However, their utility lies primarily in raising clinical suspicion rather than establishing diagnosis, reinforcing the need for longitudinal and contextual assessment.

This chapter also reviewed advances in neuroimaging, electrophysiology, peripheral biomarkers, and machine learning. Functional and structural neuroimaging studies have identified subtle but reproducible differences between bipolar and unipolar depression, particularly within frontolimbic circuits, white matter pathways, and reward-related structures. Emerging biomarker and machine learning approaches further suggest that biologically informed classification may eventually complement traditional diagnostic methods. Importantly, however, these techniques remain largely confined to the research domain. Current evidence does not support their routine clinical application, and overinterpretation of their readiness should be avoided.

Despite growing interest in novel biological markers, the most reliable diagnostic indicators at present remain clinical: a history of (hypo) manic episodes and a family history of bipolar disorder. When these factors are systematically evaluated alongside illness course, age of onset, and treatment response patterns, diagnostic confidence can be substantially improved.

In conclusion, no single symptom, test, or biomarker can adequately distinguish bipolar depression from unipolar depression. The most robust diagnostic strategy is inherently multidimensional, integrating careful longitudinal clinical assessment with judicious use of screening tools and emerging biological insights. While advances in neuroscience and data science hold promise for the future, precision psychiatry in mood disorders will depend not on replacing clinical judgment, but on enriching it through thoughtful synthesis of clinical, historical, and biological information.

References

1. American Psychiatric A. Diagnostic and statistical manual of mental disorders: DSM-5-TR. Washington, DC: American Psychiatric Association Publishing; 2022.
2. Ghaemi SN, Boiman EE, Goodwin FK. Diagnosing bipolar disorder and the effect of antidepressants: a naturalistic study. J Clin Psychiatry. 2000;61:804–8.
3. Hirschfeld RM, Lewis L, Vornik LA. Perceptions and impact of bipolar disorder: how far have we really come? Results of the national depressive and manic-depressive association 2000 survey of individuals with bipolar disorder. J Clin Psychiatry. 2003;64:161–74.
4. Goldberg JF, Truman CJ. Antidepressant-induced mania: an overview of current controversies. Bipolar Disord. 2003;5:407–20.
5. McIntyre RS, Laliberté F, Germain G, MacKnight SD, Gillard P, Harrington A. The real-world health resource use and costs of misdiagnosing bipolar I disorder. J Affect Disord. 2022;316:26–33.
6. Stensland MD, Schultz JF, Frytak JR. Diagnosis of unipolar depression following initial identification of bipolar disorder: a common and costly misdiagnosis. J Clin Psychiatry. 2008;69:749–58.
7. Angst J. On the etiology and nosology of endogenous depressive psychoses. A genetic, sociologic and clinical study. Monogr Gesamtgeb Neurol Psychiatr. 1966;112:1–118.
8. Perris C. A study of bipolar (manic-depressive) and unipolar recurrent depressive psychoses. I. Genetic investigation. Acta Psychiatr Scand Suppl. 1966;194:15–44.
9. Winokur G, Clayton P. Family history studies. I. Two types of affective disorders separated according to genetic and clinical factors. Recent Adv Biol Psychiatry. 1966;9:35–50.
10. American Psychiatric A. Diagnostic and statistical manual of mental disorders: DSM-III. Washington, DC: American Psychiatric Association; 1980.
11. American Psychiatric A, American Psychiatric Association Task Force on DI. Diagnostic and statistical manual of mental disorders: DSM-IV. Washington, DC: American Psychiatric Association; 1994.
12. Goodwin FK, Ghaemi SN. Understanding manic-depressive illness. Arch Gen Psychiatry. 1998;55:23–5.
13. Akiskal HS, Walker P, Puzantian VR, King D, Rosenthal TL, Dranon M. Bipolar outcome in the course of depressive illness. Phenomenologic, familial, and pharmacologic predictors. J Affect Disord. 1983;5:115–28.
14. Joffe RT, Young LT, MacQueen GM. A two-illness model of bipolar disorder. Bipolar Disord. 1999;1:25–30.
15. World Health Organization. International classification of diseases, 11th revision (ICD-11). Geneva: World Health Organization; 2019.
16. Regier DA, Farmer ME, Rae DS, Locke BZ, Keith SJ, Judd LL. Comorbidity of mental disorders with alcohol and other drug abuse. Results from the Epidemiologic Catchment Area (ECA) Study. JAMA. 1990;264:2511–8.
17. Merikangas KR, Akiskal HS, Angst J, Greenberg PE, Hirschfeld RM, Petukhova M. Lifetime and 12-month prevalence of bipolar spectrum disorder in the National Comorbidity Survey replication. Arch Gen Psychiatry. 2007;64:543–52.
18. Kessler RC, Berglund P, Demler O, Jin R, Koretz D, Merikangas KR. The epidemiology of major depressive disorder: results from the National Comorbidity Survey Replication (NCS-R). JAMA. 2003;289:3095–105.

19. Merikangas KR, Jin R, He JP, Kessler RC, Lee S, Sampson NA. Prevalence and correlates of bipolar spectrum disorder in the world mental health survey initiative. Arch Gen Psychiatry. 2011;68:241–51.
20. Patten SB. A major depression prognosis calculator based on episode duration. Clin Pract Epidemiol Ment Health. 2006;2:13.
21. Benazzi F. Bipolar II disorder is common among depressed outpatients. Psychiatry Clin Neurosci. 1999;53:607–9.
22. Akiskal HS, Bourgeois ML, Angst J, Post R, Möller H, Hirschfeld R. Re-evaluating the prevalence of and diagnostic composition within the broad clinical spectrum of bipolar disorders. J Affect Disord. 2000;59(Suppl 1):S5–s30.
23. Angst J, Gamma A, Benazzi F, Ajdacic V, Eich D, Rossler W. Toward a re-definition of subthreshold bipolarity: epidemiology and proposed criteria for bipolar-II, minor bipolar disorders and hypomania. J Affect Disord. 2003;73:133–46.
24. Akiskal HS, Maser JD, Zeller PJ, Endicott J, Coryell W, Keller M. Switching from 'unipolar' to bipolar II. An 11-year prospective study of clinical and temperamental predictors in 559 patients. Arch Gen Psychiatry. 1995;52:114–23.
25. Ghaemi SN, Sachs GS, Chiou AM, Pandurangi AK, Goodwin K. Is bipolar disorder still underdiagnosed? Are antidepressants overutilized? J Affect Disord. 1999;52:135–44.
26. Hantouche EG, Akiskal HS, Lancrenon S, Allilaire JF, Sechter D, Azorin JM. Systematic clinical methodology for validating bipolar-II disorder: data in mid-stream from a French national multi-site study (EPIDEP). J Affect Disord. 1998;50:163–73.
27. Kim W, Woo YS, Chae JH, Bahk WM. The diagnostic stability of DSM-IV diagnoses: an examination of major depressive disorder, bipolar I disorder, and schizophrenia in Korean patients. Clin Psychopharmacol Neurosci. 2011;9:117–21.
28. Sharma V, Khan M, Smith A. A closer look at treatment resistant depression: is it due to a bipolar diathesis? J Affect Disord. 2005;84:251–7.
29. Inoue T, Nakagawa S, Kitaichi Y, Izumi T, Tanaka T, Masui T. Long-term outcome of antidepressant-refractory depression: the relevance of unrecognized bipolarity. J Affect Disord. 2006;95:61–7.
30. Weissman MM, Bland RC, Canino GJ, Faravelli C, Greenwald S, Hwu HG. Cross-national epidemiology of major depression and bipolar disorder. JAMA. 1996;276:293–9.
31. Patella AM, Jansen K, Cardoso TA, Souza LDM, Silva RAD, Coelho F. Clinical features of differential diagnosis between unipolar and bipolar depression in a drug-free sample of young adults. J Affect Disord. 2019;243:103–7.
32. Benazzi F. Bipolar II versus unipolar chronic depression: a 312-case study. Compr Psychiatry. 1999;40:418–21.
33. Perlis RH, Brown E, Baker RW, Nierenberg AA. Clinical features of bipolar depression versus major depressive disorder in large multicenter trials. Am J Psychiatry. 2006;163:225–31.
34. Moreno C, Hasin DS, Arango C, Oquendo MA, Vieta E, Liu S. Depression in bipolar disorder versus major depressive disorder: results from the National Epidemiologic Survey on Alcohol and Related Conditions. Bipolar Disord. 2012;14:271–82.
35. Inoue T, Inagaki Y, Kimura T, Shirakawa O. Prevalence and predictors of bipolar disorders in patients with a major depressive episode: the Japanese epidemiological trial with latest measure of bipolar disorder (JET-LMBP). J Affect Disord. 2015;174:535–41.
36. Takeshima M, Oka T. A comprehensive analysis of features that suggest bipolarity in patients with a major depressive episode: which is the best combination to predict soft bipolarity. Diagnosis? J Affect Disord. 2013;147:150–5.
37. Keller MB, Lavori PW, Coryell W, Endicott J, Mueller TI. Bipolar I: a five-year prospective follow-up. J Nerv Ment Dis. 1993;181:238–45.
38. Mueller TI, Leon AC, Keller MB, Solomon DA, Endicott J, Coryell W. Recurrence after recovery from major depressive disorder during 15 years of observational follow-up. Am J Psychiatry. 1999;156:1000–6.
39. Kessing LV, Hansen MG, Andersen PK. Course of illness in depressive and bipolar disorders. Naturalistic study, 1994-1999. Br J Psychiatry. 2004;185:372–7.
40. Angst J, Gamma A, Sellaro R, Lavori PW, Zhang H. Recurrence of bipolar disorders and major depression. A life-long perspective. Eur Arch Psychiatry Clin Neurosci. 2003;253:236–40.
41. Solomon DA, Keller MB, Leon AC, Mueller TI, Lavori PW, Shea MT. Multiple recurrences of major depressive disorder. Am J Psychiatry. 2000;157:229–33.
42. Angst J, Sellaro R. Historical perspectives and natural history of bipolar disorder. Biol Psychiatry. 2000;48:445–57.
43. Liu J, Wang Y, Wilson A, Chen H, Liu P, Chen X. Anticipating Unipolar Depression and Bipolar Depression in young adult with first episode of depression using childhood trauma and personality. Front Public Health. 2022;10:1061894.
44. Palmier-Claus JE, Berry K, Bucci S, Mansell W, Varese F. Relationship between childhood adversity and bipolar affective disorder: systematic review and meta-analysis. Br J Psychiatry. 2016;209:454–9.
45. McGuffin P, Rijsdijk F, Andrew M, Sham P, Katz R, Cardno A. The heritability of bipolar affective disorder and the genetic relationship to unipolar depression. Arch Gen Psychiatry. 2003;60:497–502.
46. Sullivan PF, Neale MC, Kendler KS. Genetic epidemiology of major depression: review and meta-analysis. Am J Psychiatry. 2000;157:1552–62.
47. Smoller JW, Finn CT. Family, twin, and adoption studies of bipolar disorder. Am J Med Genet C Semin Med Genet. 2003;123C:48–58.
48. Angst J, Azorin JM, Bowden CL, Perugi G, Vieta E, Gamma A. Prevalence and characteristics of undiagnosed bipolar disorders in patients with a major

depressive episode: the BRIDGE study. Arch Gen Psychiatry. 2011;68:791–8.
49. Brockington IF, Altman E, Hillier V, Meltzer HY, Nand S. The clinical picture of bipolar affective disorder in its depressed phase. A report from London and Chicago. Br J Psychiatry. 1982;141:558–62.
50. Hantouche EG, Akiskal HS. Bipolar II vs. unipolar depression: psychopathologic differentiation by dimensional measures. J Affect Disord. 2005;84:127–32.
51. Leonhard K. Pathogenesis of manic-depressive disease. Nervenarzt. 1957;28:271–2.
52. Forty L, Smith D, Jones L, Jones I, Caesar S, Cooper C. Clinical differences between bipolar and unipolar depression. Br J Psychiatry. 2008;192:388–9.
53. Beigel A, Murphy DL. Unipolar and bipolar affective illness. Differences in clinical characteristics accompanying depression. Arch Gen Psychiatry. 1971;24:215–20.
54. Dunner DL, Dwyer T, Fieve RR. Depressive symptoms in patients with unipolar and bipolar affective disorder. Compr Psychiatry. 1976;17:447–51.
55. Katz MM, Robins E, Croughan J, Secunda S, Swann A. Behavioural measurement and drug response characteristics of unipolar and bipolar depression. Psychol Med. 1982;12:25–36.
56. Mitchell PB, Wilhelm K, Parker G, Austin MP, Rutgers P, Malhi GS. The clinical features of bipolar depression: a comparison with matched major depressive disorder patients. J Clin Psychiatry. 2001;62:212–6.
57. Agosti V, Stewart JW. Atypical and non-atypical subtypes of depression: comparison of social functioning, symptoms, course of illness, co-morbidity and demographic features. J Affect Disord. 2001;65:75–9.
58. Akiskal HS, Benazzi F. Atypical depression: a variant of bipolar II or a bridge between unipolar and bipolar II? J Affect Disord. 2005;84:209–17.
59. Angst F, Stassen HH, Clayton PJ, Angst J. Mortality of patients with mood disorders: follow-up over 34-38 years. J Affect Disord. 2002;68:167–81.
60. Benazzi F, Akiskal HS. Delineating bipolar II mixed states in the Ravenna-San Diego collaborative study: the relative prevalence and diagnostic significance of hypomanic features during major depressive episodes. J Affect Disord. 2001;67:115–22.
61. Ghaemi SN, Rosenquist KJ, Ko JY, Baldassano CF, Kontos NJ, Baldessarini RJ. Antidepressant treatment in bipolar versus unipolar depression. Am J Psychiatry. 2004;161:163–5.
62. Perugi G, Akiskal HS, Lattanzi L, Cecconi D, Mastrocinque C, Patronelli A. The high prevalence of "soft" bipolar (II) features in atypical depression. Compr Psychiatry. 1998;39:63–71.
63. Vahip S, Kesebir S, Alkan M, Yazici O, Akiskal KK, Akiskal HS. Affective temperaments in clinically-well subjects in Turkey: initial psychometric data on the TEMPS-A. J Affect Disord. 2005;85:113–25.
64. Rastelli CP, Cheng Y, Weingarden J, Frank E, Swartz HA. Differences between unipolar depression and bipolar II depression in women. J Affect Disord. 2013;150:1120–4.
65. Mitchell P, Parker G, Jamieson K, Wilhelm K, Hickie I, Brodaty H. Are there any differences between bipolar and unipolar melancholia? J Affect Disord. 1992;25:97–105.
66. Popescu C, Ionescu R, Jipescu I, Popa S. Psychomotor functioning in unipolar and bipolar affective disorders. Rom J Neurol Psychiatry. 1991;29:17–33.
67. Horwath E, Johnson J, Weissman MM, Hornig CD. The validity of major depression with atypical features based on a community study. J Affect Disord. 1992;26:117–25.
68. Robertson HA, Lam RW, Stewart JN, Yatham LN, Tam EM, Zis AP. Atypical depressive symptoms and clusters in unipolar and bipolar depression. Acta Psychiatr Scand. 1996;94:421–7.
69. Hirschfeld RMA, Williams JBW, Spitzer RL, Calabrese JR, Flynn L, Keck PE. Development and validation of a screening instrument for bipolar spectrum disorder: the Mood Disorder Questionnaire. Am J Psychiatry. 2000;157:1873–5.
70. Ghaemi SN, Miller CJ, Berv DA, Klugman J, Rosenquist KJ, Pies RW. Sensitivity and specificity of a new bipolar spectrum diagnostic scale. J Affect Disord. 2005;84:273–7.
71. Angst J, Adolfsson R, Benazzi F, Gamma A, Hantouche E, Meyer TD. The Hypomania Checklist (HCL-32): its development and external validity. J Affect Disord. 2005;88:217–33.
72. Taylor Tavares JV, Clark L, Furey ML, Williams GB, Sahakian BJ, Drevets WC. Neural basis of abnormal response to negative feedback in unmedicated mood disorders. NeuroImage. 2008;42:1118–26.
73. Almeida JR, Versace A, Mechelli A, Hassel S, Quevedo K, Kupfer DJ. Abnormal amygdala-prefrontal effective connectivity to happy faces differentiates bipolar from major depression. Biol Psychiatry. 2009;66:451–9.
74. Almeida JR, Versace A, Hassel S, Kupfer DJ, Phillips ML. Elevated amygdala activity to sad facial expressions: a state marker of bipolar but not unipolar depression. Biol Psychiatry. 2010;67:414–21.
75. Grotegerd D, Stuhrmann A, Kugel H, Schmidt S, Redlich R, Zwanzger P. Amygdala excitability to subliminally presented emotional faces distinguishes unipolar and bipolar depression: an fMRI and pattern classification study. Hum Brain Mapp. 2014;35:2995–3007.
76. Burger C, Redlich R, Grotegerd D, Meinert S, Dohm K, Schneider I. Differential abnormal pattern of anterior cingulate gyrus activation in unipolar and bipolar depression: an fMRI and pattern classification approach. Neuropsychopharmacology. 2017;42:1399–408.
77. Wang Y, Wang J, Jia Y, Zhong S, Zhong M, Sun Y. Topologically convergent and divergent functional connectivity patterns in unmedicated unipolar depression and bipolar disorder. Transl Psychiatry. 2017;7:e1165.

78. Versace A, Almeida JR, Quevedo K, Thompson WK, Terwilliger RA, Hassel S. Right orbitofrontal corticolimbic and left corticocortical white matter connectivity differentiate bipolar and unipolar depression. Biol Psychiatry. 2010;68:560–7.
79. Silverstone T, McPherson H, Li Q, Doyle T. Deep white matter hyperintensities in patients with bipolar depression, unipolar depression and age-matched control subjects. Bipolar Disord. 2003;5:53–7.
80. Savitz JB, Nugent AC, Bogers W, Roiser JP, Bain EE, Neumeister A. Habenula volume in bipolar disorder and major depressive disorder: a high-resolution magnetic resonance imaging study. Biol Psychiatry. 2011;69:336–43.
81. MacMaster FP, Leslie R, Rosenberg DR, Kusumakar V. Pituitary gland volume in adolescent and young adult bipolar and unipolar depression. Bipolar Disord. 2008;10:101–4.
82. Rosso G, Maina G, Teobaldi E, Balbo I, Di Salvo G, Montarolo F. Differential diagnosis of unipolar versus bipolar depression by GSK3 levels in peripheral blood: a pilot experimental study. Int J Bipolar Disord. 2023;11:33.
83. Wollenhaupt-Aguiar B, Librenza-Garcia D, Bristot G, Przybylski L, Stertz L, Kubiachi Burque R. Differential biomarker signatures in unipolar and bipolar depression: a machine learning approach. Aust N Z J Psychiatry. 2020;54:393–401.
84. Spironelli C, Fusina F, Bortolomasi M, Angrilli A. EEG frontal asymmetry in dysthymia, major depressive disorder and euthymic bipolar disorder. Symmetry. 2021;13:2414.
85. Tas C, Cebi M, Tan O, Hızlı-Sayar G, Tarhan N, Brown EC. EEG power, cordance and coherence differences between unipolar and bipolar depression. J Affect Disord. 2015;172:184–90.
86. Zhong BL, Xu YM, Xie WX, Li Y. Can P300 aid in the differential diagnosis of unipolar disorder versus bipolar disorder depression? A meta-analysis of comparative studies. J Affect Disord. 2019;245:219–27.
87. Vai B, Parenti L, Bollettini I, Cara C, Verga C, Melloni E. Predicting differential diagnosis between bipolar and unipolar depression with multiple kernel learning on multimodal structural neuroimaging. Eur Neuropsychopharmacol. 2020;34:28–38.
88. Rush AJ, Trivedi MH, Wisniewski SR, Nierenberg AA, Stewart JW, Warden D. Acute and longer-term outcomes in depressed outpatients requiring one or several treatment steps: a STAR*D report. Am J Psychiatry. 2006;163:1905–17.
89. Ghaemi SN, Hsu DJ, Soldani F, Goodwin FK. Antidepressants in bipolar disorder: the case for caution. Bipolar Disord. 2003;5:421–33.
90. Geddes JR, Burgess S, Hawton K, Jamison KR, Goodwin FK. Long-term lithium therapy for bipolar disorder: systematic review and meta-analysis of randomized controlled trials. Am J Psychiatry. 2004;161:217–22.
91. McElroy SL, Kemp DE, Friedman ES, Suppes T. Obesity, but not metabolic syndrome, negatively affects outcome in bipolar disorder. J Clin Psychiatry. 2010;71:215–20.
92. Suppes T, Silva R, Cucchiaro J, Baker RA, Eramo A, Gommoll C. Lurasidone for the treatment of bipolar depression: results of a 6-week, randomized, double-blind, placebo-controlled study. Am J Psychiatry. 2016;173:160–7.
93. Leverich GS, Altshuler LL, Frye MA, Suppes T, Keck PE, McElroy SL. Factors associated with suicide attempts in 648 patients with bipolar disorder in the Stanley Foundation Bipolar Network. J Clin Psychiatry. 2006;67:511–21.
94. Kupka RW, Altshuler LL, Nolen WA, Suppes T, Luckenbaugh DA, Leverich GS. Three times more days depressed than manic or hypomanic in both bipolar I and bipolar II disorder. Bipolar Disord. 2007;9:531–5.

3 Mixed Features: Challenges in Diagnosis and Treatment

In Hee Shim and Jong-Hyun Jeong

Diagnostic Challenges

Bipolar disorder is typically characterized by two distinct symptom phases: mania and depression. However, the symptoms of bipolar disorder do not always present in clearly separated forms. This has long been recognized, and in fact, some patients experience depressive symptoms alongside manic or hypomanic features. When such opposing mood states occur simultaneously, the condition is commonly referred to as a mixed state.

Historical Background

Emil Kraepelin (1856–1926) systematized mixed states by integrating clinical observations of fluctuations in mood, thought, and volition [1]. He described several clinical variants, such as depression with flight of ideas, excited depression, depressive anxious mania, unproductive mania with poverty of thought, inhibited mania, and manic stupor. Kraepelin regarded mixed states as manifestations of a hyperarousal mechanism and considered them a more severe form of bipolar disorder, emphasizing their clinical significance.

Although Kraepelin's concept was relatively well accepted in European clinical settings, it was not sufficiently reflected in formal diagnostic criteria. Before the publication of the *Diagnostic and Statistical Manual of Mental Disorders* (DSM) III [2], major depressive disorders were classified into categories such as depressive states of neurosis and those of manic-depressive illness (melancholia or endogenous depression). However, starting with DSM-III, these categories were unified under the diagnosis of major depressive disorder, and mood disorders were dichotomized into major depressive disorder and bipolar disorder. At that time, the concept of mixed states, where both poles co-occur, was not adequately addressed.

Evolution of Diagnostic Criteria

In DSM-IV, DSM-IV-TR (Text Revision) [3], and the *International Classification of Diseases* (ICD)-10 [4], the concept of mixed states was limited to manic episodes with prominent depressive features. In particular, according to the DSM-IV-TR criteria for mixed episodes, only those syndromes in which the full diagnostic criteria for both mania and depression were met for at least one week were included. Similarly, ICD-

I. H. Shim (✉)
Department of Psychiatry, Dongnam Institute of Radiological & Medical Sciences, Busan, Republic of Korea

J.-H. Jeong
Department of Psychiatry, St. Vincent's Hospital, College of Medicine, The Catholic University of Korea, Suwon, Republic of Korea
e-mail: anton3@catholic.ac.kr

W.-M. Bahk et al. (eds.), *Bipolar Disorder*, https://doi.org/10.1007/978-981-92-1323-8_3

10 defined a mixed episode as one in which both manic and depressive symptoms were present, either mixed together or rapidly alternating, for at least two weeks, regardless of symptom severity.

However, mixed episodes that strictly meet these narrow criteria are extremely rare, making it difficult to capture the full spectrum of clinically observed mixed states using such restrictive diagnostic standards [5]. Consequently, mixed states were regarded merely as an uncommon manifestation of bipolar disorder and posed significant diagnostic challenges in clinical practice.

In recent years, accumulating evidence has highlighted that subsyndromal mixed states—where features of the opposite polarity accompany a major mood episode without fulfilling the full criteria for both poles—are much more common than fully syndromal mixed episodes. Clinical studies have also reported that mixed depressive states, which were not recognized in earlier versions of the DSM, are not uncommon in real-world practice. Moreover, the presence or absence of mixed features has been found to significantly influence both treatment outcomes and the prognosis of mood disorders.

Conceptual Models of Mixed States

More recently, it has been emphasized that mixed states are not simply defined by the simultaneous or sequential presence of depressive and manic symptoms of opposite polarity, but rather represent a more complex and unstable clinical presentation with distinct pathophysiological mechanisms.

There are multiple perspectives on how to conceptualize mixed states: some view them as a severe form of manic episode; others see them as a temporary phenomenon during the transition between manic and depressive episodes. Still others consider them a distinct mood state independent from both mania and depression, or regard them as episodes in which one polarity is predominant but accompanied by subthreshold features of the opposite polarity.

Prospective studies of manic episodes have shown that the longer a severe episode persists, the more frequently dysphoric symptoms are observed [6]. Moreover, as manic episodes become more severe, symptoms such as depression, irritability, and aggression are commonly reported during this period. This evidence supports the view that mixed states can be considered a severe form of mania [7]. However, some patients experience depressive symptoms even in the absence of pronounced manic symptoms, and the presence or severity of depressive symptoms does not always correlate with the overall severity of mania [8].

Meanwhile, the argument that mixed states are transient phenomena occurring during the transition between manic and depressive episodes supports the continuum model, which posits that mania and depression lie on a single disease spectrum and vary along a continuum of severity. From this perspective, mixed states are considered temporary manifestations during the progression from milder depressive states to more severe manic states, or vice versa. However, some patients experience mixed states independently, outside of any clear transition. Mixed states can occur as the first mood episode, or as standalone episodes without preceding or subsequent manic or depressive episodes. These observations suggest that, at least for some patients, mixed states are not merely transitional phenomena [9].

Overall, the hypothesis that mixed states are distinct from both manic and depressive episodes cannot fully account for the wide range of mixed presentations. Depressive symptoms accompanying manic episodes vary considerably—from those meeting the full diagnostic criteria for a major depressive episode to those involving only subthreshold depressive symptoms [7]. These variations suggest that such presentations may reflect distinct disease entities.

DSM-V Mixed Features Specifier

In recognition of these diagnostic limitations, DSM-V introduced a broader conceptualization by distinguishing manic episodes accompanied by depressive symptoms that meet full criteria for a major depressive episode from those with only subthreshold depressive symptoms [10]. When using a manic episode as the reference point, mixed states in which mania predominates but mild depressive symptoms are present have been reported to exhibit different treatment responses compared to narrowly defined mixed episodes meeting DSM-IV-TR criteria for both mania and depression [11, 12]. This suggests that narrowly defined mixed episodes (DSM-IV-TR) and broadly defined mixed states with subclinical depressive symptoms during mania may represent distinct clinical entities.

Similarly, when using a depressive episode as the reference point, states in which depression is predominant but accompanied by subthreshold manic or hypomanic symptoms differ from narrowly defined mixed episodes. Clinical studies indicate that in depression-predominant mixed states, manic symptoms are often mild and easily overlooked [13]. Some patients exhibit hypomanic or manic symptoms only at the onset of a depressive episode [14, 15], and these cases are frequently associated with early onset, high recurrence rates, and a family history of bipolar disorder, resembling the characteristics of hypomanic episodes [16]. Moreover, patients who display manic symptoms during a depressive episode tend to have a more severe illness course compared to those with pure depressive episodes [13].

Notably, patients with major depressive disorder accompanied by subthreshold manic symptoms often show familial and longitudinal characteristics similar to those of bipolar disorder, and many are later re-diagnosed as bipolar disorder over time [17, 18]. These observations suggest that the concept of mixed states cannot be fully explained by a single definition. In clinical practice, DSM-IV-defined mixed episodes requiring full criteria for both mania and depression have shown low diagnostic prevalence. Reflecting these issues, DSM-V eliminated the separate diagnostic category of mixed episodes and instead introduced the specifier "with mixed features" within bipolar disorder. Thus, if full criteria for a manic episode are met but those for a major depressive episode are not, the condition is classified as a "manic episode with mixed features" (i.e., mania-predominant mixed state). Conversely, if full criteria for a major depressive episode are met but those for a manic or hypomanic episode are not, it is classified as a "depressive episode with mixed features" (i.e., depression-predominant mixed state).

Clinical Features

Mixed Mania

Mixed mania refers to a state where the diagnostic criteria for a manic episode are met, but the depressive symptoms do not satisfy the criteria for a major depressive episode. This represents a mixed state where manic symptoms predominate. The characteristics of manic symptoms observed in mixed mania include increased mood fluctuations and irritability compared to typical manic episodes. There is a reduced need for sleep, and symptoms such as grandiosity, euphoria, and pressured speech may be present. In mixed mania, depressive symptoms are characterized by a dysphoric mood, anxiety, excessive guilt, and suicidal tendencies [19]. These depressive symptoms in mixed mania resemble those of agitated depression without manic symptoms, but they are more severe, with greater restlessness, irritability, and cognitive impairment [20].

Mixed Depression

Mixed depression refers to a state where depressive symptoms meet the criteria for a major depressive episode, but manic symptoms do not fully satisfy the criteria for a manic episode. This represents a mixed state where depressive symptoms predominate. In mixed depression, compared to non-mixed depression, the frequency of episodes is lower, the duration of episodes is longer, and mixed episodes are more commonly observed at the onset [21, 22]. Additionally, there is less remission of symptoms between episodes, and psychotic symptoms that are incongruent with mood are more frequent [21, 22]. In mixed depression, manic symptoms may include an irritable mood, distractibility, racing thoughts, and increased speech. A study from the Systematic Treatment Enhancement Program–Bipolar Disorder study (STEP-BD), involving 1380 patients with bipolar disorder, reported that distractibility, racing thoughts, flight of ideas, and restlessness were the most commonly observed manic symptoms during depressive episodes [23]. Although reports on the specific characteristics of depressive symptoms in mixed depression are sparse, the severity of depressive symptoms seems similar to that of non-mixed depressive episodes [13, 18]. Additionally, regardless of the degree of mania or depression, mixed states are associated with worry, hyperactivity, negative self-assessment, increased vitality, and racing thoughts [24].

Non-Mood Symptoms in Mixed States

In mixed states, it is important to examine non-mood symptoms such as anxiety, restlessness, and psychotic symptoms. In manic episodes, anxiety symptoms are associated with depression and lithium resistance [12, 25]. The severity of anxiety symptoms correlates with the degree of depressive symptoms [23], but such a relationship is rarely observed in non-mixed mania [12, 20, 24]. Some researchers argue that anxiety symptoms are the most central feature of mixed states [26]. Furthermore, in mixed mania, the severity of anxiety symptoms is similar to that observed in agitated depression [20] and is associated with tension and increased affect [27]. In summary, anxiety symptoms are closely related to depressive symptoms in mixed mania and manic symptoms in mixed depression, which supports the hypothesis that mixed states arise from hyperarousal [28].

In manic episodes, the onset of psychotic symptoms is common, and their severity is reported to be lower in mixed states than in non-mixed manic episodes [12, 29]. As in manic episodes, psychosis/delusions have also been found to be associated with bipolar depressive episodes [30]. While psychotic symptoms are less frequent in depressive episodes compared to manic episodes, they are related to the severity of manic symptoms in bipolar depression [13]. Reports also suggest that psychotic symptoms are closely related to the degree of mania or depression in mixed states [24]. The psychotic manifestations in mixed states are known to be characterized by psychotic symptoms that are incongruent with the mood [21].

Suicidality and Behavioral Dysregulation

In mixed mania, impulsivity and behavioral dysregulation associated with mania are present along with depressive symptoms, and suicidal thoughts are observed at rates similar to those seen in depressive episodes, but higher than in non-mixed manic episodes [19, 31–33]. A study on patients with type I bipolar disorder found that patients with mixed states showing three or more depressive symptoms had a higher prevalence of past suicidal thoughts [34]. Furthermore, patients currently in a mixed state, regardless of their history of mixed episodes, have an increased risk of suicide compared to those currently in a non-mixed state [35].

In mixed depression, the feelings of hopelessness associated with depressive symptoms are accompanied by the impulsivity and hyperactivity characteristic of manic symptoms. Patients in this state appear to attempt suicide more frequently than those experiencing bipolar depressive episodes without manic features [23]. It is also believed that the presence of anxiety symptoms in mixed states further increases the risk of suicide [34]. Unlike manic episodes, depressive episodes already carry an elevated risk of suicide, even in the absence of mixed features. The coexistence of manic symptoms in such cases appears to further heighten this risk. Consequently, regardless of the severity of manic or depressive symptoms, mixed states should be considered high-risk for suicidal behavior due to the combination of hopelessness, impulsivity, and behavioral overactivation. The clinical course of mixed states can vary depending on several factors, including the number of episodes experienced, the presence of suicidal tendencies, comorbid conditions, and the individual's response to treatment.

Treatment Challenges

Mixed states are known to be more difficult to treat compared to pure manic or depressive episodes, and there is a lack of substantial literature supporting pharmacological treatments for mixed states. Most of the existing evidence for pharmacological treatment comes from studies that included patients with manic or mixed episodes, where post-hoc analyses or subgroup analyses were conducted to derive results. Therefore, it remains challenging to establish treatment guidelines specific to mixed states.

Treatment of Mixed Mania/Hypomania

Overview and Guidelines

The category of mixed mania/hypomania presented in DSM-V includes both mixed states where manic/hypomanic symptoms predominate and mixed states characterized by the co-occurrence of manic and depressive symptoms, mirroring the DSM-IV-TR concept of "mixed episodes." According to the Korean Medication Algorithm Project for Bipolar Disorder (KMAP-BP) guidelines, based on expert consensus, the first-line strategy for mixed mania/hypomania includes a combination of mood stabilizers and atypical antipsychotics; atypical antipsychotic monotherapy and mood stabilizer monotherapy are also considered first-line options [36]. The Canadian Network for Mood and Anxiety Treatments and International Society for Bipolar Disorders (CANMAT/ISBD) guidelines do not specify a first-line treatment but recommend second-line options such as asenapine, cariprazine, divalproex, and aripiprazole [37]. A summary of the pharmacological treatment is presented in Table 3.1.

Evidence for Asenapine Versus Olanzapine

A 3-week randomized controlled trial (RCT) plus a 9-week extension trial (asenapine n = 46 vs olanzapine n = 56) in bipolar disorder patients with DSM-IV-TR mixed episodes (analogous to DSM-V mixed mania) showed that asenapine significantly reduced Young Mania Rating Scale (YMRS) and Montgomery–Åsberg Depression Rating Scale (MADRS) scores compared to placebo, while olanzapine did not; the extension trial demonstrated sustained efficacy of asenap-

Table 3.1 Treatment of mixed mania/hypomania derived from the CANMAT-ISBD guideline update for mixed presentations [37] and supported by randomized controlled trials (RCTs) and post-hoc analyses

Medication	Evidence level/Guideline recommendation	Typical dose range (adults)	Key clinical notes
Asenapine	Second-line/moderate evidence; effective in mixed manic RCTs	5–10 mg BID (commonly used dose for mania)	Rapid antimanic effect, moderate metabolic risk
Cariprazine	Second-line/moderate; improves mania and depressive symptoms (post-hoc data)	3–6 mg/day (dose for mania)	Akathisia common; dual efficacy in mania and mixed states
Valproate	Second-line/moderate; superior or non-inferior to lithium in mixed mania	750–1500 mg/day (50–125 μg/mL)	Fast acting; hepatic/hematologic monitoring required
Aripiprazole	Second-line/moderate; limited mixed-specific RCTs	10–30 mg/day	Akathisia risk; robust antimanic effect
Olanzapine	Moderate; effective in mania ± mixed; monotherapy or adjunctive	10–20 mg/day	Metabolic risk; sedation common
Quetiapine	Low–moderate; limited direct mixed mania data	400–800 mg/day	Sedation, orthostasis; adjunctive use common

ine versus olanzapine [38]. A larger post-hoc analysis of 960 patients randomized to asenapine, olanzapine, or placebo confirmed a rapid and sustained remission advantage with asenapine: YMRS score improvements were significant from day 2 to day 21 compared to placebo, whereas olanzapine's effect was significant only at days 2 and 4 [39].

Evidence for Cariprazine

Several RCTs and pooled analyses have evaluated cariprazine in bipolar I mania or mixed episodes. Although the overall mixed-state subgroup was small, one subgroup study (≈14% of total) with 83 cariprazine versus 62 placebo patients showed significantly greater YMRS reduction after three weeks [40–43]. A pooled analysis across three trials (3–12 mg/day) also demonstrated significant improvements in mixed symptoms (hostility, irritability, agitation) by week 3 [44]. Age-stratified analysis indicated that in older bipolar patients, only the 3–6 mg/day dose was effective, while in younger patients, both 3–6 mg/day and 9–12 mg/day were effective—with the higher dose showing a stronger response—suggesting age-related dosing differences [45]. Taken together with earlier studies and subsequent pooled analyses, these findings suggest that cariprazine may be effective in treating mixed mania in bipolar I disorder.

Evidence for Quetiapine

An eight-week randomized controlled study compared adjunctive quetiapine to placebo in 55 bipolar II patients with mixed hypomania [46]. The quetiapine group demonstrated significant improvements in Clinical Global Impressions–Bipolar version severity (CGI-BP-S) and MADRS scores ($p = 0.002$, $p = 0.0138$), but there was no significant difference in YMRS scores ($p = 0.069$) [46]. A total of 55 patients with bipolar II disorder, who had been receiving stable treatment for bipolar disorder for more than two weeks, participated in the study. The quetiapine combination therapy group showed significant improvements in the CGI-BP-S total scores and in the MADRS total scores compared to the placebo combination therapy group. However, no significant differences were observed between the quetiapine and placebo groups in the YMRS total scores. This study confirmed that quetiapine combination therapy is more effective than placebo for overall symptoms and depressive symptoms in mixed hypomania in bipolar II disorder, but it does not show a difference in the improvement of hypomanic symptoms compared to placebo.

Evidence for Olanzapine

Three randomized controlled trials were integrated and analyzed post hoc to assess the effect of olanzapine in patients with mixed mania in bipolar I disorder [47]. The olanzapine group showed significant improvements in the YMRS total score compared to the placebo group, and this result was not influenced by the presence of mixed states. Additionally, there was a significant improvement in the Hamilton Depression Rating Scale (HDRS) total score in the olanzapine group compared to the placebo group, suggesting an antidepressant effect.

An eight-week randomized controlled study was conducted to compare the effects of olanzapine and divalproex combination therapy versus divalproex monotherapy in patients with bipolar disorder experiencing mixed episodes according to DSM-IV-TR criteria (which corresponds to mixed mania in DSM-V) [48]. This study was divided into two phases: Phase I (days 4–28) involved divalproex monotherapy, and patients who showed insufficient response during this period were randomized to receive either olanzapine or placebo in combination with divalproex in Phase II (6 weeks). A total of 202 patients were randomized to receive divalproex and olanzapine combination therapy or divalproex and placebo combination therapy. During Phase II (6 weeks), the olanzapine combination therapy group showed a significant reduction in HDRS total score compared to the placebo combination therapy group. The YMRS total score also showed a greater reduction in the olanzapine combination therapy group compared to the placebo combination therapy group. Furthermore, the time to achieve partial response (defined as a 25% reduction in HDRS and YMRS) and the time to achieve treatment response (defined as a 50% reduction in both scales) were significantly shorter in the olanzapine combination therapy group. This study confirmed that, in patients with mixed episodes, the combination therapy of divalproex and olanzapine led to more rapid and greater improvements in both manic and depressive symptoms compared to divalproex monotherapy.

Carbamazepine, Valproate, and Lithium

A post-hoc analysis was conducted in two similar randomized controlled trials to assess the effect of carbamazepine monotherapy in patients with manic or mixed episodes according to DSM-IV criteria [49, 50]. In one study, carbamazepine showed an effect on improving depressive symptoms in mixed episodes compared to placebo, while in another study, carbamazepine showed an effect only on improving manic symptoms. A subsequent analysis that integrated these two studies reported that carbamazepine was effective in improving both manic and depressive symptoms in patients with mixed mania compared to placebo [51]. However, there is still a lack of sufficient research reports on the combination therapy with carbamazepine.

The application of valproate and lithium in bipolar disorder mixed mania is still actively researched, but evidence supporting their efficacy remains limited. One study randomized patients with acute mania to receive lithium, valproate, or placebo to evaluate how the presence of depressive symptoms affected the treatment response [11]. Of the 179 patients, 103 were diagnosed with mixed mania. The results showed that when depressive symptoms were present during a manic episode, the antimanic effect of lithium was reduced, while valproate appeared to be more effective. However, valproate did not show a significant effect compared to placebo, and limitations such as small sample size and post-hoc analysis suggest that further studies are necessary. Additionally, an eight-week randomized controlled study of valproate monotherapy (n = 60) included patients with mild mania or hypomania, regardless of the presence of mixed symptoms, and may not be appropriate for inclusion in this section [52]. However, this study demonstrated a statistical trend for an antidepressant effect when valproate was used in combination with initial depressive symptoms (in mixed manic/hypomanic episodes), which holds some significance.

Mixed Depression

Guideline Recommendations

According to the KMAP-BP guidelines, there is no clear first-line strategy for the treatment of mixed depression. However, the first-line strategies include: mood stabilizer and atypical antipsychotic combination therapy, atypical antipsychotic and lamotrigine combination therapy, atypical antipsychotic monotherapy, mood stabilizer and lamotrigine combination therapy, and mood stabilizer monotherapy [36]. These strategies are consistent with both the 2018 and the 2022 revised versions of the guidelines. However, a notable change in the revised version is the increased preference for atypical antipsychotic monotherapy and mood stabilizer monotherapy as first-line strategies. This reflects a shift toward more diverse treatment approaches and a comprehensive consideration of the effects and safety of these medications in mixed bipolar presentations. According to the CANMAT/ISBD guidelines, there is no preferred first-line treatment strategy for mixed depression, but cariprazine and lurasidone are included as second-line treatments [37]. This highlights the variety of available treatments for mixed depression and emphasizes the need for individualized medication choices based on the patient's condition.

Antidepressant use in mixed depression remains controversial due to the risk of triggering mania or hypomania, especially in patients with bipolar disorder. While antidepressants are effective in unipolar depression, their efficacy in mixed depression is unclear, and they may exacerbate manic symptoms. The lack of robust evidence, combined with concerns about mood switching and long-term instability, makes their use more complicated. As a result, antidepressants are typically used cautiously, often in combination with mood stabilizers/antipsychotics, and only when necessary to manage depressive symptoms. A summary of the pharmacological treatment is presented in Table 3.2.

Randomized Controlled Trials for Mixed Depression

Despite this, no differences were observed in mania symptom reduction (MRS scores), and ziprasidone was well tolerated, particularly in terms of weight gain and extrapyramidal symptoms. In a six-week trial with 73 participants, ziprasidone (40–160 mg/day) showed a significantly greater reduction in MADRS scores compared to placebo by week 3, and the antidepressant effect persisted through week 6. This effect was more pronounced in patients with bipolar II disorder [53]. There was no significant difference in mania symptoms (measured by MRS), and ziprasidone had a favorable side effect profile, with minimal weight gain and extrapyramidal symptoms. However, for bipolar depression (with or without mixed features), the preponderance of evidence and major guidelines do not support ziprasidone.

A six-week trial involving 385 patients with mixed depression (185 with major depressive disorder and 200 with bipolar depression) showed that lumateperone (42 mg) led to significant improvements in MADRS and CGI-S scores compared to placebo [54]. The results were consistent across both patient groups, suggesting its broad efficacy in mixed depression.

Post-Hoc Analyses for Mixed Depression

In an eight-week trial with 788 patients, both olanzapine and olanzapine-fluoxetine combination (OFC) showed significant improvement in depressive symptoms compared to placebo, but

Table 3.2 Treatment of mixed mania/hypomania derived from the CANMAT-ISBD guideline update for mixed presentations [37] and supported by randomized controlled trials (RCTs) and post-hoc analyses

Medication	Evidence level/Guideline recommendation	Typical dose range (adults)	Key clinical notes
Lurasidone	Second-line/moderate; post-hoc analyses from bipolar depression RCTs in patients with mixed features	20–120 mg/day (with food)	Improves both depressive and mixed symptoms; low metabolic burden
Cariprazine	Second-line/moderate; post-hoc evidence in mixed depression	1.5–3 mg/day	Dual dopaminergic activity; monitor akathisia
Lumateperone	Emerging evidence/moderate; effective for bipolar I/II depression including mixed features	42 mg/day	Minimal metabolic/EPS burden; FDA-approved for bipolar depression
Olanzapine (± fluoxetine)	Low–moderate; efficacy in bipolar depression; limited mixed specific evidence	5–20 mg/day	Monitor weight gain/ metabolic effects
Quetiapine	Third-line; effective for bipolar depression overall; no direct ECT in mixed features	300–600 mg/day	Indirect evidence only; sedation and metabolic monitoring needed
Valproate	Low; limited data in mixed depression	Target trough 50–100 μg/ mL	Adjunctive role; avoid antidepressant monotherapy in mixed states
Lithium	Low; limited data in acute mixed depression; maintenance benefit	0.6–1.0 mEq/L (maintenance)	Monitor renal/thyroid; caution in acute mixed depression

ECT electroconvulsive therapy, *EPS* extrapyramidal symptoms, *FDA* Food and Drug Administration

OFC did not demonstrate superior efficacy. Additionally, no significant difference in mania switch rates was observed between the treatment and placebo groups, indicating both options were similarly effective in managing mixed depression [55].

A separate post-hoc analysis of 1214 patients showed that olanzapine monotherapy significantly improved MADRS scores compared to placebo after six weeks. This study further supports olanzapine as an effective option for treating mixed depression in bipolar I disorder [56].

In a six-week trial with 272 patients, lurasidone (20–120 mg) significantly reduced MADRS scores compared to placebo, confirming its antidepressant effect in mixed bipolar depression. Mania switch rates were not significantly different between the lurasidone and placebo groups [57].

An analysis of 1383 patients demonstrated that cariprazine (1.5 mg and 3 mg) significantly improved MADRS scores compared to placebo after six weeks, highlighting its potential as a treatment option for mixed depression in bipolar I disorder [58].

A post-hoc analysis of 376 patients with mixed depression (from a larger study) showed significant improvements in both MADRS and CGI-BP-S scores. This analysis further supports lumateperone's efficacy, with minimal side effects reported [59].

Summary and Limitations

Post-hoc analyses of randomized controlled trials targeting mixed depression (including subsyndromal manic symptoms in major depressive episodes) based on DSM-V are limited to olanzapine, lurasidone, asenapine, cariprazine, and lumateperone, and only a few randomized controlled trials have been conducted with ziprasidone and lumateperone. Furthermore, similar to mixed mania/hypomania, the focus has been primarily on atypical antipsychotics. Therefore, there is currently insufficient research to discuss the treatment of mixed depression, making it difficult to draw a definitive conclusion.

Declarations

Competing Interests The author(s) has no competing interests to declare that are relevant to the content of this manuscript.

Ethics Approval The author(s) declares that this manuscript does not include primary research with human participants.

The author(s) declares that this manuscript does not include primary studies involving animals.

References

1. Kraepelin E. Manic-depressive illness and paranoia. Edinburgh: E&S Livingstone; 1921.
2. American Psychiatric Association. Diagnostic and statistical manual of mental disorders, 3rd ed. Washington, DC: American Psychiatric Association; 1980.
3. American Psychiatric Association. Diagnostic and statistical manual of mental disorders, 4th ed, Text Rev. Washington, DC: American Psychiatric Association; 2000.
4. World Health Organization. The ICD-10 classification of mental and Behavioural disorders: diagnostic criteria for research. Geneva: World Health Organization; 1993.
5. Suppes T, Mintz J, McElroy SL, Altshuler LL, Kupka RW, Frye MA, et al. Mixed hypomania in 908 patients with bipolar disorder evaluated prospectively in the Stanley Foundation Bipolar Treatment Network: a sex-specific phenomenon. Arch Gen Psychiatry. 2005;62(10):1089–96. https://doi.org/10.1001/archpsyc.62.10.1089.
6. Carlson GA, Goodwin FK. The stages of mania: a longitudinal analysis of the manic episode. Arch Gen Psychiatry. 1973;28(2):221–8. https://doi.org/10.1001/archpsyc.1973.01750320053009.
7. Post RM, Rubinow DR, Uhde TW, Roy-Byrne PP, Linnoila M, Rosoff A, et al. Dysphoric mania: clinical and biological correlates. Arch Gen Psychiatry. 1989;46(4):353–8.
8. Secunda SK, Swann A, Katz MM, Koslow SH, Croughan J, Chang S. Diagnosis and treatment of mixed mania. Am J Psychiatry. 1987;144(1):96–8.
9. McElroy SL, Keck PE Jr, Pope HG Jr, Hudson JI, Faedda GL, Swann AC. Clinical and research implications of the diagnosis of dysphoric or mixed mania or hypomania. Am J Psychiatry. 1992;149(12):1633–44.
10. American Psychiatric Association. Diagnostic and statistical manual of mental disorders, 5th ed. Washington, DC: American Psychiatric Association; 2013.
11. Swann AC, Bowden CL, Morris D, Calabrese JR, Petty F, Small J, et al. Depression during mania: treatment response to lithium or divalproex. Arch

Gen Psychiatry. 1997;54(1):37–42. https://doi.org/10.1001/archpsyc.1997.01830130041008.
12. Swann AC, Secunda SK, Katz MM, Koslow SH, Maas JW, Chang S, et al. Lithium treatment of mania: clinical characteristics, specificity of symptom change, and outcome. Psychiatry Res. 1986;18(2):127–41. https://doi.org/10.1016/0165-1781(86)90025-9.
13. Swann AC, Moeller FG, Steinberg JL, Schneider L, Barratt ES, Dougherty DM. Manic symptoms and impulsivity during bipolar depressive episodes. Bipolar Disord. 2007;9(3):206–12.
14. Akiskal HS, Benazzi F, Perugi G, Rihmer Z. Agitated "unipolar" depression reconceptualized as a depressive mixed state: implications for the antidepressant–suicide controversy. J Affect Disord. 2005;85(2–3):245–58.
15. Benazzi F, Akiskal HS. Delineating bipolar II mixed states in the Ravenna–San Diego collaborative study: the relative prevalence and diagnostic significance of hypomanic features during major depressive episodes. J Affect Disord. 2001;67(1–2):115–22.
16. Akiskal HS, Benazzi F. Family history validation of the bipolar nature of depressive mixed states. J Affect Disord. 2003;73(1–2):113–22.
17. Fiedorowicz JG, Endicott J, Leon AC, Solomon DA, Keller MB, Coryell WH. Subthreshold hypomanic symptoms in progression from unipolar major depression to bipolar disorder. Am J Psychiatry. 2011;168(1):40–8.
18. Zimmermann P, Brückl T, Nocon A, Pfister H, Lieb R, Wittchen HU, et al. Heterogeneity of DSM-IV major depressive disorder as a consequence of subthreshold bipolarity. Arch Gen Psychiatry. 2009;66(12):1341–52.
19. Cassidy F, Murry E, Forest K, Carroll BJ. Signs and symptoms of mania in pure and mixed episodes. J Affect Disord. 1998;50(3):187–201.
20. Swann AC, Secunda SK, Katz MM, Koslow SH, Croughan J, Bowden CL, et al. Specificity of mixed affective states: clinical comparison of dysphoric mania and agitated depression. J Affect Disord. 1993;28(2):81–9.
21. Perugi G, Akiskal HS, Micheli C, Toni C, Madaro D. Clinical characterization of depressive mixed state in bipolar-I patients: Pisa-San Diego collaboration. J Affect Disord. 2001;67(1–3):105–14. https://doi.org/10.1016/S0165-0327(01)00443-8.
22. Chung YI. Emerging concepts of bipolar disorder: focus on mixed states. J Korean Neuropsychiatr Assoc. 2008;47(2):119–25.
23. Goldberg JF, Perlis RH, Bowden CL, Thase ME, Miklowitz DJ, Marangell LB, et al. Manic symptoms during depressive episodes in 1,380 patients with bipolar disorder: findings from the STEP-BD. Am J Psychiatry. 2009;166(2):173–81.
24. Swann AC, Steinberg JL, Lijffijt M, Moeller GF. Continuum of depressive and manic mixed states in patients with bipolar disorder: quantitative measurement and clinical features. World Psychiatry. 2009;8(2):166–72.
25. González-Pinto A, Aldama A, Mosquera F, González Gómez C. Epidemiology, diagnosis and management of mixed mania. CNS Drugs. 2007;21(8):611–26. https://doi.org/10.2165/00023210-200721080-00001.
26. Cassidy F. Anxiety as a symptom of mixed mania: implications for DSM-5. Bipolar Disord. 2010;12(4):437–9. https://doi.org/10.1111/j.1399-5618.2010.00824.x.
27. Henry C, M'Baïlara K, Poinsot R, Casteret AA, Sorbara F, Leboyer M, et al. Evidence for two types of bipolar depression using a dimensional approach. Psychother Psychosom. 2007;76(5):325–31.
28. Bertschy G, Gervasoni N, Favre S, Liberek C, Ragama-Pardos E, Aubry JM, et al. Frequency of dysphoria and mixed states. Psychopathology. 2008;41(4):187–93.
29. González-Pinto A, Aldama A, Pinto AG, Mosquera F, Pérez de Heredia JL, Ballesteros J, et al. Dimensions of mania: differences between mixed and pure episodes. Eur Psychiatry. 2004;19(5):307–10.
30. Sato T, Bottlender R, Kleindienst N, Möller HJ. Irritable psychomotor elation in depressed inpatients: a factor validation of mixed depression. J Affect Disord. 2005;84(2–3):187–96.
31. Hantouche EG, Akiskal HS, Azorin JM, Châtenet-Duchêne L, Lancrenon S. Clinical and psychometric characterization of depression in mixed mania: a report from the French National Cohort of 1090 manic patients. J Affect Disord. 2006;96(3):225–32. https://doi.org/10.1016/j.jad.2005.01.005.
32. Strakowski SM, McElroy SL, Keck PE Jr, West SA. Suicidality among patients with mixed and manic bipolar disorder. Am J Psychiatry. 1996;153(5):674–6.
33. Goldberg JF, Garno JL, Leon AC, Kocsis JH, Portera L. Association of recurrent suicidal ideation with nonremission from acute mixed mania. Am J Psychiatry. 1998;155(12):1753–5.
34. Diefenbach GJ, Woolley SB, Goethe JW. The association between self-reported anxiety symptoms and suicidality. J Nerv Ment Dis. 2009;197(2):92–7.
35. Pacchiarotti I, Mazzarini L, Kotzalidis GD, Valenti M, Nivoli AM, Sani G, et al. Mania and depression: mixed, not stirred. J Affect Disord. 2011;133(1–2):105–13. https://doi.org/10.1016/j.jad.2011.03.037.
36. Kim W, Bahk WM, Woo YS, Jeong JH, Seo JS, Choo IH, et al. Korean medication algorithm project for bipolar disorder 2022: mixed features. J Korean Neuropsychiatr Assoc. 2022;61(2):133–42. https://doi.org/10.4306/jknpa.2022.61.2.133.
37. Yatham LN, Chakrabarty T, Bond DJ, Schaffer A, Beaulieu S, Parikh SV, et al. Canadian Network for Mood and Anxiety Treatments (CANMAT) and International Society for Bipolar Disorders (ISBD) recommendations for the management of patients with bipolar disorder with mixed presentations. Bipolar Disord. 2021;23(8):767–88. https://doi.org/10.1111/bdi.13135.

38. Azorin J, Sapin C, Weiller E. Effect of asenapine on manic and depressive symptoms in bipolar I patients with mixed episodes: results from post hoc analyses. J Affect Disord. 2013;145(1):62–9.
39. McIntyre RS, Tohen M, Berk M, Zhao J, Weiller E. DSM-5 mixed specifier for manic episodes: evaluating the effect of depressive features on severity and treatment outcome using asenapine clinical trial data. J Affect Disord. 2013;150(2):378–83. https://doi.org/10.1016/j.jad.2013.04.025.
40. Calabrese JR, Keck PE Jr, Starace A, Lu K, Ruth A, Laszlovszky I, et al. Efficacy and safety of low- and high-dose cariprazine in acute and mixed mania associated with bipolar I disorder: a double-blind, placebo-controlled study. J Clin Psychiatry. 2015;76(3):284–92. https://doi.org/10.4088/JCP.14m09081.
41. Durgam S, Starace A, Li D, Migliore R, Ruth A, Nemeth G, et al. The efficacy and tolerability of cariprazine in acute mania associated with bipolar I disorder: a phase II trial. Bipolar Disord. 2015;17(1):63–75. https://doi.org/10.1111/bdi.12238.
42. Sachs GS, Greenberg WM, Starace A, Lu K, Ruth A, Laszlovszky I, et al. Cariprazine in the treatment of acute mania in bipolar I disorder: a double-blind, placebo-controlled, phase III trial. J Affect Disord. 2015;174:296–302. https://doi.org/10.1016/j.jad.2014.11.018.
43. Vieta E, Durgam S, Lu K, Ruth A, Debelle M, Zukin S. Effect of cariprazine across the symptoms of mania in bipolar I disorder: analyses of pooled data from phase II/III trials. Eur Neuropsychopharmacol. 2015;25(11):1882–91. https://doi.org/10.1016/j.euroneuro.2015.08.001.
44. Citrome L, Li C, Yu J, Kramer K, Nguyen HB. Effects of cariprazine on reducing symptoms of irritability, hostility, and agitation in patients with manic or mixed episodes of bipolar I disorder. J Affect Disord. 2024;(358):353–60. https://doi.org/10.1016/j.jad.2024.04.084.
45. Garel N, Dols A, Yu J, Cresce CD, Rej S, Sajatovic M. Effect of Cariprazine on outcomes in older-aged and younger-aged patients with bipolar I disorder: a post-hoc analysis. Am J Geriatr Psychiatry. 2025;33(4):372–86.
46. Suppes T, Ketter TA, Gwizdowski IS, Dennehy EB, Hill SJ, Fischer EG, et al. First controlled treatment trial of bipolar II hypomania with mixed symptoms: quetiapine versus placebo. J Affect Disord. 2013;150(1):37–43. https://doi.org/10.1016/j.jad.2013.02.031.
47. Tohen M, McIntyre RS, Kanba S, Fujikoshi S, Katagiri H. Efficacy of olanzapine in the treatment of bipolar mania with mixed features defined by DSM-5. J Affect Disord. 2014;(168):136–41. https://doi.org/10.1016/j.jad.2014.06.039.
48. Houston JP, Tohen M, Degenhardt EK, Jamal HH, Liu LL, Ketter TA. Olanzapine-divalproex combination versus divalproex monotherapy in the treatment of bipolar mixed episodes: a double-blind, placebo-controlled study. J Clin Psychiatry. 2009;70(11):1540–7. https://doi.org/10.4088/JCP.08m04895yel.
49. Weisler RH, Kalali AH, Ketter TA; SPD417 Study Group. A multicenter, randomized, double-blind, placebo-controlled trial of extended-release carbamazepine capsules as monotherapy for bipolar disorder patients with manic or mixed episodes. J Clin Psychiatry. 2004;65(4):478–84. https://doi.org/10.4088/JCP.v65n0405.
50. Weisler RH, Keck PE Jr, Swann AC, Cutler AJ, Ketter TA, Kalali AH; SPD417 Study Group. Extended-release carbamazepine capsules as monotherapy for acute mania in bipolar disorder: a multicenter, randomized, double-blind, placebo-controlled trial. J Clin Psychiatry. 2005;66(3):323–30. https://doi.org/10.4088/JCP.v66n0308.
51. Weisler RH, Hirschfeld R, Cutler AJ, Gazda T, Ketter TA, Keck PE Jr, et al. Extended-release carbamazepine capsules as monotherapy in bipolar disorder. CNS Drugs. 2006;20(3):219–31. https://doi.org/10.2165/00023210-200620030-00004.
52. McElroy SL, Martens BE, Creech RS, Welge JA, Jefferson L, Guerdjikova AI, et al. Randomized, double-blind, placebo-controlled study of divalproex extended-release loading monotherapy in ambulatory bipolar spectrum disorder patients with moderate-to-severe hypomania or mild mania. J Clin Psychiatry. 2010;71(5):557–65. https://doi.org/10.4088/JCP.08m04854yel.
53. Patkar A, Gilmer W, Pae CU, Vohringer PA, Ziffra M, Pirok E, et al. A 6-week randomized, double-blind, placebo-controlled trial of ziprasidone for the acute depressive mixed state. PLoS One. 2012;7(4):e34757. https://doi.org/10.1371/journal.pone.0034757.
54. Durgam S, Kozauer SG, Earley WR, Chen C, Huo J, Lakkis H, et al. Lumateperone for the treatment of major depressive disorder with mixed features or bipolar depression with mixed features: a randomized placebo-controlled trial. J Clin Psychopharmacol. 2025;45(2):67–75. https://doi.org/10.1097/JCP.0000000000001964.
55. Benazzi F, Berk M, Frye MA, Wang W, Barraco A, Tohen M. Olanzapine/fluoxetine combination for the treatment of mixed depression in bipolar I disorder: a post hoc analysis. J Clin Psychiatry. 2009;70(9):1424–31. https://doi.org/10.4088/JCP.08m04414.
56. Tohen M, Kanba S, McIntyre RS, Fujikoshi S, Katagiri H. Efficacy of olanzapine monotherapy in the treatment of bipolar depression with mixed features. J Affect Disord. 2014;164:57–62. https://doi.org/10.1016/j.jad.2014.04.033.
57. McIntyre RS, Cucchiaro J, Pikalov A, Kroger H, Loebel A. Lurasidone in the treatment of bipolar depression with mixed (subsyndromal hypomanic) features: post hoc analysis of a randomized placebo-controlled trial. J Clin Psychiatry. 2015;76(4):398–405. https://doi.org/10.4088/JCP.14m09128.

58. McIntyre RS, Suppes T, Earley W, Patel M, Stahl SM. Cariprazine efficacy in bipolar I depression with and without concurrent manic symptoms: post hoc analysis of 3 randomized, placebo-controlled studies. CNS Spectr. 2020;25(4):502–10. https://doi.org/10.1017/S1092852920000756.
59. McIntyre RS, Durgam S, Huo J, Kozauer SG, Stahl SM. The efficacy of lumateperone in patients with bipolar depression with mixed features. J Clin Psychiatry. 2023;84(3):22m14739. https://doi.org/10.4088/JCP.22m14739.

Cognitive Dysfunction in Bipolar Disorder: A Comprehensive Review of Clinical Evidence and Implications

4

Kang Soo Lee and Young-Min Park

Since Emil Kraepelin first distinguished dementia praecox and manic-depressive insanity as two distinct entities, the presence of inter-episodic periods of normal functioning has been considered a defining feature differentiating bipolar disorder (BD) from schizophrenia. Recent studies, however, indicate that patients with bipolar disorder can retain some degree of cognitive dysfunction even during the remission phase. Moreover, cognitive impairments have been reported in biological relatives of patients diagnosed with bipolar disorder. There is substantial evidence supporting these findings, particularly that patients with bipolar disorder exhibit abnormal brain structure from an early stage, characterized by enlarged ventricles, atrophy in the temporal and frontal lobes, and alterations in white matter integrity.

This review aims to synthesize current findings related to cognitive dysfunction in patients with bipolar disorder, thereby broadening the understanding of the disorder's implications beyond mere mood disturbances.

K. S. Lee (✉)
Department of Psychiatry, CHA Bundang Medical Center, CHA University, Seongnam, Republic of Korea
e-mail: antiaging@chamc.co.kr

Y.-M. Park
Brain and Mind Mental Health Clinic, Goyang, Republic of Korea

Brain and Mind Institute, Goyang, Republic of Korea

Assessment of Cognitive Function in Patients with Bipolar Disorder

Multiple instruments exist for assessing cognitive function in individuals with bipolar disorder. The most well-known among these is the Measurement and Treatment Research to Improve Cognition in Schizophrenia (MATRICS) Consensus Cognitive Battery (MCCB) [1]. This instrument was originally developed for evaluating cognitive function in schizophrenia but is increasingly utilized to assess bipolar disorder. The MCCB encompasses seven domains: (1) processing speed, (2) attention/vigilance, (3) working memory, (4) verbal learning, (5) visual learning, (6) reasoning and problem-solving, and 7) social cognition. The International Society for Bipolar Disorders (ISBD) recommends that patients undergo at least two screening tests, the first being the Screen for Cognitive Impairment in Psychiatry (SCIP) and the second, the Cognitive Complaints in Bipolar Disorder Rating Scale (COBRA). The SCIP is a brief instrument to test cognitive function that takes approximately 15 minutes to complete; it evaluates immediate and delayed verbal learning, working memory, verbal fluency, and processing speed. COBRA functions as a self-report scale concentrating on overall cognitive functions, specifically in bipolar disorder. The ISBD recommends that all patients with bipolar disorder in remission undergo cognitive testing two to three months after achieving remission and at five-year intervals thereafter.

W.-M. Bahk et al. (eds.), *Bipolar Disorder*, https://doi.org/10.1007/978-981-92-1323-8_4

Premorbid Cognitive Functioning and Genetic Effects in Patients with Bipolar Disorder

Compelling evidence indicates cognitive dysfunction in children, adolescents, and adults diagnosed with bipolar disorder [2]. However, limited research has examined the premorbid cognitive function of these patients. The following were the relevant studies [3–5]. In one study, 74 children of patients with bipolar disorder, those with depression, and healthy persons were assessed for premorbid intelligence and executive function. Among the nine individuals who developed bipolar disorder in adulthood demonstrated average intelligence quotient (IQ) but significantly lower executive function scores compared to the others. Another study reported that children who developed bipolar disorder demonstrated significantly lower executive function and visuospatial ability compared to those who did not develop this disorder.

Two recent meta-analyses revealed that families of individuals with bipolar disorder consistently exhibit cognitive dysfunction relative to healthy individuals [6, 7]. In the first meta-analysis, family members of bipolar disorder patients displayed the most significant discrepancies in response inhibition, followed by executive function, with verbal learning and memory ranking next. The second meta-analysis corroborated similar findings; however, some cognitive domains did not show statistically significant differences, suggesting that not all aspects of cognitive function were equally affected. An intriguing recent twin study indicated that healthy twins of parents with bipolar disorder demonstrated superior verbal fluency and verbal learning compared to those with non-affected parents, implying variability in cognitive function among relatives of patients with bipolar disorder.

Unlike mood-related symptoms, cognitive impairments are not state-dependent. Since such abnormalities appear in the biological relatives of patients with bipolar disorder and persist during remissions, they may serve as biological markers for bipolar disorder.

Cognitive Profiles Across Illness Phases

A comprehensive study indicated that patients with bipolar disorder exhibit deficits across all cognitive domains, including verbal memory, working memory, psychomotor speed, verbal fluency, attention, and executive function [8]. The participants included those experiencing manic, depressive, or mixed episodes, as well as individuals in remission. These findings have been replicated in multiple studies. Some researchers contend that impaired sustained attention is the most characteristic cognitive dysfunction distinguishing individuals with bipolar disorder from healthy controls. Further investigations examined whether cognitive dysfunction correlates with variables such as sex, age, or educational background [9, 10]. However, these factors did not produce significant alterations in cognitive performance between healthy subjects and those with bipolar disorder.

A meta-analysis published in 2006 classified patients with bipolar disorder in remission based on the effect size of cognitive function differences compared to healthy individuals [8]. Cognitive domains yielding the largest effect sizes included category fluency, mental manipulation, and verbal learning, whereas psychomotor speed, response inhibition, abstraction, verbal memory, and sustained attention reflected moderate effect sizes. Domains associated with small effect sizes included verbal fluency and immediate memory. The observed effects were independent of premorbid IQ, educational levels, and cultural or regional factors. However, although participants were in remission, the influence of residual symptoms could not be entirely ruled out, as statistical significance vanished in some analyses when residual symptoms were considered [11, 12]. Conversely, other studies maintained significant differences regardless of residual symptoms [11–13]. These inconsistencies may stem from differing definitions of remission across studies [8]. Given that some investigations document cognitive dysfunction even in the early stages of the disease, such dysfunction may be regarded as a trait marker for bipolar disorder. Further complexities arise from the potential impact of pharmacological treatments. In one study, comparison of cognitive function between patients with bipolar disorder in remission who were taking mood regulators and those who were not revealed no significant difference [14]. This means that cognitive dysfunction in bipolar disorder cannot be solely attributed to medication. However, owing to the scarcity of studies excluding the effects of drugs, drug-related effects cannot be completely ruled out, emphasizing the need for further exploration regarding the effects on cognition of benzodiazepines and antipsychotics.

As previously noted, significant differences in cognitive function exist between individuals with bipolar disorder and healthy controls during manic, depressive, and mixed episodes, as well as in remission phases. Therefore, it is essential to consider whether cognitive dysfunction varies by episode type or if specific episode types present distinctive cognitive profiles. In one study, patients in a manic episode exhibited the lowest scores in executive function, affecting verbal memory, reasoning, and problem-solving capabilities [15]. Another investigation reported substantial executive dysfunction, particularly in reasoning and problem-solving, while yet another emphasized that impaired working memory characterizes manic episodes [16, 17]. Conversely, some researchers argue that impaired attention is central to manic episodes, with compromised verbal memory affecting working memory on a secondary level [13]. Others suggest that psychomotor speed represents the most pronounced cognitive dysfunction among manic patients, characterized by high error rates [15]. However, researchers have also suggested that medication with antipsychotics or benzodiazepines may influence these cognitive patterns at the time of testing.

During depressive episodes, reductions in verbal fluency and psychomotor speed have been documented in multiple studies [18, 19]. One study found that verbal fluency exhibited the most significant impairment, while another indicated that psychomotor speed was more adversely affected. A third study linked depressive symptoms, particularly related to psychomotor speed and attention, to severe cognitive dysfunction [20].

Research on mixed episodes reveals impairments in executive function, encompassing working memory, reasoning, and problem-solving, alongside decreased attention and processing speed [15]. These patterns resemble those observed during manic episodes. Some researchers have argued that in manic episodes, impaired working memory is exacerbated by the presence of mixed symptoms [21].

Patients with bipolar disorder in remission consistently score significantly higher on cognitive function tests compared to those experiencing manic, depressive, or mixed episodes. However, they score lower than healthy controls [15, 22].

In summary, patients with bipolar disorder show cognitive dysfunction regardless of episode type or whether they are experiencing an active episode, although the specific profiles of cognitive dysfunction differ depending on the type of episode. In addition, patients in remission demonstrate better cognitive functions than those currently experiencing episodes, yet their cognitive function remains impaired when compared to healthy individuals.

Some studies comparing cognitive function between patients with type 1 and type 2 bipolar disorder suggest that type 1 patients exhibit more severe cognitive dysfunction than type 2 patients, and meta-analyses have corroborated these findings [22]. However, another research posits that these differences may arise from type 1 patients being prescribed more antipsychotics than type 2 patients [23]. Conversely, certain studies report no cognitive performance differences between type 1 and type 2 bipolar disorder [24]. Shared features include deficits in psychomotor speed, working memory, and executive function compared to healthy individuals. In contrast, type 2 patients do not exhibit issues with verbal learning and delayed memory, while deficits in visual/constructional abilities are noted. Future research should further investigate comparative differences between types 1 and 2 while controlling for medication effects.

Recently, cognitive function was assessed between individuals with type 2 bipolar disorder and unipolar depression, specifically excluding medication effects [25]. Patients with unipolar depression scored poorly on cognitive speed and cognitive flexibility, while type 2 bipolar disorder patients unexpectedly demonstrated no cognitive dysfunction. Notably, type 2 bipolar disorder patients exhibited a decrement in verbal memory correlated with the duration of their illness.

A meta-analysis comparing cognitive function between patients with bipolar disorder exhibiting psychopathological symptoms and those not exhibiting the symptoms22 revealed overall decreased cognitive function in the former. In addition, patients with psychopathological symptoms demonstrated higher rates of hospitalization, markedly worse verbal memory, and slower executive function compared to patients without psychopathological symptoms. However, this study reported that the use of antipsychotics did not affect cognitive function. Therefore, future studies comparing cognitive function by clinical presentation subtypes should utilize more homogeneous patient groups while controlling for medication variables.

Differences in Cognitive Function Between Patients with Schizophrenia and Those with Bipolar Disorder

Some meta-analyses have analyzed cognitive function in the families of patients with schizophrenia, revealing that psychomotor slowing and reduced verbal fluency serve as significant endophenotypes for schizophrenia [26, 27]. In addition, the families of patients with schizophrenia demonstrated more severe general cognitive dysfunction than the families of patients with bipolar disorder. However, they did not demonstrate the clear impairment of response inhibition observed in the families of patients with bipolar disorder. Another characteristic is that families of individuals with schizophrenia experience overall declines in sustained attention, whereas families of patients with bipolar disorder show primarily reduced abilities in target detection. Given the shared genetic underpinnings of schizophrenia and bipolar disorder, verbal memory and shifting attention may represent trait markers for patients with a discernible psychiatric history, while impaired response inhibition has been suggested as an endophenotype. Reduced verbal memory and shifting attention may also act as endophenotypes associated with psychiatric disorders, independent of diagnosis [22].

Etiologies for Cognitive Dysfunction in Bipolar Disorder

Childhood Trauma

Numerous studies have reported associations between childhood trauma, such as abuse or neglect, and cognitive dysfunction in individuals with bipolar disorder [28–30]. A study involving patients with bipolar disorder and psychosis found that those with a history of childhood trauma exhibited worse cognitive outcomes than those without such experiences. In another analysis adhering to the same standards, irrespective of the presence of psychosis, similar results were observed; cognitive domains demonstrating discrepancies differed, indicating the potential effect of psychosis. One hypothesized mechanism involves a decrease in brain-derived neurotrophic factor (BDNF), which plays a critical role in cognitive function. Evidence supports the notion that patients with bipolar disorder who experienced childhood trauma demonstrate significantly lower BDNF levels. A second hypothesis is associated with the hypothalamic–pituitary–adrenal (HPA) axis. Persistent activation of the HPA axis due to childhood trauma results in hypersecretion of cortisol, promoting inflammatory responses and glutamate activation in the brain, ultimately leading to neurobiological damage. Changes in brain structure consequent to childhood trauma have also been suggested. However, reliance on retrospective accounts of childhood trauma makes findings susceptible to mood fluctuations and memory distortions during assessments.

Obesity

Bipolar disorder exhibits a close relationship with metabolic syndrome. Interestingly, studies indicate that obese patients with bipolar disorder display more severe cognitive dysfunction than their non-obese counterparts [31–33]. Brain imaging studies have also indicated that increasing body mass index (BMI) correlates with decreased gray and white matter [34]. Nevertheless, cognitive dysfunction is evident in non-obese patients with bipolar disorder, suggesting that obesity acts more as an exacerbating factor than a primary cause of cognitive impairments.

Inflammation

Inflammation and neuroplasticity are hypothesized to play roles in the pathology of both depressive and bipolar disorders [35–37]. Prolonged stress leads to activation of the HPA axis, cortisol secretion, which in turn induces inflammatory cytokines. These cytokines affect the brain by stimulating phagocytes, secreting further cytokines, leading to a state of cerebral inflammation. Consequently, synthesis of serotonin from tryptophan diminishes, increasing levels of quinolinic acid, which possesses glutamate-like properties, potentially causing neurodegeneration, including hippocampal atrophy, ultimately resulting in mood disorders.

Abnormalities of Brain Structure and Function

Numerous consistent findings have emerged from brain imaging studies in patients with bipolar disorder [38, 39]. The typical presentation often includes decreased frontal lobe activation and increased limbic system activation, including the amygdala. Additionally, aberrations in connectivity between the limbic system and frontal lobes impair emotional regulation. Patients with bipolar disorder frequently demonstrate white matter changes and reduced gray matter volume, corroborating findings of abnormal connectivity between the frontal lobe and the limbic system [40, 41]. Disruptions in connectivity impact emotional regulation and cognitive impairment, illustrating that cognitive dysfunction in bipolar disorder cannot be separated from broader health concerns. Reports have detailed findings such as enlarged ventricles and cerebellar or temporal lobe atrophy. Collectively, these structural and functional abnormalities in the brain are hypothesized to affect cognitive dysfunction (Fig. 4.1).

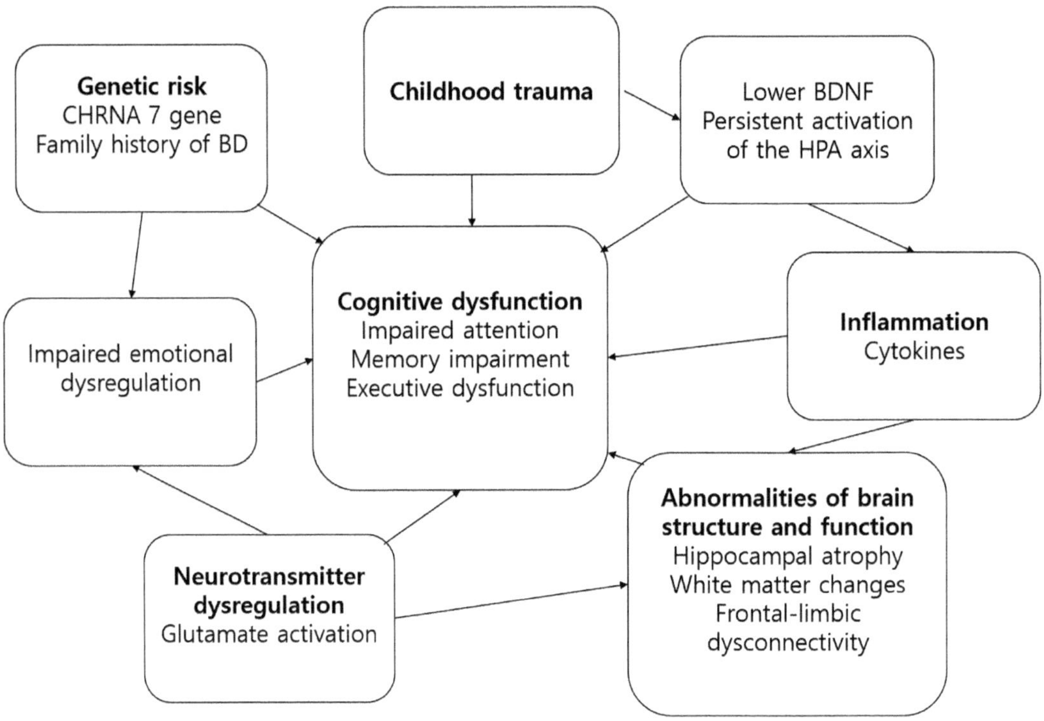

Fig. 4.1 An integrative conceptual framework of cognitive dysfunction in bipolar disorder

Mechanisms of Cognitive Dysfunction in Bipolar Disorder

Impaired Attention

Attention refers to the cognitive capacity for selecting and integrating information in the brain through perception and understanding for use in cognitive tasks, memory, perception, planning, and behavior. Compared to a healthy control group, patients with bipolar disorder exhibit significantly diminished attention, regardless of whether they are experiencing mania, depression, or a euthymic state.

Studies have documented that persistent attention deficits in patients with euthymic bipolar disorder are related to the CHRNA7 gene, abnormal brain metabolism in the hippocampus or temporal lobe, or white matter injury.

Memory Impairment

In studies utilizing the MCCB to evaluate cognitive function in bipolar disorder, one study assessed 27 family members of patients with asymptomatic bipolar disorder, 47 healthy controls, and 28 patients with bipolar disorder. Learning, processing speed, and working memory emerged as potential endophenotypes for the genetic risk associated with bipolar disorder.

Impairment of Executive Function

Longitudinal follow-up studies have demonstrated impaired executive function in patients with euthymic bipolar disorder; however, cognitive dysfunction is not reported to worsen over time. Presently, the literature indicates that executive function in patients with bipolar disorder is impaired in the acute phase, but conclusions on whether executive function is impaired in remission remain inconsistent, necessitating further large-scale, long-term follow-up studies. The mechanisms underlying executive function impairment in bipolar disorder have been explained through neurobiological models involving frontotemporal and subcortical circuits. In adolescents with bipolar disorder, serum lipid peroxide levels regulated by BDNF exhibited a negative correlation with executive function. Therefore, lipid peroxides and BDNF could serve as informative biological indicators linked to executive dysfunction in this population. Consistent findings confirm impaired executive function and reduced BDNF levels in patients with bipolar disorder relative to healthy controls during both euthymia and active manic episodes [42].

Effects of Drugs on Cognitive Function in Bipolar Disorder

Lithium

Some studies have reported impairments in attention and memory within 14 days of initiating lithium treatment; however, these findings have not been consistently replicated in subsequent investigations [43]. Furthermore, some studies have failed to demonstrate cognitive function disparities between bipolar disorder patients receiving pharmacotherapy, including lithium, and those not undergoing treatment. Conversely, a meta-analysis indicated that patients on lithium experienced heightened difficulties in learning, encoding, and cognitive flexibility compared to those not on lithium [44]. Nevertheless, long-term lithium use is generally considered to have minimal adverse effects on cognition. In a six-year follow-up study, patients with bipolar disorder receiving lithium therapy did not demonstrate impairments in memory performance. A similar four-year follow-up study indicated no differences in attention, verbal memory, visual memory, or executive function between patients receiving lithium and those not undergoing treatment or compared to healthy controls [45].

Anticonvulsants

When psychomotor speed, memory, attention, and executive function were compared between patients with bipolar disorder taking valproic acid, lamotrigine, carbamazepine, or lithium, results indicate that those taking lamotrigine demonstrated marginally better cognitive function compared to those taking other drugs [46]. Although research on the effects of valproic acid and carbamazepine on cognitive function in patients with bipolar disorder is limited, decreased psychomotor speed and impaired memory and attention were generally observed compared to healthy controls or patients suffering from convulsions.

Antipsychotics

Antipsychotics can impair verbal memory in patients with euthymic bipolar disorder. However, since patients receiving antipsychotics are likely to have previously exhibited psychotic symptoms, undergone inpatient treatment, or experienced more severe manic symptoms, the effects of their previous clinical courses on cognitive function cannot be excluded. The effects of atypical antipsychotics on cognitive function remain inconclusive; reports vary, with one study reporting that quetiapine impairs cognitive function more than risperidone, one reporting superiority in terms of long-term cognitive function compared to other drugs, and one reporting that long-term use resulted in a mild improvement in cognitive function.

Effects of Cognitive Dysfunction on Functional Impairment and Prognosis in Bipolar Disorder

It is unclear whether the cognitive dysfunction observed in patients with bipolar disorder can adequately explain their functional impairment. In an analysis of 52 studies, both cross-sectional and longitudinal studies repeatedly confirmed that bipolar disorder is associated with cognitive impairment [47]. In a meta-analysis, cognitive impairment was shown to be closely associated with functional decline. Among the areas showing cognitive dysfunction, the most severe dysfunction was observed in working memory [48].

In addition, more severe cognitive dysfunction after a manic episode was associated with worse quality of life six months later. Over a six-year evaluation period, quality of life deteriorated more rapidly than cognitive dysfunction progressed.

Social cognition is defined as the ability to perceive and judge the intentions and behaviors of others and to respond appropriately. It can be divided into the following five domains: theory of mind, social perception, social knowledge, attributional bias, and emotional processing. Relatively substantial research has focused on social cognitive function in bipolar disorder when compared to autism or schizophrenia. One study posited that social cognitive function is essential for differentiating low-functioning from high-functioning patients with bipolar disorder [49]. Among the components of social cognition, the theory of mind was shown to be a strong predictor of overall cognitive dysfunction in bipolar disorder. However, research on social cognition remains sparser than for neurocognitive function, leading to a lack of consistent findings. Therefore, further studies are warranted.

Trajectory of Cognitive Function in Patients with Bipolar Disorder

Cognitive dysfunction may arise before the onset of bipolar disorder, become less evident with acute mood episodes, and persist even after remission in many patients. Cognitive impairment in bipolar disorder is genetic and also appears to be affected by abnormalities in neurodevelopmental processes. Despite patients being in a euthymic state following the onset of bipolar disorder, impairment is still observed in all areas of cognitive function after recovery from the first episode. The severity of cognitive impairment can vary based on the age of onset; verbal learning and processing speed may be more adversely affected in adolescent-onset bipolar disorder compared to adult-onset bipolar disorder. In addition, cognitive dysfunction becomes increasingly severe with repeated episodes, indicating that cognitive impairment may progress due to cumulative biological toxicity linked with repeated mood episodes. Some commentators suggest that severe cognitive impairment could signify a phenotype characteristic of severe bipolar disorder, characterized by frequent recurrences and genetic susceptibility, rather than being a consequence of disease progression itself. However, recent meta-analyses examining long-term outcomes found no definitive worsening of cognitive function over time among patients with bipolar disorder, complicating conclusions.

Treatment of Cognitive Dysfunction in Patients with Bipolar Disorder

The first drugs used to treat cognitive dysfunction in bipolar disorder were cholinesterase inhibitors, utilized primarily in Alzheimer's disease and other forms of dementia, but the effects were minimal. Although conclusions remain limited due to insufficient rigor in existing studies, it can be inferred that cognitive dysfunction in bipolar disorder is associated with non-cholinergic neurotransmitter systems.

Memantine, which is used for Alzheimer's disease, and acts as an N-methyl-D-aspartate (NMDA) receptor agonist employed in Alzheimer's treatment, has shown efficacy in acute mania within both preclinical and clinical investigations. Some studies have reported positive effects of memantine on cognitive function in patients with bipolar disorder, yet evidence regarding improvements in mood symptoms and independent cognitive performance remains uncertain. Attempts involving intranasal insulin, pramipexole, and antioxidants have similarly failed to yield definitive results. In addition to pharmacotherapy, electroconvulsive therapy has demonstrated effects comparable to pharmacological interventions in enhancing cognitive function, while repetitive transcranial magnetic stimulation (rTMS) has shown promise for addressing both mood symptoms and cognitive improvements independently. Cognitive rehabilitation or functional rehabilitation therapies are also commonly employed and are anticipated to contribute to enhancements in cognitive functioning.

Beyond pharmacological interventions, several non-pharmacological interventions should also be considered. Transcranial direct current stimulation (tDCS) upregulates long-term potentiation (LTP) and genes responsible for neuroplasticity and the regulation of neurotrophic factors and inflammatory mediators. These cellular and molecular mechanisms of action would suggest a possible procognitive effect, which has been demonstrated in bipolar depressed patients as well as euthymic BD patients [50]. One other neurostimulation technique that has demonstrated efficacy for cognitive impairment in BD is repetitive transcranial magnetic stimulation (rTMS). Two randomized controlled trials have found that rTMS enhances several domains of cognitive functioning without improving depressive symptoms [51, 52]. Cognitive remediation is another non-pharmacological intervention that may prove to be effective for cognitive impairment in BD. A randomized proof of concept trial demonstrated that a 12-week cognitive remediation therapy (CRT) program is feasible for individuals with BD and that it may enhance IQ, working memory, executive function, and psychosocial functioning [53].

Conclusion

Cognitive dysfunction associated with bipolar disorder is evident irrespective of whether patients are in manic, depressive, or mixed episodes and persists even after remission. Additionally, cognitive impairment can manifest before the onset of bipolar disorder and has also been identified in the families of patients with bipolar disorder. Therefore, this cognitive dysfunction likely constitutes an endophenotype characteristic of bipolar disorder. Although cognitive dysfunction profiles show differences between schizophrenia and bipolar disorder, further studies are required to elucidate specific distinctions. The underlying causes of cognitive dysfunction in bipolar disorder include childhood trauma, obesity, inflammation, and abnormalities in brain structure and function. In summary, cognitive dysfunction in bipolar disorder does not improve during remission and is a characteristic trait present irrespective of episodes. This characteristic holds substantial clinical significance, as it is closely associated with demonstrated patients' quality of life and serves as a critical predictor of overall occupational and social functioning. Future research should pursue more detailed investigations to facilitate individualized assessments of cognitive functioning in bipolar disorder and to inform the development of tailored therapeutic strategies. Clinicians must routinely assess cognitive impairments in patients with bipolar disorder and provide appropriate treatments to mitigate the risk of further cognitive decline due to recurrence, while continuously exploring additional intervention strategies.

Declarations

Competing Interests The author(s) has no competing interests to declare that are relevant to the content of this manuscript.

Ethics Approval The author(s) declares that this manuscript does not include primary research with human participants.

The author(s) declares that this manuscript does not include primary studies involving animals.

References

1. Burdick KE, Goldberg TE, Cornblatt BA, Keefe RS, Gopin CB, Derosse P, et al. The MATRICS consensus cognitive battery in patients with bipolar I disorder. Neuropsychopharmacology. 2011;36:1587–92.
2. Lima IMM, Peckham AD, Johnson SL. Cognitive deficits in bipolar disorders: implications for emotion. Clin Psychol Rev. 2018;59:126–36.
3. Gale CR, Batty GD, McIntosh AM, Porteous DJ, Deary IJ, Rasmussen F. Is bipolar disorder more common in highly intelligent people? A cohort study of a million men. Mol Psychiatry. 2013;18:190–4.
4. Tiihonen J, Haukka J, Henriksson M, Cannon M, Kieseppa T, Laaksonen I, et al. Premorbid intellectual

functioning in bipolar disorder and schizophrenia: results from a cohort study of male conscripts. Am J Psychiatry. 2005;162:1904–10.
5. Meyer SE, Carlson GA, Wiggs EA, Martinez PE, Ronsaville DS, Klimes-Dougan B, et al. A prospective study of the association among impaired executive functioning, childhood attentional problems, and the development of bipolar disorder. Dev Psychopathol. 2004;16:461–76.
6. Arts B, Jabben N, Krabbendam L, van Os J. Meta-analyses of cognitive functioning in euthymic bipolar patients and their first-degree relatives. Psychol Med. 2008;38:771–85.
7. Bora E, Yucel M, Pantelis C. Cognitive endophenotypes of bipolar disorder: a meta-analysis of neuropsychological deficits in euthymic patients and their first-degree relatives. J Affect Disord. 2009;113:1–20.
8. Robinson LJ, Thompson JM, Gallagher P, Goswami U, Young AH, Ferrier IN, et al. A meta-analysis of cognitive deficits in euthymic patients with bipolar disorder. J Affect Disord. 2006;93:105–15.
9. Kolur US, Reddy YC, John JP, Kandavel T, Jain S. Sustained attention and executive functions in euthymic young people with bipolar disorder. Br J Psychiatry. 2006;189:453–8.
10. Ferrier IN, Chowdhury R, Thompson JM, Watson S, Young AH. Neurocognitive function in unaffected first-degree relatives of patients with bipolar disorder: a preliminary report. Bipolar Disord. 2004;6:319–22.
11. Ferrier IN, Stanton BR, Kelly TP, Scott J. Neuropsychological function in euthymic patients with bipolar disorder. Br J Psychiatry. 1999;175:246–51.
12. Clark L, Iversen SD, Goodwin GM. Sustained attention deficit in bipolar disorder. Br J Psychiatry. 2002;180:313–9.
13. Thompson JM, Gallagher P, Hughes JH, Watson S, Gray JM, Ferrier IN, et al. Neurocognitive impairment in euthymic patients with bipolar affective disorder. Br J Psychiatry. 2005;186:32–40.
14. Joffe RT, MacDonald C, Kutcher SP. Lack of differential cognitive effects of lithium and carbamazepine in bipolar affective disorder. J Clin Psychopharmacol. 1988;8:425–8.
15. Vrabie M, Marinescu V, Talasman A, Tautu O, Drima E, Miclutia I. Cognitive impairment in manic bipolar patients: important, understated, significant aspects. Ann General Psychiatry. 2015;14:41.
16. Clark L, Iversen SD, Goodwin GM. A neuropsychological investigation of prefrontal cortex involvement in acute mania. Am J Psychiatry. 2001;158:1605–11.
17. McGrath J, Chapple B, Wright M. Working memory in schizophrenia and mania: correlation with symptoms during the acute and subacute phases. Acta Psychiatr Scand. 2001;103:181–8.
18. Martinez-Aran A, Vieta E, Reinares M, Colom F, Torrent C, Sanchez-Moreno J, et al. Cognitive function across manic or hypomanic, depressed, and euthymic states in bipolar disorder. Am J Psychiatry. 2004;161:262–70.
19. Wolfe J, Granholm E, Butters N, Saunders E, Janowsky D. Verbal memory deficits associated with major affective disorders: a comparison of unipolar and bipolar patients. J Affect Disord. 1987;13:83–92.
20. van der Werf-Eldering MJ, Burger H, Holthausen EA, Aleman A, Nolen WA. Cognitive functioning in patients with bipolar disorder: association with depressive symptoms and alcohol use. PLoS One. 2010;5:e13032.
21. Zubieta JK, Huguelet P, Lajiness-O'Neill R, Giordani BJ. Cognitive function in euthymic bipolar I disorder. Psychiatry Res. 2001;102:9–20.
22. Bora E. Neurocognitive features in clinical subgroups of bipolar disorder: a meta-analysis. J Affect Disord. 2018;229:125–34.
23. Palsson E, Figueras C, Johansson AG, Ekman CJ, Hultman B, Ostlind J, et al. Neurocognitive function in bipolar disorder: a comparison between bipolar I and II disorder and matched controls. BMC Psychiatry. 2013;13:165.
24. Sole B, Martinez-Aran A, Torrent C, Bonnin CM, Reinares M, Popovic D, et al. Are bipolar II patients cognitively impaired? A systematic review. Psychol Med. 2011;41:1791–803.
25. ADP M, DTY L, AKW C, SHW S, Leung O, SLY W, et al. Cognitive impairment in treatment-naive bipolar II and unipolar depression. Sci Rep. 2018;8:1905.
26. Sitskoorn MM, Aleman A, Ebisch SJ, Appels MC, Kahn RS. Cognitive deficits in relatives of patients with schizophrenia: a meta-analysis. Schizophr Res. 2004;71:285–95.
27. Snitz BE, Macdonald AW 3rd, Carter CS. Cognitive deficits in unaffected first-degree relatives of schizophrenia patients: a meta-analytic review of putative endophenotypes. Schizophr Bull. 2006;32:179–94.
28. Bucker J, Muralidharan K, Torres IJ, Su W, Kozicky J, Silveira LE, et al. Childhood maltreatment and corpus callosum volume in recently diagnosed patients with bipolar I disorder: data from the Systematic Treatment Optimization Program for Early Mania (STOP-EM). J Psychiatr Res. 2014;48:65–72.
29. Bucker J, Kozicky J, Torres IJ, Kauer-Sant'anna M, Silveira LE, Bond DJ, et al. The impact of childhood trauma on cognitive functioning in patients recently recovered from a first manic episode: data from the Systematic Treatment Optimization Program for Early Mania (STOP-EM). J Affect Disord. 2013;148:424–30.
30. Blanco L, Nydegger LA, Camarillo G, Trinidad DR, Schramm E, Ames SL. Neurological changes in brain structure and functions among individuals with a history of childhood sexual abuse: a review. Neurosci Biobehav Rev. 2015;57:63–9.
31. Yim CY, Soczynska JK, Kennedy SH, Woldeyohannes HO, Brietzke E, McIntyre RS. The effect of overweight/obesity on cognitive function in euthymic individuals with bipolar disorder. Eur Psychiatry. 2012;27:223–8.

32. Mora E, Portella MJ, Martinez-Alonso M, Teres M, Forcada I, Vieta E, et al. The impact of obesity on cognitive functioning in euthymic bipolar patients: a cross-sectional and longitudinal study. J Clin Psychiatry. 2017;78:e924–32.
33. Liu CS, Carvalho AF, Mansur RB, McIntyre RS. Obesity and bipolar disorder: synergistic neurotoxic effects? Adv Ther. 2013;30:987–1006.
34. Bond DJ, Ha TH, Lang DJ, Su W, Torres IJ, Honer WG, et al. Body mass index-related regional gray and white matter volume reductions in first-episode mania patients. Biol Psychiatry. 2014;76:138–45.
35. Arnone D, Saraykar S, Salem H, Teixeira AL, Dantzer R, Selvaraj S. Role of Kynurenine pathway and its metabolites in mood disorders: a systematic review and meta-analysis of clinical studies. Neurosci Biobehav Rev. 2018;92:477–85.
36. Rosenblat JD, McIntyre RS. Bipolar disorder and immune dysfunction: epidemiological findings, effectsd pathophysiology and clinical implications. Brain Sci. 2017;7:144.
37. Data-Franco J, Singh A, Popovic D, Ashton M, Berk M, Vieta E, et al. Beyond the therapeutic shackles of the monoamines: new mechanisms in bipolar disorder biology. Prog Neuro-Psychopharmacol Biol Psychiatry. 2017;72:73–86.
38. Phillips ML, Swartz HA. A critical appraisal of neuroimaging studies of bipolar disorder: toward a new conceptualization of underlying neural circuitry and a road map for future research. Am J Psychiatry. 2014;171:829–43.
39. Wessa M, Kanske P, Linke J. Bipolar disorder: a neural network perspective on a disorder of emotion and motivation. Restor Neurol Neurosci. 2014;32:51–62.
40. Selvaraj S, Arnone D, Job D, Stanfield A, Farrow TF, Nugent AC, et al. Grey matter differences in bipolar disorder: a meta-analysis of voxel-based morphom etry studies. Bipolar Disord. 2012;14:135–45.
41. Nortje G, Stein DJ, Radua J, Mataix–Cols D, Horn N. Systematic review and voxel-based meta-analysis of diffusion tensor imaging studies in bipolar disorder. J Affect Disord. 2013;150:192–200.
42. Stip E, Dufresne J, Lussier I, et al. A double-blind, placebo-controlled study of the effects of lithium on cognition in healthy subjects: mild and selective effects on learning. J Affect Disord. 2000;60:147–57.
43. Pavuluri MN, Schenkel LS, Aryal S, et al. Neurocognitive function in unmedicated manic and medicated euthymic pediatric bipolar patients. Am J Psychiatry. 2006;163:286–93.
44. Wingo AP, Wingo TS, Harvey PD, et al. Effects of lithium on cognitive performance: a meta-analysis. J Clin Psychiatry. 2009;70:1588–97.
45. López-Jaramillo C, Lopera-Vásquez J, Ospina-Duque J, et al. Lithium treatment effects on the neuropsychological functioning of patients with bipolar I disorder. J Clin Psychiatry. 2010;71:1055–60.
46. Gualtieri CT, Johnson LG. Comparative neurocognitive effects of 5 psychotropic anticonvulsants and lithium. MedGenMed. 2006;8:46.
47. Baune BT, Li X, Beblo T. Short- and long-term relationships between neurocognitive performance and general function in bipolar disorder. J Clin Exp Neuropsychol. 2013;35:759–74.
48. Depp CA, Mausbach BT, Harmell AL, Savla GN, Bowie CR, Harvey PD, et al. Meta-analysis of the association between cognitive abilities and everyday functioning in bipolar disorder. Bipolar Disord. 2012;14:217–26.
49. Thaler NS, Sutton GP, Allen DN. Social cognition and functional capacity in bipolar disorder and schizophrenia. Psychiatry Res. 2014;220:309–14.
50. D'Urso G, Toscano E, Barone A, et al. Transcranial direct current stimulation for bipolar depression: systematic reviews of clinical evidence and biological underpinnings. Neuropsychopharmacol Biol Psychiatry. 2023;121:110672.
51. Yang L-L, Zhao D, Kong L-L, et al. High-frequency repetitive transcranial magnetic stimulation (rTMS) improves neurocognitive function in bipolar disorder. J Affect Disord. 2019;246:851–6.
52. Myczkowski ML, Fernandes A, Moreno M, et al. Cognitive outcomes of TMS treatment in bipolar depression: safety data from a randomized controlled trial. J Affect Disord. 2018;235:20–6.
53. Strawbridge R, Tsapekos D, Hodsoll J, et al. Cognitive remediation therapy for patients with bipolar disorder: a randomised proof-of-concept trial. Bipolar Disord. 2021;23:196–208.

Normal, Hypomanic, and Manic States: Key Differences and Their Implications

5

Jeongwan Hong and Moon-Doo Kim

Mood disorders can be categorized into depressive disorder and bipolar disorder. The main difference between the two disorders is the presence of manic/hypomanic episodes. If a patient experiences manic/hypomanic episodes even once, a diagnosis of bipolar disorder can be made. Clinicians can differentiate between bipolar disorder and depressive disorder based on the presence of manic/hypomanic episodes. Recognizing manic/hypomanic symptoms will be an essential skill for mental health practitioners who treat mood disorders. In this chapter, you will learn about hypomanic and manic symptoms.

Normal

To understand the psychopathology of mood disorders, we need to define normal mood states. In general, being mentally healthy is defined as being stable, flexible, and adaptable, with no mental disorders and no obvious abnormalities in behavior. Euthymia is also defined as the absence of overt symptoms of depression or mania. However, this definition of "normal in the absence of a mental disorder" falls into a circular logic when combined with the definition of mental disorder as "a pathological condition that is not normal." The most widely used version of the American Psychiatric Association's Diagnostic and Statistical Manual of Mental Disorders, fifth Edition (DSM-V) states, "Mental disorders are usually associated with significant distress or disability in social, occupational, or other important activities" [1]. Applying this definition to mood disorders, mood disturbance that do not impair social, occupational, or daily functioning would be considered normal. Euthymia is allostasis (stability through change) of mood rather than homeostasis (stability despite change).

The term "euthymia" originates from Greek, combining "eu" meaning "well" and "thymos" meaning "soul, emotion." The concept of euthymia is generally attributed to Democritus, who described it as being content with what is present and available, paying little attention to those who are envied or admired, and observing the lives of those who suffer yet endure. It represents a state of quiet satisfaction—a balance of emotions that overcomes fear. The Latin philosopher Seneca translated the Greek term "euthymia" as "tranquillitas animi (a state of internal calm and contentment)" and associated it with psychological well-being as a process of learning.

The broader concept of euthymia, as defined by Fava and Bech [2], is characterized by the following features:

J. Hong (✉)
Department of Psychiatry, Iksan Hospital, Iksan, Republic of Korea
e-mail: taz67621@gmail.com

M.-D. Kim
Department of Psychiatry, Jeju National University Hospital, School of Medicine, Jeju National University, Jeju, Republic of Korea
e-mail: mdkim66@jejunu.ac.kr

W.-M. Bahk et al. (eds.), *Bipolar Disorder*, https://doi.org/10.1007/978-981-92-1323-8_5

(a) Absence of mood disturbances that meet diagnostic criteria; if the subject has a prior history of mood disorder, they should be in full remission. Any experiences of sadness, anxiety, or irritability are typically brief, situation-specific, and do not significantly impact daily functioning.
(b) The subject feels cheerful, calm, and active, is interested in things, and experiences refreshing or restorative sleep.
(c) The subject demonstrates balance and integration of psychic forces (flexibility), a unifying outlook on life that guides actions and feelings to shape the future accordingly, and resilience, including tolerance to stress, anxiety, and frustration.

Mania

Elevated mood and grandiosity, increased psychomotor speed, flight of ideas, distractibility, and decreased need for sleep are the hallmarks of euphoric mania, and unstable mood and hostility are also common clinical features. In manic episodes, irritable mood is the most common mood state (71%), followed by euphoric (63%) or expansive mood (60%), and labile mood (49%) [3]. Psychomotor activation is a prominent feature of manic episodes, manifesting as excessive energy and activity, talkativeness, rapid speech, and pressured speech. Thought processes may also be accelerated, resulting in symptoms such as flight of ideas and distractibility. Along with these psychomotor activation, decreased need for sleep is present in about 80% of manic patients. In addition, the content of thoughts in manic episodes is overly positive, optimistic, and exaggerated.

The DSM-V describes manic episodes as "abnormally and persistently elevated, expansive, or irritable mood and abnormally and persistently increased goal-directed activity or energy, lasting at least 1 week and present most of the day, nearly everyday" and is diagnosed when three or more of the seven manic symptoms are present and result in significant impairment of social or occupational functioning [1].

Hypomania

Hypomania, as the name suggests, is a mild form of mania. It is a condition that exceeds the level of normal mood swings but is not severe enough (hypo-) to be diagnosed as mania. Hypomania is usually defined as a state where the mood is elevated or energy is increased, but control is not impaired. Patients with hypomania are not bothered by these changes and may even enjoy their increased abilities (supernormal), but hypomania is an abnormal state.

In the DSM-V diagnostic criteria, the symptoms of hypomania are identical to the seven symptoms of mania, but the duration is shorter than that of mania, at 4 days or more. If psychotic symptoms are accompanied, it is diagnosed as a manic episode regardless of the period. There is a clue that the functional impairment of hypomanic episodes does not cause significant impairment and does not necessitate hospitalization. However, these mood disturbances are accompanied by changes in function that are clearly different from when there are no symptoms, and these changes in function can be observable by others. Mania and hypomania differ in four key ways according to criteria outlined in the DSM-V as shown in Table 5.1.

The International Classification of Diseases, 11th Edition (ICD-11) also describes mania as an "extreme mood state" and hypomania as a mild elevation that lasts for several days.

Table 5.1 Differences between hypomania and mania

	Hypomania	Mania
Duration	At least 4 consecutive days	At least 1 week
Severity of episode	Not severe enough to significantly affect social or occupational functioning	Causes severe impact on social or occupational functioning
Need for hospitalization	No	Possibly
Psychotic features	Can't be present for a diagnosis of hypomania	Is among possible symptoms

Current diagnostic systems, the DSM and ICD, use categorical diagnoses, which are based on the type and number of symptoms. While these categorical classifications are effective in identifying illnesses, the symptoms of mental disorders are often dimensional rather than categorical. Due to the dimensional nature of mental disorders, the boundary between normal and abnormal is ambiguous, and there are cases where conditions below the threshold of the diagnostic criteria must be re-diagnosed.

In the diagnosis of bipolar disorder, how to define hypomania has also been a key issue, and accordingly, bipolar disorder has been divided into types I and II. Hypomania can occur as a single, isolated episode or as a temporary episode on a continuum between normal mood and the most severe manic state. In the United Kingdom, it is not uncommon for patients hospitalized with mania to have their diagnosis changed to hypomania when they improve and are ready to be discharged [4].

Because of the impression given by the name, "a state less severe than mania," hypomania was the last to be recognized as a mental disorder in the field of mood disorders. It was not until the DSM-IV era that bipolar II disorder was included in the diagnostic classification system. However, bipolar II disorder is no longer considered a milder condition than bipolar I disorder, and it is known that chronic depression and mood instability eventually lead to impairment in occupational and social functions over time.

Although many clinicians now consider bipolar II disorder to be a milder form of bipolar I disorder and believe it can progress to bipolar I disorder, classical views have supported the diagnostic stability of bipolar II disorder. The prevalence of bipolar II disorder is estimated to be 0.5–1% in the United States and 3–6% in Europe, with the difference in prevalence being attributed to the use of broader diagnostic criteria in Europe than in the United States [5]. Bipolar disorder typically begins in adolescence, around the average age of 18, and is often initially diagnosed as unipolar depression, adjustment disorder, or personality disorder. It is characterized by mild mood disturbance that gradually increases in severity and frequency until the threshold for mood episodes is crossed [6]. It is estimated that it takes about 10 years from the first symptom to the final diagnosis [7]. Compared to bipolar I disorder, bipolar II disorder is characterized by more frequent mood episodes, shorter episodes of euphoria and more frequent episodes of depression, and a chronic course.

Recent thinking has tended to lump the various existing bipolar disorders together under the umbrella of bipolar spectrum disorder. The discussion on the diagnosis of bipolar spectrum disorders is still ongoing, and the current diagnostic system can be said to be provisional. Hypomania has also been referred to as a hypomania spectrum disorder and is often categorized into full-syndromal hypomania, which meets diagnostic criteria, brief-episode hypomania, which has a sufficient number of symptoms but lasts less than 4 days, and subsyndromal hypomania, which has fewer symptoms and an unspecified duration [8]. Once the distinction between mania and hypomania is more clearly defined and it is known whether these two conditions share the same properties or have independent properties that distinguish them, it may be possible to reorganize the diagnosis.

Is It Necessary to Distinguish Between Hypomania and Mania?

Although the distinction between bipolar I disorder and bipolar II disorder (mania vs. hypomania) was clarified in the 1994 DSM-IV, and this categorical diagnostic criterion has persisted to the present day, some argue that it is more helpful to combine hypomania and mania into a single diagnosis. Gitilin and Malhi and others [9] said that the combined diagnosis of hypomania and mania as a single symptom fits the reality of the clinical dimensions of bipolar disorder. The only differences are in the degree of severity (marked impairment of function vs. obvious change in function) and duration (7 vs. 4 days), and if they are mental disorders with the same symptoms, it would be reasonable to classify them as mild, moderate, and severe. Just as the diagnosis of major depressive disorder is categorized by the severity of symptoms. The DSM-V even suggests short-duration hypomania as a "conditions for further study" with a duration of "at least 2 days but less than 4 consecutive days." The subdivision of manic symptoms suggests that a diagnosis is needed for hypomanic symptoms that do not meet the criteria for a hypomanic episode. It is unclear whether this breakdown into smaller and smaller diagnoses of normal/short-duration hypomania/hypomania/mania is the right way to go for a dimensional approach.

The use of unified diagnostic criteria for mania would allow for a more active discussion of bipolar spectrum disorders. In the current situation where the distinction between bipolar I and bipolar II disorders is divided into vague diagnostic categories, patients with agitated states in which depressive symptoms are the predominant mood symptom but do not meet the diagnostic criteria for a hypomanic episode cannot be diagnosed with either major depressive disorder or bipolar disorder.

Of course, there are many more researchers who said against the unification of bipolar disorders. Vieta [10] said that if the two disorders are integrated because there are no distinct biomarkers, genetic or imaging findings between bipolar I and bipolar II disorders, the distinction between schizophrenia and bipolar disorder, major depressive disorder, and bipolar disorder will also become unclear. Psychiatry is a dimensional approach, but in clinical practice, a categorical distinction is needed for effective treatment and prognosis management.

Antidepressant-Induced Hypomania

How to interpret antidepressant-induced hypomania in patients without a history of hypomania or mania while taking antidepressants has been a matter of interest to many clinicians. In the DSM-III-R, this was considered part of the bipolar spectrum, but in the DSM-IV, it was diagnosed as a substance-induced mood disorder. However, many subsequent studies have shown that it is correct to diagnose bipolar disorder in patients who develop hypomania while taking antidepressant treatments. An analysis of 98 antidepressant clinical trials found that in 89% of the trials, neither mania nor hypomania occurred, suggesting that drug-induced hypomania is not common in patients with depression. Furthermore, the family histories of patients who developed mania or hypomania while taking antidepressant treatments were similar to those of patients with bipolar disorder [11]. Therefore, the current consensus is that if a patient with depression develops hypomania or mania while taking antidepressant treatments, the diagnosis should be revised to bipolar disorder. Based on these findings, the DSM-V allows the diagnosis of hypomania episode as a hypomanic symptoms if it occurs during treatment for depression, such as medication or electroconvulsive therapy. However, if a person is taking an antidepressant medication and experiences symptoms such as feeling irritable, nervous, or agitated, but does not meet the criteria for mania or hypomania, this is considered a nonspecific side effect and is not diagnostic of bipolar disorder.

Differential Diagnosis

Because bipolar disorder is still diagnosed based on symptoms alone, it is often difficult to differentiate bipolar disorder from other conditions with similar symptoms. Careful differentiation of these similar conditions is the first step in preventing misdiagnosis and providing appropriate treatment.

A common clinical concern is whether elevated mood, hyperactivity, and expanded self-confidence in a person with a normally extroverted temperament should be viewed as changes within the normal range or as hypomania [12].. The heightened emotional expression that is common in patients with cluster B personality disorders such as borderline personality disorder (BPD) and the hyperactivity, disinhibition, and inattention that are often seen in attention-deficit/hyperactivity disorder (ADHD) can also be mistaken for hypomania [13]. In such cases, a judgment should be made by comprehensively considering factors such as affect and sleep state. Symptoms similar to hypomania can also appear when taking psychostimulants or in internal diseases such as hyperthyroidism. Patients with substance use disorders often have bipolar disorder, and symptoms of substance abuse can make the diagnosis of bipolar disorder difficult.

The most important thing in differential diagnosis is to investigate not only the current condition but also the past history, including the family history, to see if there are any recurring patterns or characteristics. In particular, when a patient diagnosed with major depressive disorder is carefully investigated for a history of hypomania, it was found that 45% of them can be diagnosed with bipolar disorder. This fact shows the importance of evaluating the past history in diagnosing bipolar disorder [14]. The original concept of bipolar disorder was that there were distinct mood episodes that were separated from normal, with a return to normal in between episodes, but in many cases, symptoms are present in between episodes, and these residual symptoms affect psychosocial functioning. In particular, a study that prospectively followed patients with bipolar II disorder for 13.4 years found that the long-term course of bipolar II disorder was dominated even more by depressive symptoms (50.9% of weeks), with patients experiencing very few follow-up weeks of hypomania or cycling or mixed affective symptoms (1.3% of weeks with hypomanic and 2.3% with mixed cycling symptoms; an approximately 30 to 1 ratio) [15]. Furthermore, patients are more likely to visit to clinics with depressive episodes and less likely to talk about their experience of manic episodes. For these reasons, It is easy to misdiagnose bipolar disorder as depressive disorder unless an accurate history is collected from multiple caregivers in addition to the patient.

Hypomania and Borderline Personality Disorder (BPD)

There is much debate about whether borderline personality disorder and bipolar disorder are independent or interdependent conditions. Some researchers said that borderline personality disorder is an "ultra-rapid cycling" form of bipolar disorder and should be included in the bipolar spectrum [16]. In both disorders, mood disturbances, intentional self-injurious behaviors, and suicide attempts are common, and impulsive behaviors such as sexual disinhibition, overspending, and alcohol or drug misuse are frequent. Affective instability and impulsivity are common features of both disorders, and the affective instability of patients with borderline personality disorder is similar to hypomania [17]. In general, bipolar I disorder is easier to differentiate from borderline personality disorder because it is more severe and often includes psychotic symptoms during manic episodes. However, hypomanic episodes are more difficult to differentiate from borderline personality disorder because of the absence of psychotic symptoms, shorter duration of episodes, and milder symptoms. The differential diagnosis of bipolar II disorder and borderline personality disorder is summarized in Table 5.2.

Table 5.2 Clinical differences between bipolar II disorder and borderline personality disorder

	Bipolar II disorder	Borderline personality disorder
Triggers	Usually internal	Triggered by interpersonal problems
Psychotic symptoms	None	Common in stressful situations
Expressions of "heightened" states	Exaggerated, extreme feelings, often with decreased anxiety	Few or brief episodes of extreme emotion, but anxiety is prominent
Depressive features	Melancholic	Not melancholic
Maladaptive behaviors	Not severe	Severe
Self-injurious, suicidal behavior	Relatively few	Relatively severe
Impulsivity	Severe during hypomania	Unplanned impulsivity, present regardless of mood state
Relationships	Relatively stable relationships	Relationship problems are prominent
Self-identity	Affected by mood state	Painfully inconsistent

Assessments

Because patients with bipolar II disorder typically visit to psychiatry in a depressed mood state, and a history of mixed hypomania or hypomania may be overlooked, utilizing an assessment tool that screens for bipolar disorder is helpful in diagnosis.

The most widely used tool is the self-report mood disorder questionnaire (MDQ). The MDQ can screen for a history of mania if a patient reports at least seven of the 13 manic symptoms in the past, that they occurred at the same time, and that they caused moderate or greater problems, but it is not sensitive enough to screen for a history of hypomania [18].

The Bipolar Spectrum Diagnostic Scale (BSDS) was developed to address the shortcomings of the MDQ in screening for bipolar II disorder. The BSDS is a 19-item mood symptom scale with a score of 1 for each item and 0–6 for how much the symptom applies to the individual. It has a sensitivity of 0.76 and specificity of 0.85 using a cutoff of 12 [19].

A screening test more specific to hypomania is the Hypomania Symptom Checklist-32 (HCL-32). This 32-item self-report questionnaire is designed to identify hypomanic symptoms in past depressive episodes and to differentiate bipolar spectrum disorder [20].

There is a Hypomanic Personality Scale as a tool to measure hypomanic tendencies that do not exceed the diagnostic threshold. It is a self-report scale consisting of 48 items on personality factors that can be seen in daily life rather than emphasizing the pathological symptoms themselves. It has a two-factor structure of "social vitality and self-confidence" and "hypomanic-like symptoms." The higher the total score, the more active the person is in social relationships and open to new experiences. In addition, borderline personality traits, impulsivity, stimulation-seeking tendencies, grandiosity, and mood symptoms were reported more [21].

The Young Mania Rating Scale (YMRS) is a clinical interview scale to assess the severity of manic states primarily used for research. Although not sensitive to hypomania, it can be used to assess the severity of current manic or hypomanic symptoms. The depressive and bipolar disorders of Structural Clinical Interview for DSM-V-Clinical Version (SCID-V-CV) can also be used to identify hypomanic episodes.

Treatment

Treatment for hypomania is the same as treatment for mania in most guidelines, although clinical studies are lacking. The general principles are stop any existing antidepressant medications and start a mood modulator or antipsychotic. In the acute phase, aripiprazole, asenapine, carbamazepine, olanzapine, quetiapine, ziprasidone, and valproate (divalproex) are preferred, and combination therapy may be used in severe case [22].

There is also not much information on maintenance treatment for bipolar II disorder. The drugs mainly used in the maintenance treatment phase are lithium and lamotrigine, which are known to be more effective for depressive symptoms. Lithium maintenance treatment reduced depressive episodes in both bipolar I and II disorders, and was more effective in bipolar II disorder. The complete remission rate was approximately 25%, and the earlier lithium was administered, the better the long-term treatment response [23]. In the case of antipsychotic drugs, monotherapy with olanzapine and quetiapine or combination therapy with lithium/divalproex was effective for maintenance treatment [22].

There are no definitive conclusions about prescribing antidepressants to patients with bipolar disorder. Caution is warranted in the use of antidepressants in patients with bipolar disorder due to the potential to cause a change to mania or hypomania or to accelerate the cycle of episodes. However, short-term antidepressants are often used in combination with mood stabilizers to treat and prevent depressive episodes [24]. Compared with bipolar I disorder, bipolar II disorder had a lower risk of mood changes due to antidepressants and a lower incidence of hypomania [25]. For atypical antipsychotics, quetiapine monotherapy was effective in depressive episodes and rapid cycling in bipolar II disorder

[26]. The olanzapine–fluoxetine combination was effective in depressive episodes in bipolar I disorder, but its effectiveness was not clear in bipolar II disorder [27].

Conclusion

Although hypomania was officially recognized in the current diagnostic system in 1994, the limitations of the current diagnostic criteria may lead to overlooked or misdiagnosed cases. Bipolar II disorder may be the most common phenotype of bipolar disorder. The study of hypomania in its various forms, including mixed, antidepressant-induced, and unipolar, has the potential to improve our understanding of the types of bipolar disorder, the characteristics of people who are susceptible to bipolar disorder, and the pathways by which bipolar disorder develops. Although there are various practical limitations, in the future, in addition to the current scale-based research, studies with more biological and objective indicators should be added.

Declarations

Competing Interests The author(s) has no competing interests to declare that are relevant to the content of this manuscript.

Ethics Approval The author(s) declares that this manuscript does not include primary research with human participants.

The author(s) declares that this manuscript does not include primary studies involving animals.

References

1. American Psychiatric Association D, Association AP. Diagnostic and statistical manual of mental disorders: DSM-5. Washington, DC: American Psychiatric Association; 2013.
2. Fava GA, Bech P. The concept of euthymia. Psychother Psychosom. 2016;85(1):1–5.
3. Goodwin FK, Jamison KR. Manic-depressive illness: bipolar disorders and recurrent depression. Oxford University Press; 2007.
4. Goodwin G. Hypomania: what's in a name? Br J Psychiatry. 2002;181(2):94–5.
5. Merikangas KR, Lamers F. The 'true'prevalence of bipolar II disorder. Curr Opin Psychiatry. 2012;25(1):19–23.
6. Shain BN. Pediatric bipolar disorder and mood dysregulation: diagnostic controversies. Adolesc Med State Art Rev. 2014;25(2):398–408.
7. Hirschfeld RM, Lewis L, Vornik LA. Perceptions and impact of bipolar disorder: how far have we really come? Results of the national depressive and manic-depressive association 2000 survey of individuals with bipolar disorder. J Clin Psychiatry. 2003;64(2):161–74.
8. Päären A, Bohman H, von Knorring A-L, von Knorring L, Olsson G, Jonsson U. Hypomania spectrum disorder in adolescence: a 15-year follow-up of non-mood morbidity in adulthood. BMC Psychiatry. 2014;14:1–15.
9. Gitlin M, Malhi GS. The existential crisis of bipolar II disorder. Int J Bipolar Disord. 2020;8(1):5.
10. Vieta E. Bipolar II disorder: frequent, valid, and reliable. Can J Psychiatry. 2019;64(8):541–3.
11. Baldessarini RJ, Faedda GL, Offidani E, Vazquez GH, Marangoni C, Serra G, et al. Antidepressant-associated mood-switching and transition from unipolar major depression to bipolar disorder: a review. J Affect Disord. 2013;148(1):129–35.
12. Zeschel E, Bingmann T, Bechdolf A, Krueger-Oezguerdal S, Correll CU, Leopold K, et al. Temperament and prodromal symptoms prior to first manic/hypomanic episodes: results from a pilot study. J Affect Disord. 2015;173:39–44.
13. Mistry S, Zammit S, Price V-E, Jones HJ, Smith DJ. Borderline personality and attention-deficit hyperactivity traits in childhood are associated with hypomanic features in early adulthood. J Affect Disord. 2017;221:246–53.
14. Allilaire J, Hantouche E, Sechter D, Bourgeois M, Azorin J, Lancrenon S, et al. Frequency and clinical aspects of bipolar II disorder in a French multicenter study: EPIDEP. L'encephale. 2001;27(2):149–58.
15. Judd LL, Akiskal HS. Depressive episodes and symptoms dominate the longitudinal course of bipolar disorder. Curr Psychiatry Rep. 2003;5(6):417–8.
16. MacKinnon DF, Pies R. Affective instability as rapid cycling: theoretical and clinical implications for borderline personality and bipolar spectrum disorders. Bipolar Disord. 2006;8(1):1–14.
17. Kernberg OF, Yeomans FE. Borderline personality disorder, bipolar disorder, depression, attention deficit/hyperactivity disorder, and narcissistic personality disorder: practical differential diagnosis. Bull Menn Clin. 2013;77(1):1–22.
18. Miller CJ, Klugman J, Berv DA, Rosenquist KJ, Ghaemi SN. Sensitivity and specificity of the mood disorder questionnaire for detecting bipolar disorder. J Affect Disord. 2004;81(2):167–71.
19. Ghaemi SN, Miller CJ, Berv DA, Klugman J, Rosenquist KJ, Pies RW. Sensitivity and specificity of a new bipolar spectrum diagnostic scale. J Affect Disord. 2005;84(2–3):273–7.

20. Angst J, Adolfsson R, Benazzi F, Gamma A, Hantouche E, Meyer TD, et al. The HCL-32: towards a self-assessment tool for hypomanic symptoms in outpatients. J Affect Disord. 2005;88(2):217–33.
21. Terrien S, Stefaniak N, Morvan Y, Besche-Richard C. Factor structure of the French version of the hypomanic personality scale (HPS) in non-clinical young adults. Compr Psychiatry. 2015;62:105–13.
22. Takeshima M. Treating mixed mania/hypomania: a review and synthesis of the evidence. CNS Spectr. 2017;22(2):177–85.
23. Tondo L, Baldessarini RJ, Hennen J, Floris G. Lithium maintenance treatment of depression and mania in bipolar I and bipolar II disorders. Am J Psychiatry. 1998;155(5):638–45.
24. Pacchiarotti I, Bond DJ, Baldessarini RJ, Nolen WA, Grunze H, Licht RW, et al. The International Society for Bipolar Disorders (ISBD) task force report on antidepressant use in bipolar disorders. Am J Psychiatry. 2013;170(11):1249–62.
25. Suppes T, Mintz J, McElroy SL, Altshuler LL, Kupka RW, Frye MA, et al. Mixed hypomania in 908 patients with bipolar disorder evaluated prospectively in the Stanley Foundation bipolar treatment network: a sex-specific phenomenon. Arch Gen Psychiatry. 2005;62(10):1089–96.
26. Suppes T, Hirschfeld RM, Vieta E, Raines S, Paulsson B. Quetiapine for the treatment of bipolar II depression: analysis of data from two randomized, double-blind, placebo-controlled studies. World J Biol Psychiatry. 2008;9(3):198–211.
27. Tohen M, Vieta E, Calabrese J, Ketter TA, Sachs G, Bowden C, et al. Efficacy of olanzapine and olanzapine-fluoxetine combination in the treatment of bipolar I depression. Arch Gen Psychiatry. 2003;60(11):1079–88.

Part II

Bipolar Disorder in Diverse Populations and Clinical Contexts

The Significance of Bipolar Disorder in Women

6

Hangoeunbi Kang, Jyeheon Song, and Beomwoo Nam

Clinical Characteristics of Bipolar Disorder in Women

The prevalence, clinical presentation, long-term course, and comorbidity patterns of bipolar disorder differ by sex. Biological factors—including hormones, menstruation, menopause, pregnancy, and childbirth—as well as variations in psychosocial stressors, influence the clinical characteristics of the disorder.

The overall prevalence of bipolar disorder is generally reported to be similar in men and women [1, 2]. However, in contrast to bipolar I disorder, bipolar II disorder demonstrates clear sex differences, with a higher prevalence observed in women [3].

The age at onset of bipolar disorder has generally been reported to show no sex differences [4]. However, in bipolar I disorder, men with an initial manic episode tend to have an earlier onset age compared with women [2, 5, 6].

Sex differences have been reported in both the type of initial episode and the predominant polarity of bipolar disorder. The total number of episodes does not appear to differ substantially between men and women. Over the long-term course, men are more likely to show a predominance of manic episodes, whereas women more often demonstrate a predominance of depressive episodes. In both sexes, the cumulative duration of depressive symptoms exceeds that of (hypo)manic episodes, underscoring the prognostic importance of managing depression. However, women are reported to experience depressive episodes more frequently and to spend a greater proportion of the illness course in depression [7–9].

Women with bipolar disorder are often first diagnosed with unipolar depression. When the initial episode is depressive, they are usually treated with antidepressants until a (hypo)manic episode appears. Because women more frequently present with depression as the first episode, they are at higher risk of delayed diagnosis, longer antidepressant exposure, and associated effects on the long-term course of illness. Antidepressant-induced (hypo)mania is also reported more commonly in women [7].

The characteristics of mood episodes differ by sex. Depressive episodes in women more often present with atypical features compared with those in men, and mixed episodes are also more common. The proportion of (hypo)manic episodes with mixed features has likewise been reported to be higher in women [10, 11]. In addition, rapid cycling occurs more frequently in women than in men. A meta-analysis of 2057 patients with bipolar disorder found that the prevalence of rapid cycling was approximately twice as high in women as in men (30 vs. 17%) [12].

H. Kang · J. Song
Department of Psychiatry, Naju National Hospital, Naju, Republic of Korea

B. Nam (✉)
Dr. Nam's Psychiatric Clinic, Chungju, Republic of Korea
e-mail: nempty@daum.net

W.-M. Bahk et al. (eds.), *Bipolar Disorder*, https://doi.org/10.1007/978-981-92-1323-8_6

Although some debate remains as to whether rapid cycling is truly more common in women, it has been linked to bipolar II disorder, mixed features, early onset, antidepressant use, comorbid alcohol abuse, hypothyroidism, and sex hormones, which may help explain its higher prevalence in women.

Comorbidity with other psychiatric disorders is reported to be higher in women with bipolar disorder than in men. In men, substance use disorders, conduct disorder, and attention-deficit/hyperactivity disorder are more common, whereas in women, comorbid anxiety disorders—including posttraumatic stress disorder—as well as phobias and eating disorders are more frequently observed. Women with bipolar disorder also have higher rates of comorbid medical conditions such as thyroid disease and migraine [3, 4, 13, 14]. The risk of alcohol misuse is particularly elevated in women with bipolar disorder. In the general population, the lifetime prevalence of alcohol use disorder is higher in men than in women (49 vs. 29%). However, in bipolar disorder, the sex-specific pattern differs: compared with individuals without bipolar disorder, the prevalence of alcohol use disorder is reported to be 2.77 times higher in men and 7.35 times higher in women [15].

Bipolar disorder is associated with a substantially increased risk of suicide, estimated to be approximately 15 times higher than in the general population. In the general population, suicide attempts are more common among women, whereas completed suicides are more frequent among men. However, this sex-specific pattern appears to differ in bipolar disorder. Women with bipolar disorder attempt suicide more often than men, but unlike in the general population, their rates of completed suicide are reported to be comparable to—or even higher than—those of men [16, 17].

Women with bipolar disorder are reported to have been more frequently exposed to physical and sexual abuse during childhood and adolescence than men. Patients with a history of childhood abuse tend to have a longer course of illness and a poorer treatment response for a variety of reasons [18].

The Impact of the Menstrual Cycle on Bipolar Disorder

Estrogen, the primary female sex hormone, regulates the menstrual cycle, prepares the body for pregnancy, and plays key roles in the central nervous system. It decreases the activity of monoamine oxidase, an enzyme that metabolizes serotonin and dopamine, thereby exerting serotonergic agonist–like effects. By modulating serotonin transport between cells, estrogen also increases synaptic serotonin levels, enhancing serotonergic transmission and contributing to mood improvement [19]. In addition, estrogen increases noradrenergic activity, exerts cholinergic agonist effects, and reduces the sensitivity of dopamine D2 receptors. Postpartum psychosis has been associated with increased sensitivity of hypothalamic dopamine receptors, a change that may be triggered by the sharp decline in estrogen levels after childbirth [20]. The antimanic effects of tamoxifen, a selective estrogen receptor modulator, are thought to result from its inhibition of protein kinase C as well as its mixed agonist/antagonist actions at estrogen receptors [21]. In women with postpartum psychosis, estrogen treatment has been reported to produce marked symptom improvement, and women with bipolar disorder treated with tamoxifen demonstrated a significant increase in serum estradiol levels. These findings highlight the important role of estrogen in the pathophysiology of bipolar disorder in women [22].

Many women report mood changes associated with the menstrual cycle, and such fluctuations are also commonly observed in women with bipolar disorder. A retrospective study found that 66% of women with bipolar I disorder experienced a worsening of mood symptoms during the premenstrual or menstrual phase. Another study reported that oral contraceptives alleviated cycle--related mood symptoms in 50% of women with bipolar disorder [1, 23]. These findings suggest that hormonal changes across the menstrual cycle may influence mood. However, interpretation of these results remains limited by factors such as retrospective study designs, heterogeneity of study populations, lack of objective confirmation of ovulation, and unclear methodologies. To date, research on the relationship between the menstrual cycle and mood fluctuations in women with bipolar disorder produced inconsistent findings [24].

The menopausal and perimenopausal transitions are recognized as particularly vulnerable periods for women with bipolar disorder. Data from the Systematic Treatment Enhancement Program for Bipolar Disorder (STEP-BD) indicate an increased risk of worsening depressive symptoms during the perimenopausal transition. Another study found higher rates of depressive episodes and overall mood episodes in perimenopausal women with bipolar disorder. These outcomes may reflect the combined influence of hormonal fluctuations, sleep disturbances, shifting midlife roles, and experiences of loss that are common during this stage of life [23, 25].

Considerations in the Pharmacological Treatment of Women with Bipolar Disorder

In the treatment of women with bipolar disorder, it is important to account for sex-specific pharmacokinetic and pharmacodynamic factors, such as lower hepatic metabolic rates and the influence of the menstrual cycle.

Among women receiving valproate, a higher prevalence of polycystic ovary syndrome (PCOS) and more frequent menstrual irregularities have been reported. Weight gain associated with valproate may contribute to metabolic disturbances such as hyperinsulinemia, hyperandrogenism, and ultimately the development of PCOS [26]. Adverse effects such as weight gain and alopecia can be particularly concerning in women and should be carefully considered when selecting this medication.

Lithium-associated hypothyroidism is reported more frequently in women, with the risk particularly elevated in middle-aged and older populations [27].

In women with bipolar disorder, antipsychotics such as risperidone, which can cause hyperprolactinemia, should be used with caution, as they may lead to anovulation, menstrual irregularities, and osteoporosis. Antipsychotics associated with a high risk of weight gain, including olanzapine and clozapine, should likewise be prescribed with particular caution in women.

The Impact of Pregnancy on the Course of Bipolar Disorder

Research on the impact of pregnancy and childbirth on the course of bipolar disorder in women consistently indicates that the postpartum period is strongly associated with the onset and worsening of mood episodes. The elevated risk of recurrence during this time has been attributed to rapid hormonal changes following delivery as well as sleep disruption related to childcare and breastfeeding. Importantly, this association between parenthood and recurrence risk has not been observed in men [23, 28, 29]. Studies comparing periods before, during, and after pregnancy further suggest that recurrence risk is higher in the pre-pregnancy and postpartum periods than during pregnancy itself, with large register-based studies from Denmark and the United Kingdom showing that the first three months postpartum—particularly the first weeks—represent the period of greatest vulnerability [30, 31]. Notably, pregnancy itself does not appear to be uniformly protective against mood episode recurrence in women with bipolar disorder.

Evidence from a meta-analysis encompassing multiple studies indicates that discontinuation of pharmacological treatment during pregnancy is associated with a substantially higher risk of relapse compared with maintenance treatment, underscoring the protective role of continued therapy, particularly lithium, in preventing both antenatal and postpartum recurrence. [32] Across observational studies, additional factors associated with recurrence include a history of illness recurrence during previous pregnancies, prior psychiatric illness, family history, and obstetric complications [32].

Large cohort and prospective observational studies further demonstrate that mood episodes occur more frequently in the postpartum period than during pregnancy across bipolar subtypes, with manic or psychotic episodes tending to recur earlier than depressive episodes [33, 35]. Studies examining lithium discontinuation highlight that relapse risk increases following withdrawal, particularly when discontinuation is abrupt, and that postpartum recurrence rates are markedly higher among women who discontinue lithium during pregnancy [28, 34]. Recurrence risk has also been reported to be higher in women with bipolar II disorder, early illness onset, frequent prior episodes, recent mood episodes, and antidepressant use, whereas maintenance treatment—especially with lithium—appears to confer relative protection [34].

Parity has been proposed as a potential modifier of recurrence risk, with some studies suggesting greater vulnerability during first pregnancies and others reporting lower recurrence rates with subsequent deliveries [36, 37]. However, these findings are inconsistent and may be confounded by treatment effects and reproductive decision--making, and the independent influence of parity on postpartum relapse in bipolar disorder remains difficult to establish [32].

Key studies summarizing recurrence rates and risk factors for bipolar disorder during pregnancy and the postpartum period are presented in Table 6.1.

Overall, evidence summarized in Table 6.1 indicates that pregnancy does not confer reliable protection against mood episode recurrence in women with bipolar disorder. Rather, relapse risk during pregnancy is strongly influenced by treatment-related factors, particularly the discontinuation of maintenance pharmacotherapy, with abrupt withdrawal consistently associated with higher relapse rates, earlier recurrence, and increased vulnerability in the postpartum period. This pattern is further supported by meta-analytic evidence demonstrating a substantially higher relapse risk among women who discontinue treatment during pregnancy compared with those who maintain pharmacotherapy [32].

Despite these consistent findings, uncertainty remains regarding the extent to which pregnancy-related biological changes independently affect relapse risk, as most available data are derived from observational studies and are confounded by illness severity, treatment history, and indication bias. In addition, the modifying roles of bipolar subtype, parity, and psychosocial stressors have not been fully elucidated [32, 36, 37].

Clinically, these findings underscore that routine discontinuation of maintenance treatment during pregnancy may expose women to substantial relapse risk without proportionate fetal benefit. Treatment decisions should, therefore, be individualized, balancing maternal illness history and relapse vulnerability against medication-specific fetal risks rather than adopting a uniform approach to medication withdrawal [32, 34].

Table 6.1 Research findings on recurrence and risk factors of bipolar disorder during pregnancy

Author (year)	Study objective	Study design	Patients (N, diagnosis)	Recurrence rate	Other findings	Risk factors for recurrence
Rosso et al. (2016) [38]	To evaluate the preventive effect of lithium on recurrence during pregnancy in a high-risk group	Prospective observational	17 women (17 lithium-responsive BD I)	During pregnancy: 11% ($n = 2$) Postpartum recurrence: 27.8% ($n = 5$)		- Immediate postpartum period - Discontinuation of maintenance therapy - Abrupt discontinuation - BD II - Early onset of illness - History of frequent relapses - Recent mood episode - Antidepressant use - Use of anticonvulsants (vs. lithium) - First pregnancy with prior mood episode - Depressive symptoms during pregnancy
Di Florio et al. (2013) [33]	To investigate the frequency and timing of perinatal mood episodes in women with bipolar disorder	Retrospective observational	1212 women (BD I: 980; BD II: 232; RMD: 573)	During pregnancy BD 1:4.3%, BD 2: 7.8%, Recurrent major depression (RDM): 4.7% Recurrence postpartum BD 1: 45.7% BD II: 34.4% RDM: 38%		
Viguera et al. (2011) [35]	To compare the risk of mood episodes during pregnancy and postpartum	Retrospective observational	1162 women (BD I: 283; BD II: 338; MDD: 541)	Postpartum: 51.5% (BD) During pregnancy: 21.7% (BD)	Postpartum: 29.8% During (MDD) pregnancy: 4.6% (MDD)	
Viguera et al. (2007) [34]	To compare recurrence rates between maintenance and discontinuation groups during pregnancy	Prospective observational	89 women (BD I: 61; BD II: 28)	Discontinuation group: 85.5% Maintenance group: 37.0%	Overall recurrence during pregnancy: 71%	
Akdeniz et al. (2003) [39]	To investigate the impact of pregnancy and childbirth on the course of bipolar disorder	Retrospective observational	72 women (BD; 252 pregnancies observed)	32% experienced a mood episode during pregnancy or within 1 month postpartum		
Freeman et al. (2002) [23]	To examine the impact of menstruation, pregnancy, and childbirth on the course of bipolar disorder	Retrospective observational	50 women (BD I: 36; BD II: 13; BD NOS: 1)	67% of women experienced a postpartum mood episode		
Viguera et al. (2000) [28]	To compare recurrence rates after lithium discontinuation between pregnant and non-pregnant women	Retrospective observational	101 women (BD I: 68; BD II: 33)	Pregnant group: 52% Non-pregnant control group: 58%	Recurrence rate before lithium discontinuation: 21%	

BD bipolar disorder, *BD I* bipolar I disorder, *BD II* bipolar II disorder, *BD NOS* bipolar disorder not otherwise specified, *MDD* major depressive disorder, *RMD* recurrent major depression

Treatment of Bipolar Disorder During Pregnancy

The primary goal in treating bipolar disorder during pregnancy is to provide the safest possible care for the fetus while preventing relapse and maintaining stability in the mother. A comprehensive relapse-prevention plan should include preconception counseling and planned pregnancy, pharmacological treatment during pregnancy and the postpartum period, close monitoring for early signs of recurrence, management of fetal drug exposure during pregnancy and breastfeeding, and careful attention to postpartum risk factors such as adequate sleep, stable circadian rhythms, stress reduction, and promotion of maternal–infant bonding.

Discontinuation of medication during pregnancy increases the risk of relapse in women with bipolar disorder. When risks are compared, recurrence in untreated mothers is generally considered to pose a greater threat to the fetus than medication exposure, making continued treatment relatively safer. With careful preconception planning, attention to factors influencing fetal drug risk, and appropriate dose adjustments as pregnancy progresses, pharmacological treatment for bipolar disorder during pregnancy should not be viewed with undue concern. The potential risks of medication use must always be weighed against the risks associated with treatment discontinuation. [34]

If discontinuation of medication during pregnancy is being considered, the decision should be made with caution and based on an individualized risk–benefit analysis that incorporates the patient's clinical characteristics and treatment response. Several factors have been identified as predictors of a higher risk of recurrence following discontinuation. For example, women receiving combination therapy have a 2.3-fold greater risk of recurrence compared with those on monotherapy. Other predictors of increased recurrence risk include early onset, bipolar II disorder, rapid cycling, recent mood episodes, frequent prior episodes, a history of suicide attempts, comorbid psychiatric disorders, antidepressant use, and abrupt discontinuation of maintenance medication [34]. In women with these risk factors, discontinuation should be carefully reconsidered.

Abrupt discontinuation of medication during pregnancy increases the risk of relapse; therefore, tapering should be planned in advance whenever discontinuation is considered. Even in cases of unplanned pregnancy, a gradual taper is preferable. Because unplanned pregnancies are often not recognized until after the period of greatest teratogenic risk from drug exposure has passed, sudden discontinuation at that stage may increase maternal relapse risk without substantially reducing fetal risk. The teratogenic potential of psychotropic medications depends primarily on dosage, duration, and timing of exposure. Accordingly, treatment planning for pregnant women with bipolar disorder should consider maternal clinical status, gestational age, the specific medication used, and patient preferences. Close monitoring for early signs of relapse is essential after discontinuation. Given the particularly high risk of recurrence in the postpartum period, resumption of medication immediately after delivery is recommended [40].

Fetal Effects of Medication Use During Pregnancy

The U.S. Food and Drug Administration (FDA) previously classified medications into five categories (A, B, C, D, and X) according to their teratogenic risk during pregnancy. This system, in place since 1979, has since been gradually phased out and replaced by the Pregnancy and Lactation Labeling Rule (PLLR). The PLLR, implemented on June 30, 2015, was designed to provide more detailed and transparent information on the potential risks of medication use during pregnancy and lactation. Instead of offering a simple "yes" or "no" regarding risk, the new labeling requires data-driven, individualized clinical interpretation to guide treatment decisions. Its intent is to support pregnant women who require pharmacological therapy in making informed choices in consultation with their physicians.

Information provided under the FDA's PLLR is available through DailyMed. The labeling is divided into three sections: 8.1 Pregnancy, 8.2 Lactation, and 8.3 Females and Males of Reproductive Potential. These sections offer evidence-based guidance that considers gestational age and timing of drug exposure. They include the rationale for use or avoidance of a medication, the risks of adverse effects in breastfeeding mothers and infants, recommendations on the duration of breastfeeding, and guidance regarding pregnancy testing and contraception.

Exposure to antidepressants during pregnancy has been associated with an increased risk of miscarriage and impaired fetal growth. Some neonates exposed to antidepressants in utero may exhibit transient symptoms at birth. Bupropion is classified as category B, whereas most selective serotonin reuptake inhibitors (SSRIs), with the exception of paroxetine, are classified as category C. Paroxetine, however, was reclassified from category C to category D by the FDA in 2005 after reports suggested that first-trimester exposure was linked to an increased risk of congenital cardiac malformations, including atrial and ventricular septal defects. Accordingly, the use of paroxetine during the first trimester should be undertaken with caution [41, 42].

Evidence regarding the association between lamotrigine and the risk of oral clefts, such as cleft lip and cleft palate, has been inconsistent. Lamotrigine is classified as category C, and since the overall risk of major malformations is not considered high, its use during pregnancy may be appropriate. In neonates, potential risks include hepatotoxicity and skin rash. During pregnancy, increased drug clearance leads to lower serum concentrations compared with pre-pregnancy levels. Therefore, therapeutic drug monitoring of lamotrigine is recommended. Ideally, a baseline serum concentration should be established prior to conception, with dose adjustments made as pregnancy progresses [43–45].

Lithium is classified as category D, and its use during pregnancy requires careful consideration based on gestational age. Lithium has long been associated with an increased risk of Ebstein's anomaly, which historically led to restrictions on its use in the treatment of bipolar disorder during pregnancy [46]. More recent evidence, however, suggests that this risk may have been overstated. Studies indicate that while lithium exposure is associated with an increased risk of cardiovascular malformations, the absolute risk is lower than previously believed [47]. In a large cohort study of 1,325,563 live births, cardiac malformations were identified in 16 of 663 infants (2.41%) exposed to lithium, compared with 15,251 of 1,322,955 infants (1.15%) not exposed [48]. The adjusted risk ratio for cardiac malformations in lithium-exposed infants was 1.65 (95% confidence interval [CI], 1.02–2.68) relative to unexposed infants. Risk also varied by dose: 1.11 (95% CI, 0.46–2.64) for ≤600 mg/day, 1.60 (95% CI, 0.67–3.80) for 601–900 mg/day, and 3.22 (95% CI, 1.47–7.02) for >900 mg/day [48]. In other words, maternal lithium exposure during the first trimester is associated with approximately one additional case of cardiac malformation per 100 births, and this risk appears to be dose-dependent.

Carbamazepine is classified as category D, and its use during the first trimester of pregnancy has been associated with a risk of craniofacial defects of up to 11% and spina bifida of about 1%. It may be considered when no safer alternative is available. Because carbamazepine can cause vitamin K deficiency in the neonate, vitamin K supplementation is recommended in late pregnancy and after delivery.

Valproate is classified as category D and should be avoided whenever possible. Registry studies from multiple countries have shown that daily doses of lamotrigine ≤300 mg or carbamazepine ≤400 mg are not associated with an increased risk of major congenital malformations compared with the general population. In contrast, the risk of fetal malformations with valproate exposure is substantially higher than with other anticonvulsants, leading to strong recommendations against its use during pregnancy. The risk of major congenital malformations is determined not only by the specific agent but also by the dosage [49]. A study evaluating the risk of major congenital malformations with valproate monotherapy versus combination therapy found that the prevalence at one year after birth was 10.0% with valproate monotherapy, 11.3% with valproate plus lamotrigine, and 11.7% with valproate combined with other anticonvulsants. In all three groups, the prevalence of major congenital malformations increased with higher valproate doses, suggesting that the risk was attributable to the dosage of valproate itself rather than to the concomitant use of other anticonvulsants [50]. An important finding from follow-up studies of neurodevelopmental outcomes after in utero exposure to anticonvulsants is the reduction in intelligence quotient (IQ) observed in children exposed to valproate during pregnancy. This effect appears to be irreversible and may affect educational achievement and occupational functioning later in life. Therefore, valproate should not be considered a first-line treatment option during pregnancy [51, 52].

Antipsychotics are generally considered safer than mood stabilizers during pregnancy and are useful when maintenance treatment is necessary or in the event of relapse. Typical antipsychotics such as chlorpromazine have well-established safety profiles supported by extensive clinical experience. Clozapine is classified as category B, whereas aripiprazole, olanzapine, quetiapine, risperidone, and ziprasidone are classified as category C. In recent years, atypical antipsychotics have been increasingly preferred because of their lower risk of anticholinergic side effects and extrapyramidal symptoms [53]. Use of atypical antipsychotics is associated with weight gain and metabolic syndrome, which theoretically could increase the risk of insulin resistance, gestational diabetes, and preeclampsia; however, the available data remain limited. An analysis from the Massachusetts General Hospital Pregnancy Registry found no increased risk of diabetes during pregnancy among women without preexisting diabetes, despite exposure to atypical antipsychotics during gestation [54].

Fetal exposure to benzodiazepines during pregnancy has been reported to increase the risk of congenital malformations, particularly cleft lip and cleft palate, and these agents are classified as category D. Although benzodiazepines can be useful for the acute management of symptoms, their potential benefits and risks should be carefully weighed. More recent studies, however, have found no increased risk of malformations associated with benzodiazepine exposure during the first trimester [55]. A study comparing outcomes including birth weight, respiratory distress, feeding difficulties, head circumference, Apgar scores, admission to intensive care, and preterm birth between infants exposed to benzodiazepines in utero and control groups found that intrauterine exposure to benzodiazepines was associated with an increased risk of admission to intensive care units and microcephaly. No increased risk of other congenital malformations was observed [56].

Preconception Management

Planned pregnancy can reduce both the risk of teratogenic effects from psychotropic medications and the risk of recurrence in the mother. Establishing a pregnancy and delivery plan before conception is, therefore, essential. Ideally, the patient should be in remission at the time of planning to enable informed, collaborative decision-making with the clinician. Involving the partner in prenatal planning may also be beneficial. Counseling should highlight the benefits of planned pregnancy, include education on contraception, and address potential drug–drug interactions between mood stabilizers and oral contraceptives. Nevertheless, unintended pregnancies occur 40–50% more frequently in women with bipolar disorder [47]. Even in such cases, patients should be reassured that the absolute risk of congenital malformations from medication exposure is generally low.

In women of reproductive age using contraception, carbamazepine or topiramate can induce cytochrome P450 enzymes, leading to increased metabolism of oral contraceptives and reduced plasma concentrations. In such cases, higher dose contraceptives or alternative contraceptive methods should be considered. Oral contraceptives can also reduce lamotrigine plasma levels, thereby diminishing its therapeutic efficacy, and dose adjustment may be required. Plasma concentrations of lamotrigine have been reported to be approximately 50% lower in women taking oral contraceptives compared with those not using them [57]. This interaction is primarily attributable to ethinyl estradiol, which induces lamotrigine metabolism. In contrast, progestogens do not lower lamotrigine plasma concentrations, suggesting that progestogen-only contraceptives may avoid this interaction. Given these drug–drug interactions, non-hormonal contraceptive devices may be a useful option for preventing unintended pregnancies [58].

Women with bipolar disorder often discontinue pharmacotherapy before or during pregnancy because they perceive the potential effects of medication on the fetus as more serious than the risk of recurrence. However, recurrence after discontinuation exposes the fetus to maternal anxiety and stress. Recurrence of mood episodes in the mother may also result in poor nutrition, neglect of physical health, smoking, alcohol misuse, increased risk of violence, and even suicide, all of which can endanger fetal health. Patients should be counseled that maternal recurrence may pose a greater risk to fetal well-being than potential medication exposure.

In women who experience infrequent relapses and maintain full remission between episodes, it may be reasonable to gradually taper maintenance medication and plan pregnancy after discontinuation. However, in patients with a history of frequent relapses or a tendency to relapse quickly after stopping medication, continuation of maintenance therapy with a lower-risk agent should be prioritized. If past relapses have been mild or symptoms resolved rapidly after restarting treatment, discontinuation with close monitoring may be a reasonable option. When maintenance therapy is discontinued, patients and their families should be informed of both the potential benefits and risks for mother and fetus and should be actively involved in the decision-making process [47, 59].

Management During Pregnancy

The first trimester of pregnancy is the critical period of organogenesis and carries the highest risk of teratogenic effects from medication exposure. Whenever possible, medication should be discontinued during this time. If maintenance treatment is absolutely necessary or recurrence occurs during pregnancy, efforts should be made to avoid periods of greatest teratogenic risk, and treatment should be limited to the lowest effective dose and preferably monotherapy. The timing of maximal risk varies by medication. Neural tube defects associated with anticonvulsant exposure are most likely to occur between 17 and 30 days after conception. The risk of spina bifida increases after day 23, while lithium exposure is associated with the highest risk of Ebstein's anomaly between 21 and 56 days after conception.

During the first trimester, lithium, lamotrigine, or antipsychotics are generally preferred over valproate for the treatment of bipolar disorder. In pregnant women exposed to valproate, prenatal diagnostic evaluations such as alpha-fetoprotein testing and ultrasound should be offered, along with counseling regarding the risk of congenital malformations, and high-dose folic acid supplementation (4 mg/day) should be prescribed [60]. However, even with high-dose folic acid, the preventive effect against valproate-associated spina bifida is limited [61]. For women receiving lithium, fetal ultrasound examinations are recommended. Lithium should be administered in divided doses to maintain stable serum concentrations, and therapeutic drug monitoring is essential during pregnancy, as increased renal clearance may lower serum levels.

The second and third trimesters of pregnancy carry a relatively lower risk of major congenital malformations compared with the first trimester. During these stages, the potential effects of medication exposure are more likely to include minor malformations, behavioral effects, low birth weight, or preterm delivery rather than severe structural anomalies [47].

During the second trimester, the fetus undergoes skeletal and lung development. Valproate exposure is associated not only with congenital malformations from early pregnancy but also with neurotoxic effects on the developing central nervous system. High-dose valproate use during pregnancy (≥1000 mg/day) has been linked to adverse effects on cognitive development, with exposed children demonstrating IQ scores approximately 7–10 points lower. Therefore, its use should be avoided whenever possible [51].

In women taking atypical antipsychotics during this period, monitoring for metabolic syndrome is recommended, and screening for gestational diabetes should be conducted. However, increases in abdominal circumference and serum lipid levels are normal physiological changes of pregnancy and should not be mistaken for metabolic syndrome.

The third trimester is primarily a period of fetal growth and maturation rather than organ development, and the risk of major malformations is, therefore, relatively low. However, medication exposure during this stage has been associated with neonatal withdrawal syndromes after delivery. Antipsychotic use has been linked to abnormal motor symptoms and withdrawal signs in newborns, while benzodiazepine use during the third trimester has also been associated with neonatal withdrawal [56].

During this stage, glomerular filtration rate increases, resulting in approximately a twofold increase in lithium clearance. Accordingly, serum lithium levels should be monitored every one to two weeks, and the dosage adjusted as needed to maintain therapeutic concentrations. In contrast, immediately after delivery, reductions in maternal fluid volume can elevate serum lithium levels, necessitating dose adjustment to avoid toxicity. To minimize neonatal serum lithium exposure at birth, lithium should be discontinued 24–48 h before the onset of labor or cesarean delivery and restarted immediately postpartum [62].

Postpartum Management

The postpartum period represents the most consistently high-risk phase for recurrence in women with bipolar disorder, with the greatest vulnerability occurring during the first weeks after delivery. Evidence across multiple cohort and register-based studies demonstrates that postpartum relapse rates substantially exceed those observed during pregnancy, regardless of bipolar subtype. Manic and psychotic episodes tend to occur earlier than depressive episodes, highlighting the need for heightened vigilance immediately after childbirth.

While the magnitude of postpartum risk is well established, uncertainty persists regarding the relative contributions of hormonal withdrawal, sleep deprivation, and psychosocial stressors. Furthermore, optimal prophylactic strategies—particularly the choice and timing of pharmacotherapy—remain informed primarily by observational data rather than randomized trials.

From a clinical standpoint, these findings strongly support proactive postpartum relapse-prevention strategies. Initiation or resumption of maintenance treatment immediately after delivery, guided by prior treatment response, should be considered standard practice for women at high risk, rather than a reactive approach following symptom emergence.

Accordingly, the immediate postpartum period—particularly the first week after childbirth—carries the greatest risk of recurrence. During this period, it is recommended that maintenance therapy be guided by the medication that has previously been most effective for the patient. In cases of postpartum recurrence, treatment should be selected according to the type of mood episode that has occurred. Furthermore, because most medications are excreted in breast milk, potential effects on the infant should be carefully considered when choosing pharmacotherapy during breastfeeding.

Postpartum women are at particularly high risk of sleep deprivation and emotional disturbances while caring for a newborn. Even without a prior history of bipolar disorder, it is not uncommon for women to experience a first episode of postpartum psychosis, which typically emerges within two to three weeks after delivery. Postpartum psychosis should be considered a psychiatric emergency, and pharmacological treatment with antipsychotics, benzodiazepines, or lithium has been shown to be effective [40].

When prescribing pharmacotherapy during breastfeeding, medication choice should be made in collaboration with the patient, taking into

Table 6.2 Bipolar disorder pharmacotherapy: Concentrations in breast milk and safety during lactation

Drug		Relative infant dose (%) [63]	Note [64, 65]
Mood stabilizers	Carbamazepine	5.9	Generally considered safe
	Lamotrigine	9.2–18.3	Use with caution; lowest effective dose; monitor infant
	Lithium	12–30.1	Use with close monitoring / not absolutely contraindicated
	Valproic acid	1.4–1.7	Generally considered safe
Selective serotonin reuptake inhibitors	Citalopram	3.6	Considered safe
	Escitalopram	5.3	
	Fluvoxamine	1.6	
	Fluoxetine	5–9	
	Paroxetine	1.4	
	Sertraline	0.54	
Serotonin and norepinephrine reuptake inhibitors	Venlafaxine	8.1	Limited data; use with caution and monitor infant
	Desvenlafaxine	6.8	
	Duloxetine	0.1	
Antipsychotics	Olanzapine	1.6	Considered safe; first-line option
	Risperidone	4.3	Generally safe with close monitoring
	Quetiapine	0.09	Considered safe; first-line option

account potential effects on the infant. Recent studies have provided updated evidence on drug concentrations and safety during lactation (Table 6.2). Selective serotonin reuptake inhibitors (SSRIs) generally have a low relative infant dose (RID) and are considered first-line treatments for depressive and anxiety symptoms in breastfeeding women. Among SSRIs, sertraline is the most extensively studied and is preferred because concentrations in both breast milk and infant serum are very low. Fluoxetine, by contrast, has a higher RID and is, therefore, less favored. For antipsychotics, atypical agents are preferred. Quetiapine and olanzapine are regarded as the most suitable options during lactation, whereas risperidone may be used with close monitoring. Clozapine is contraindicated because it is excreted into breast milk at high concentrations and has been associated with agranulocytosis in infants. Amisulpride is likewise contraindicated due to high levels of excretion into breast milk. Among mood stabilizers, valproate and carbamazepine have low RIDs and are generally considered compatible with breastfeeding, whereas lamotrigine may be used with careful monitoring of infant serum levels. Lithium, although historically contraindicated due to its high RID and classification as L4, has more recently been reported in some studies to be a viable option, and in certain contexts even a first-line choice, provided that infant serum concentrations are closely monitored [63–66].

Summary

Understanding sex differences in bipolar disorder provides important insights into its clinical characteristics in women, aids in estimating morbidity risk, and informs the development of appropriate treatment strategies. The prevalence of bipolar I disorder does not differ by sex, but bipolar II disorder is more common in women. Compared with men, women with bipolar disorder experience depressive episodes more frequently and spend a greater proportion of the illness course in depression. Because depressive episodes are often the initial presentation in women, diagnosis of bipolar disorder is frequently delayed, increasing the likelihood of prolonged antidepressant exposure and adversely influencing long-term outcomes. Women are also more likely to exhibit mixed episodes and rapid cycling, and they have higher rates of comorbid psychiatric conditions such as anxiety disorders (including alcohol misuse and eating disorders) as well as medical illnesses such as thyroid disease and migraine. When treating women with bipolar disorder, it is important to consider biological differences, including lower hepatic metabolic capacity and the influence of the menstrual cycle and pregnancy.

During pregnancy, it is essential to select the safest possible treatment for the fetus while also preventing recurrence and maintaining stability in the mother. Discontinuation of maintenance therapy during pregnancy is associated with increased recurrence rates. When weighing risks, maternal recurrence can pose greater harm to the fetus than medication exposure, making continued treatment relatively safer in many cases. The potential risks of medication use should always be evaluated alongside the risks of treatment discontinuation.

Decisions about discontinuation during pregnancy should be made collaboratively with the patient, based on an individualized risk–benefit analysis that considers clinical characteristics and prior treatment response. Women with early onset, frequent prior recurrence, or abrupt discontinuation of medication are at particularly high risk of recurrence and require special caution. The first trimester, a critical period of organogenesis with the highest risk of congenital malformations, may warrant consideration of discontinuing medication if clinically feasible. Planned pregnancy can help minimize both teratogenic risks from medication and the risk of recurrence, as treatment tapering can be done gradually with close monitoring for recurrence.

The postpartum period, particularly the first three months, carries an exceptionally high risk of recurrence. Therefore, initiating maintenance therapy immediately after delivery is strongly recommended to reduce this risk. Regarding specific agents, evidence suggests that valproate should generally be avoided during pregnancy, whereas antipsychotics, lithium, and lamotrigine are relatively safer alternatives. During breastfeeding, quetiapine and olanzapine are considered among the safer options.

These conclusions are supported by observational and register-based studies summarized in Tables 6.1 and 6.2

Declarations

Competing Interests The author(s) has no competing interests to declare that are relevant to the content of this manuscript.

Ethics Approval The author(s) declares that this manuscript does not include primary research with human participants.

The author(s) declares that this manuscript does not include primary studies involving animals.

References

1. Blehar MC, DePaulo JR Jr, Gershon ES, Reich T, Simpson SG, Nurnberger JI Jr. Women with bipolar disorder: findings from the NIMH genetics initiative sample. Psychopharmacol Bull. 1998;34:239–43.
2. Kennedy N, Boydell J, Kalidindi S, Fearon P, Jones PB, van Os J, et al. Gender differences in incidence and age at onset of mania and bipolar disorder over a 35-year period in Camberwell, England. Am J Psychiatry. 2005;162:257–62.
3. Baldassano CF, Marangell LB, Gyulai L, Ghaemi SN, Joffe H, Kim DR, et al. Gender differences in bipolar disorder: retrospective data from the first 500 STEP-BD participants. Bipolar Disord. 2005;7:465–70.
4. Suppes T, Leverich GS, Keck PE, Nolen WA, Denicoff KD, Altshuler LL, et al. The Stanley Foundation bipolar treatment outcome network. II. Demographics and illness characteristics of the first 261 patients. J Affect Disord. 2001;67:45–59.
5. Grant BF, Stinson FS, Hasin DS, Dawson DA, Chou SP, Ruan WJ, et al. Prevalence, correlates, and comorbidity of bipolar I disorder and axis I and II disorders: results from the National Epidemiologic Survey on alcohol and related conditions. J Clin Psychiatry. 2005;66:1205–15.
6. Azorin JM, Belzeaux R, Kaladjian A, Adida M, Hantouche E, Lancrenon S, et al. Risks associated with gender differences in bipolar I disorder. J Affect Disord. 2013;151:1033.
7. Leibenluft E. Women with bipolar illness: clinical and research issues. Am J Psychiatry. 1996;153:163–73.
8. Judd LL, Akiskal HS, Schettler PJ, Endicott J, Maser J, Solomon DA, et al. The long-term natural history of

the weekly symptomatic status of bipolar I disorder. Arch Gen Psychiatry. 2002;59:530–7.
9. Altshuler LL, Kupka RW, Hellemann G, Frye MA, Sugar CA, McElroy SL, et al. Gender and depressive symptoms in 711 patients with bipolar disorder evaluated prospectively in the Stanley Foundation bipolar treatment outcome network. Am J Psychiatry. 2010;167:708–15.
10. Benazzi F. Gender differences in bipolar-II disorder. Eur Arch Psychiatry Clin Neurosci. 2006;256:67–71.
11. Suppes T, Mintz J, McElroy SL, Altshuler LL, Kupka RW, Frye MA, et al. Mixed hypomania in 908 patients with bipolar disorder evaluated prospectively in the Stanley Foundation Bipolar Treatment Network: a sex-specific phenomenon. Arch Gen Psychiatry. 2005;62:1089–96.
12. Kupka RW, Luckenbaugh DA, Post RM, Leverich GS, Nolen WA. Rapid and non-rapid cycling bipolar disorder: a meta-analysis of clinical studies. J Clin Psychiatry. 2003;64:1483–94.
13. Arnold LM. Gender differences in bipolar disorder. Psychiatr Clin North Am. 2003;26:595–620.
14. Kawa I, Carter JD, Joyce PR, Doughty CJ, Frampton CM, Wells JE, et al. Gender differences in bipolar disorder: age of onset, course, comorbidity, and symptom presentation. Bipolar Disord. 2005;7:119–25.
15. Frye MA, Altshuler LL, SL ME, Suppes T, Keck PE, Denicoff K, et al. Gender differences in prevalence, risk, and clinical correlates of alcoholism comorbidity in bipolar disorder. Am J Psychiatry. 2003;160:883–9.
16. Osby U, Brandt L, Correia N, Ekbom A, Sparen P. Excess mortality in bipolar and unipolar disorder in Sweden. Arch Gen Psychiatry. 2001;58:844–50.
17. Baldessarini RJ, Tondo L. Suicide risk and treatments for patients with bipolar disorder. JAMA. 2003;290:1517–9.
18. Leverich GS, McElroy SL, Suppes T, PE K Jr, Denicoff KD, Nolen WA, et al. Early physical and sexual abuse associated with an adverse course of bipolar illness. Biol Psychiatry. 2002;51:288–97.
19. Payne JL. The role of estrogen in mood disorders in women. Int Rev Psychiatry. 2003;15:280–90.
20. Wieck A, Davies RA, Hirst AD, Brown N, Papadopoulos A, Marks MN, et al. Menstrual cycle effects on hypothalamic dopamine receptor function in women with a history of puerperal bipolar disorder. J Psychopharmacol. 2003;17:204–9.
21. Yildiz A, Guleryuz S, Ankerst DP, Ongur D, Renshaw PF. Protein kinase C inhibition in the treatment of mania: a double-blind, placebo-controlled trial of tamoxifen. Arch Gen Psychiatry. 2008;65:255–63.
22. Ahokas A, Aito M, Rimon R. Positive treatment effect of estradiol in postpartum psychosis: a pilot study. J Clin Psychiatry. 2000;61:166–9.
23. Freeman MP, Smith KW, Freeman SA, SL ME, Kmetz GE, Wright R, et al. The impact of reproductive events on the course of bipolar disorder in women. J Clin Psychiatry. 2002;63:284–7.
24. Sit D, Seltman H, Wisner KL. Menstrual effects on mood symptoms in treated women with bipolar disorder. Bipolar Disord. 2011;13:310–7.
25. Marsh WK, Ketter TA, Rasgon NL. Increased depressive symptoms in menopausal age women with bipolar disorder: age and gender comparison. J Psychiatr Res. 2009;43:798–802.
26. Isojarvi JI, Laatikainen TJ, Pakarinen AJ, Juntunen KT, Myllyla VV. Polycystic ovaries and hyperandrogenism in women taking valproate for epilepsy. N Engl J Med. 1993;329:1383–8.
27. Kirov G, Tredget J, John R, Owen MJ, Lazarus JH. A cross-sectional and a prospective study of thyroid disorders in lithium-treated patients. J Affect Disord. 2005;87:313–7.
28. Viguera AC, Nonacs R, Cohen LS, Tondo L, Murray A, Baldessarini RJ. Risk of recurrence of bipolar disorder in pregnant and nonpregnant women after discontinuing lithium maintenance. Am J Psychiatry. 2000;157:179–84.
29. Lewis KJS, Di Florio A, Forty L, Gordon-Smith K, Perry A, Craddock N, et al. Mania triggered by sleep loss and risk of postpartum psychosis in women with bipolar disorder. J Affect Disord. 2018;225:624–9.
30. Grof P, Robbins W, Alda M, Berghoefer A, Vojtechovsky M, Nilsson A, et al. Protective effect of pregnancy in women with lithium-responsive bipolar disorder. J Affect Disord. 2000;61:31–9.
31. Munk-Olsen T, Laursen TM, Pedersen CB, Mors O, Mortensen PB. New parents and mental disorders: a population-based register study. JAMA. 2006;296:2582–9.
32. Wesseloo R, Kamperman AM, Munk-Olsen T, Pop VJ, Kushner SA, Bergink V. Risk of postpartum relapse in bipolar disorder and postpartum psychosis: a systematic review and meta-analysis. Am J Psychiatry. 2016;173:117–27.
33. Di Florio A, Forty L, Gordon-Smith K, Heron J, Jones L, Craddock N, et al. Perinatal episodes across the mood disorder spectrum. JAMA Psychiatry. 2013;70:168–75.
34. Viguera AC, Whitfield T, Baldessarini RJ, Newport DJ, Stowe Z, Reminick A, et al. Risk of recurrence in women with bipolar disorder during pregnancy: prospective study of mood stabilizer discontinuation. Am J Psychiatry. 2007;164:1817–24. quiz 1923.
35. Viguera AC, Tondo L, Koukopoulos AE, Reginaldi D, Lepri B, Baldessarini RJ. Episodes of mood disorders in 2,252 pregnancies and postpartum periods. Am J Psychiatry. 2011;168:1179–85.
36. Di Florio A, Jones L, Forty L, Gordon-Smith K, Blackmore ER, Heron J, et al. Mood disorders and parity - a clue to the aetiology of the postpartum trigger. J Affect Disord. 2014;152–154:334–9.
37. Munk-Olsen T, Jones I, Laursen TM. Birth order and postpartum psychiatric disorders. Bipolar Disord. 2014;16:300–7.
38. Rosso G, Albert U, Di Salvo G, Scata M, Todros T, Maina G. Lithium prophylaxis during pregnancy and the postpartum period in women with

lithium-responsive bipolar I disorder. Arch Womens Ment Health. 2016;19:429–32.
39. Akdeniz F, Vahip S, Pirildar S, Vahip I, Doganer I, Bulut I. Risk factors associated with childbearing-related episodes in women with bipolar disorder. Psychopathology. 2003;36:234–8.
40. Yatham LN, Kennedy SH, Parikh SV, Schaffer A, Bond DJ, Frey BN, et al. Canadian Network for Mood and Anxiety Treatments (CANMAT) and International Society for Bipolar Disorders (ISBD) 2018 guidelines for the management of patients with bipolar disorder. Bipolar Disord. 2018;20:97–170.
41. Kallen BA, Otterblad OP. Maternal use of selective serotonin re-uptake inhibitors in early pregnancy and infant congenital malformations. Birth Defects Res A Clin Mol Teratol. 2007;79:301–8.
42. Yonkers KA, Blackwell KA, Glover J, Forray A. Antidepressant use in pregnant and postpartum women. Annu Rev Clin Psychol. 2014;10:369–92.
43. Paulzen M, Lammertz SE, Veselinovic T, Goecke TW, Hiemke C, Grunder G. Lamotrigine in pregnancy - therapeutic drug monitoring in maternal blood, amniotic fluid, and cord blood. Int Clin Psychopharmacol. 2015;30:249–54.
44. Wesseloo R, Liu X, Clark CT, Kushner SA, Munk-Olsen T, Bergink V. Risk of postpartum episodes in women with bipolar disorder after lamotrigine or lithium use during pregnancy: a population-based cohort study. J Affect Disord. 2017;218:394–7.
45. Clark CT, Wisner KL. Treatment of peripartum bipolar disorder. Obstet Gynecol Clin N Am. 2018;45:403–17.
46. Nora JJ, Nora AH. Editorial: can the pill cause birth defects? N Engl J Med. 1974;291:731–2.
47. Yonkers KA, Wisner KL, Stowe Z, Leibenluft E, Cohen L, Miller L, et al. Management of bipolar disorder during pregnancy and the postpartum period. Am J Psychiatry. 2004;161:608–20.
48. Patorno E, Huybrechts KF, Bateman BT, Cohen JM, Desai RJ, Mogun H, et al. Lithium use in pregnancy and the risk of cardiac malformations. N Engl J Med. 2017;376:2245–54.
49. Tomson T, Battino D, Bonizzoni E, Craig J, Lindhout D, Sabers A, et al. Dose-dependent risk of malformations with antiepileptic drugs: an analysis of data from the EURAP epilepsy and pregnancy registry. Lancet Neurol. 2011;10:609–17.
50. Tomson T, Battino D, Bonizzoni E, Craig J, Lindhout D, Perucca E, et al. Dose-dependent teratogenicity of valproate in mono- and polytherapy: an observational study. Neurology. 2015;85:866–72.
51. Adab N, Kini U, Vinten J, Ayres J, Baker G, Clayton-Smith J, et al. The longer term outcome of children born to mothers with epilepsy. J Neurol Neurosurg Psychiatry. 2004;75:1575–83.
52. Bromley R, Weston J, Adab N, Greenhalgh J, Sanniti A, McKay AJ, et al. Treatment for epilepsy in pregnancy: neurodevelopmental outcomes in the child. Cochrane Database Syst Rev. 2014:CD010236.
53. Huybrechts KF, Hernandez-Diaz S, Patorno E, Desai RJ, Mogun H, Dejene SZ, et al. Antipsychotic use in pregnancy and the risk for congenital malformations. JAMA Psychiatry. 2016;73:938–46.
54. Panchaud A, Hernandez-Diaz S, Freeman MP, Viguera AC, SC MD, Sosinsky AZ, et al. Use of atypical antipsychotics in pregnancy and maternal gestational diabetes. J Psychiatr Res. 2017;95:84–90.
55. Ban L, West J, Gibson JE, Fiaschi L, Sokal R, Doyle P, et al. First trimester exposure to anxiolytic and hypnotic drugs and the risks of major congenital anomalies: a United Kingdom population-based cohort study. PLoS One. 2014;9:e100996.
56. Freeman MP, Goez-Mogollon L, McInerney KA, Davies AC, Church TR, Sosinsky AZ, et al. Obstetrical and neonatal outcomes after benzodiazepine exposure during pregnancy: results from a prospective registry of women with psychiatric disorders. Gen Hosp Psychiatry. 2018;53:73–9.
57. Sidhu J, Job S, Singh S, Philipson R. The pharmacokinetic and pharmacodynamic consequences of the co-administration of lamotrigine and a combined oral contraceptive in healthy female subjects. Br J Clin Pharmacol. 2006;61:191–9.
58. Winner B, Peipert JF, Zhao Q, Buckel C, Madden T, Allsworth JE, et al. Effectiveness of long-acting reversible contraception. N Engl J Med. 2012;366:1998–2007.
59. Sharma V. Management of bipolar II disorder during pregnancy and the postpartum period--Motherisk Update 2008. Can J Clin Pharmacol. 2009;16:e33–41.
60. Kennedy D, Koren G. Valproic acid use in psychiatry: issues in treating women of reproductive age. J Psychiatry Neurosci. 1998;23:223–8.
61. Patel N, Viguera AC, Baldessarini RJ. Mood-stabilizing anticonvulsants, spina bifida, and folate supplementation: commentary. J Clin Psychopharmacol. 2018;38:7–10.
62. Newport DJ, Viguera AC, Beach AJ, Ritchie JC, Cohen LS, Stowe ZN. Lithium placental passage and obstetrical outcome: implications for clinical management during late pregnancy. Am J Psychiatry. 2005;162:2162–70.
63. Rowe H, Baker T, Hale TW. Maternal medication, drug use, and breastfeeding. Child Adolesc Psychiatr Clin N Am. 2015;24:1–20.
64. Pacchiarotti I, Leon-Caballero J, Murru A, Verdolini N, Furio MA, Pancheri C, et al. Mood stabilizers and antipsychotics during breastfeeding: focus on bipolar disorder. Eur Neuropsychopharmacol. 2016;26:1562–78.
65. Uguz F, Sharma V. Mood stabilizers during breastfeeding: a systematic review of the recent literature. Bipolar Disord. 2016;18:325–33.
66. Galbally M, Bergink V, Vigod SN, Buist A, Boyce P, Chandra P, et al. Breastfeeding and lithium: is breast always best? Lancet Psychiatry. 2018;5:534–6.

Characteristics and Treatment of Bipolar Disorder in the Elderly

7

Eunsoo Moon and Jung goo Lee

Bipolar disorder is common in young people, but it can recur throughout life, making it a serious condition that requires clinical attention even in older age. On the other hand, there may be cases where there is no significant mood disorder in youth, but bipolar disorder develops in old age. Considering various clinical situations, bipolar disorder in elderly can be classified into several clinical subtypes (see Table 7.1) [1, 2]. There may be cases where bipolar disorder has gone into remission but treatment continues into old age to prevent recurrence. Some individuals receive an initial diagnosis of bipolar disorder in early adulthood and continue to experience recurrent manic or depressive episodes throughout later life. There is also a subset of patients with a longstanding history of major depressive disorder who subsequently develop mania/hypomania in late life, prompting a revised diagnosis of bipolar disorder. This progression may reflect the natural illness trajectory, wherein depressive episodes precede the emergence of mania or hypomania in older age. In some cases, the onset of manic or hypomanic symptoms may be precipitated by antidepressant treatment.

Bipolar disorder may also first emerge in older adulthood, without any prior history of mood episodes earlier in life. This is commonly referred to as *late-onset bipolar disorder*. While the term "late onset" suggests an onset in old age, it is often used more broadly to denote what is sometimes called *geriatric bipolar disorder* [1]. The distinction between *late-onset* and *early-onset* bipolar disorder is conceptually important, though the specific age cutoff used to define late onset varies across studies. Some define late-onset bipolar disorder as beginning at age 50 or older [3], while others use thresholds of 60 [4] or even 65 years [5]. Similarly, the definitions of "elderly," "geriatric," and "older adults" vary in the literature. Many studies consider individuals aged 60 and older to fall into these categories [6], while others use slightly younger age ranges (e.g., 50–55 years) to define "older adults" [6]. Despite these variations in terminology and classification, patients labeled as having elderly [7], geriatric [3], late life [6], late-life-onset [8], late-onset [1], older age [9], or older adults [10] bipolar disorder (see Table 7.2) generally exhibit similar clinical features. It is also important to note that the onset of manic or hypomanic symptoms in late life may occasionally be secondary to underlying physical illness, medication effects, substance use, or structural brain abnormalities. In such cases, the clinical presentation can differ significantly from that of primary late-life bipolar disorder.

E. Moon (✉)
Department of Psychiatry, Pusan National University School of Medicine, Yangsan, Republic of Korea
e-mail: esmun0124@pusan.ac.kr

J. g. Lee
Department of Psychiatry, Inje University Haeundae Paik Hospital, Busan, Republic of Korea

W.-M. Bahk et al. (eds.), *Bipolar Disorder*, https://doi.org/10.1007/978-981-92-1323-8_7

Table 7.1 Clinical subtypes of bipolar disorder in the elderly

Category	Description
A. Onset in youth (persistence into old age)	1. Mania onset in youth (a) Remission achieved and maintenance therapy continued into old age (b) Recurrent manic or depressive episodes persisting into old age 2. Depression onset in youth, later manic episode in old age – This pattern can occur spontaneously or may be triggered by antidepressant treatment
B. Onset in old age	1. Primary mania or hypomania developing in old age without any prior mood disorder 2. Secondary mania or hypomania developing in old age without any prior mood disorder, often related to medical or neurological causes 3. Mania in old age with an uncertain etiology (primary vs. secondary)

The clinical presentation of bipolar disorder in late life is, therefore, heterogeneous, encompassing both primary and secondary forms. Primary late-onset bipolar disorder refers to idiopathic cases in which manic or hypomanic episodes first appear in late adulthood, typically without evident medical, neurological, or pharmacological precipitating factors. These individuals generally exhibit minimal structural or metabolic abnormalities and are thought to represent a delayed expression of an intrinsic bipolar diathesis. In contrast, secondary mania arises in association with identifiable organic causes, such as cerebrovascular disease, endocrine or metabolic dysregulation, systemic medical illness, or exposure to specific pharmacologic agents. Distinguishing between these subtypes is essential for accurate diagnosis, elucidation of underlying pathophysiology, and formulation of individualized treatment strategies in late-life populations.

Prevalence and Incidence of Bipolar Disorder in Late Life

Compared to younger adults, the prevalence of bipolar disorder in late life is considerably lower. Epidemiological studies in community samples estimate the point prevalence of late-life bipolar disorder to range from 0.1 to 0.5%, with lifetime prevalence estimates between 0.5 and 1% [3]. According to the National Institute of Mental Health Epidemiologic Catchment Area (NIMH ECA) study, the 12-month prevalence of bipolar disorder was 1.4% among individuals aged 18–44, but only 0.1% in those aged 65 and older [11]. Similarly, a study utilizing a mood disorder questionnaire reported a point prevalence of 9.3% in individuals aged 18–24, compared to just 0.5% in those over 65 [12]. Collectively, these data demonstrate a clear declining trend in both point and lifetime prevalence with increasing age. Findings from the United States National Comorbidity Survey further corroborate this trend, showing a combined lifetime prevalence of bipolar I and II disorders at 5.9% in those aged 18–29, decreasing to 1% in individuals aged 60 or older [13].

Several hypotheses have been proposed to explain this age-related decline in prevalence [3, 10, 13]. One possibility is that bipolar disorder most commonly manifests earlier in life, rendering late-onset cases relatively rare. Another explanation is that early-onset bipolar disorder is associated with an elevated risk of suicide, which may reduce the number of affected individuals surviving into old age. A third consideration is that mood symptoms in older adults may often be attributed to general medical conditions or substance use and thus may not be classified as bipolar disorder in epidemiological surveys.

Despite its low prevalence in the general population, bipolar disorder is not uncommon among older adults receiving psychiatric care. Studies indicate that 4–8% of geriatric psychiatric inpatients carry a diagnosis of bipolar disorder [14], and approximately 17% of older adults presenting to psychiatric emergency services meet criteria for the disorder [15]. Furthermore, an

Table 7.2 Similar terms of bipolar disorder in elderly

Elderly bipolar disorder
Geriatric bipolar disorder
Late-life bipolar disorder
Late-life-onset bipolar disorder
Late-onset bipolar illness
Older age bipolar disorder

estimated 20–25% of patients receiving treatment for bipolar disorder are aged 60 or older [16]. Notably, this proportion appears to be increasing over time [5].

Several factors may account for this trend [5, 14–16]. First, the proportion of older adults within the general population is growing, naturally resulting in a higher number of older patients receiving treatment. Second, increased life expectancy has extended the period during which treatment can be accessed. Third, reduced stigma and improved public awareness of mental health issues have likely increased the willingness of older adults with bipolar disorder to seek psychiatric care. Finally, manic episodes in late life often necessitate specialized psychiatric treatment, in contrast to certain other psychiatric conditions in the elderly that may be managed outside of psychiatric settings.

Diagnostic Features of Bipolar Disorder in Late Life

The diagnostic criteria for bipolar disorder in late life are fundamentally consistent with those applied to adults in other age groups. According to the *Diagnostic and Statistical Manual of Mental Disorders, Fifth Edition, Text Revision* (DSM-5-TR), bipolar and related disorders encompass several categories, including bipolar I disorder, bipolar II disorder, cyclothymic disorder, substance/medication-induced bipolar and related disorder, bipolar and related disorder due to another medical condition, other specified bipolar and related disorder, and unspecified bipolar and related disorder. To capture the heterogeneity of bipolar presentations more comprehensively, the concept of a bipolar spectrum has been proposed. Akiskal and Pinto [17] introduced a classification model encompassing up to nine bipolar subtypes. Notably, bipolar disorder type III describes patients initially diagnosed with depression who subsequently develop hypomanic or manic symptoms following antidepressant treatment, electroconvulsive therapy (ECT), or medical interventions [17]. Bipolar disorder type III½ refers to mood disturbances induced by substance or alcohol use [17]. Furthermore, some researchers have suggested a subtype termed bipolar disorder type VI to characterize cases in which bipolar symptoms in late life may represent early manifestations of dementia, highlighting a potential continuum between affective and cognitive disorders [1].

Table 7.3 Medical causes of secondary mania

Category	Examples
Physical illness	Autoimmune hypothyroidism, autoimmune thrombocytopenia, Cushing syndrome, dialysis, hyperthyroidism, hypercalcemia, hyponatremia, influenza, pancreatic cancer, papillary thyroid carcinoma, postoperative state, systemic infection, uremia, vitamin B12 deficiency
Brain disease	Brain hemorrhage, brain tumor, cerebral infarction, Creutzfeldt-Jakob disease, cryptococcus meningitis, dementia (Alzheimer's dementia, frontotemporal dementia, vascular dementia), epilepsy, Huntington's disease, multiple sclerosis, neurosyphilis, pituitary adenoma, traumatic brain injury, viral encephalitis

Older adults with bipolar disorder frequently present with comorbid physical and neurological conditions and are often prescribed multiple medications. Consequently, this population has a higher likelihood than younger patients of meeting criteria for substance/medication-induced bipolar disorder or bipolar disorder due to another medical condition. Differentiating primary from secondary bipolar symptoms can be challenging, and ambiguous cases with insufficient information to make an accurate diagnosis may be classified as unspecified bipolar and related disorder. Therefore, clinicians evaluating older adults with new-onset mania or bipolar symptoms must conduct thorough assessments to exclude secondary causes (see Tables 7.3 and 7.4) [2, 18–24].

Table 7.4 Pharmacological causes of secondary mania

Category	Examples
Substance	Alcohol, amphetamine, cocaine, hallucinogens, opiate, phencyclidine (PCP)
Medication	Anticholilnergics, antidepressants, baclofen, benzodiazepines, bromocriptine, captopril, carbotaxel, cimetidine, cisplatin, corticosteroids, cyclosporin, docetaxel, fentanyl, hydralazine, isoniazid, levodopa, methylphenidate, metrizamide, procarbazine, procyclidine, rivastigmine, yohimbine

The risk of medical comorbidities, polypharmacy, and cerebrovascular disease increases with advancing age, all of which can contribute substantially to the development of bipolar-like syndromes. Importantly, even in individuals with minimal genetic vulnerability, structural brain damage—such as that caused by stroke or trauma in regions critical to mood regulation—may precipitate the emergence of bipolar symptoms in late life.

Clinical Features of Late-Onset Mania

Mania with onset in late life presents with several clinical and etiological distinctions compared to early-onset cases. One of the most notable differences is the relatively weaker association with genetic predisposition [18]. Early-onset bipolar disorder is generally more strongly influenced by hereditary factors, whereas late-onset cases are more frequently linked to physical, environmental, or external contributors [14, 25, 26]. Nevertheless, even among individuals with late-onset mania, the likelihood of an underlying genetic vulnerability remains higher than in age-matched elderly individuals without psychiatric disorders [18]. In other words, while the genetic influence is attenuated relative to early-onset cases, it is still notable when compared to the general older population.

Structural brain abnormalities are more commonly observed in older adults with mania. Neuroimaging studies comparing older patients with late-onset mania to healthy elderly controls have demonstrated significant reductions in both cortical and subcortical brain volumes [19–21]. Additionally, the presence of cerebrovascular disease and localized brain lesions has been more frequently reported in patients with late-onset mania [18].

Furthermore, older adults presenting with mania are more likely to have comorbid general medical conditions and to be taking medications that may contribute to the emergence of manic symptoms [18]. These findings underscore the importance of conducting a thorough medical and pharmacological evaluation when assessing mood dysregulation in geriatric populations.

Age- and Sex-Related Differences in Bipolar Disorder

As individuals with bipolar disorder age into later life, notable changes in symptom presentation are frequently observed [18, 27–31]. Compared to younger patients, older adults tend to exhibit less severe manic symptoms, although the duration of manic episodes may be somewhat prolonged. Euphoric mood becomes less common in late-life mania; instead, presentations are often characterized by irritability, mixed states, and pronounced anger or hostility. The typical expansiveness and elevated mood seen in younger bipolar patients is frequently replaced by more dysphoric and agitated presentations, and mood infectivity is generally reduced. Speech and cognitive features of mania also differ with age. Older adults are less likely to exhibit pressured speech in younger patients. Grandiose delusions occur less frequently, while mood-incongruent paranoid delusions are more commonly reported. Thought content tends to include fewer religious themes, with derailment and tangentiality being more prominent. Psychomotor activity, energy levels, and sexual interest are typically diminished in older manic patients. Psychomotor retardation is frequently observed, contrasting with the hyperactivity and goal-directed behavior often seen in younger individuals. Taken together, these findings suggest that the classical manic features—euphoria, hyperactivity, pressured speech, and grandiosity—are attenuated in late life.

Depressive symptoms in older adults with bipolar disorder also tend to be milder compared to those in younger populations, and suicidal ideation may occur less frequently [30]. However, symptom severity does not necessarily decline linearly with age [31]. There was no significant difference in daily function between patients with late-onset bipolar disorder compared with those with early-onset [32]. Cognitive impairment, delirium, and disorientation are more commonly observed in older adults with bipolar disorder, and insight is often reduced likely due to age-related neurobiological decline. Moreover, older patients are more likely to have coexisting medical conditions, such as cardiovascular or musculoskeletal diseases, underscoring the need for integrated medical and psychiatric care [30, 32].

Sex differences in the clinical presentation of elderly bipolar disorder are also well-documented [32, 33]. Female patients tend to experience an earlier age of onset compared to male patients and are more likely to present with anxiety symptoms, somatic preoccupations, and more severe mood disturbances. They also exhibit higher rates of psychiatric hospitalization. In contrast, male patients are more likely to have a lifetime history of comorbid substance use disorders. These findings underscore the need for individualized, age- and sex-sensitive approaches to the diagnosis and management of bipolar disorder in elderly.

Cognitive Function in Late-Life Bipolar Disorder

Cognitive impairment is commonly observed in older adults with bipolar disorder [34], and several factors may contribute to this decline. One possibility is that some individuals exhibit cognitive deterioration prior to the onset of bipolar symptoms in later life [1]. Given the age-related increase in the risk of Alzheimer's disease, it is plausible that older adults presenting with mania may already be in a prodromal phase of neurodegeneration. In cases where mania is associated with cerebrovascular pathology or other structural brain abnormalities, cognitive deficits may precede the onset of affective symptoms.

Second, mania itself may contribute to cognitive decline. Manic episodes are linked to elevated dopamine and glutamate activity, which can induce excitotoxicity and neuronal apoptosis. These neurotoxic effects may be especially detrimental in older adults, whose brain reserve capacity is diminished due to age-related neuronal loss. Even in the absence of overt dementia, mania-induced neurobiological changes may be sufficient to impair cognitive function. Additionally, bipolar disorder has been associated with mitochondrial and endoplasmic reticulum dysfunction, as well as dysregulation of apoptosis—all of which may exacerbate neurodegenerative processes [35, 36].

Third, depressive episodes are also implicated in cognitive dysfunction. Repeated depressive episodes in late-life bipolar disorder have been associated with impairments in memory and executive functioning, which may be present during both acute phases and residual periods. Persisting subthreshold symptoms, sleep disturbances, and neuroinflammatory mechanisms may further contribute to long-term cognitive decline [37, 38]. Chronic stress and elevated cortisol levels associated with recurrent mood episodes may also damage the hippocampus, a region critical for memory processing [39]. Given these risks, comprehensive cognitive assessments should be an integral component of the evaluation and management of bipolar disorder in older adults.

Does Late-Life Bipolar Disorder Increase the Risk of Dementia?

The relationship between late-life bipolar disorder and dementia has emerged as a significant focus of clinical research, with three key areas drawing particular attention. First, a major concern is whether recurrent mood episodes—particularly manic and depressive relapses—may contribute to long-term cognitive decline and increase the risk of dementia. Longitudinal studies suggest this may be the case. For example, in one five- to seven-year follow-up study, approximately 32% of older adults with a history of manic episodes scored below 24 on the Mini-Mental State Examination (MMSE), indicating clinically significant cognitive impairment [40]. Similarly, the prevalence of dementia among older individuals with bipolar disorder has been reported at 19%, compared to just 6% in age-matched controls [41]. A meta-analysis further supports this association, reporting an odds ratio of 2.96 for the development of dementia in this population [42]. Some comparative studies of bipolar disorder and late-life depression have yielded mixed results [42–46].

The second area of inquiry concerns the potential influence of pharmacologic treatment on dementia risk. Although a Danish study reported a higher prevalence of dementia among individuals who had ever used lithium, those receiving long-term lithium therapy exhibited a reduced risk [47]. While subsequent research has produced mixed findings [41, 48], more recent data suggest that sustained lithium use may exert a protective effect against cognitive decline in patients with bipolar disorder [42, 49]. In contrast, other mood stabilizers—such as anticonvulsants, antidepressants, and antipsychotics—have not demonstrated similar neuroprotective effects [49]. Taken together, these findings indicate that the elevated risk of dementia in older adults with bipolar disorder is more likely attributable to the underlying illness itself rather than its pharmacologic treatment. Notably, lithium appears to be an exception, with evidence pointing toward its potential role in mitigating this risk.

A third area of interest involves the hypothesis that late-onset bipolar disorder may, in some cases, represent an early manifestation of a neurodegenerative process. As dementia progresses, patients may develop behavioral and mood disturbances that mimic bipolar symptoms, complicating diagnostic clarity. Although this hypothesis has important clinical implications, current pathophysiological evidence remains limited and inconsistent, and no definitive causal link has been established [34, 50, 51].

Pharmacological Treatment in Late-Life Bipolar Disorder

The overall pharmacological approach to treating late-life bipolar disorder does not differ substantially from that used in younger adults [44, 47, 48]. However, several studies have noted important differences in prescription patterns and treatment responses among older patients. Interestingly, the number of medications prescribed to older adults with bipolar disorder is generally similar to that in younger individuals. Nevertheless, the dosages are typically lower in the elderly, particularly for agents such as lithium, valproate, and risperidone.

Among these medications, valproate appears to be the most commonly prescribed in older adults, whereas lithium is used less frequently. Despite its lower rate of use, lithium has shown surprisingly favorable outcomes in this population. In one study, the remission rate with lithium monotherapy in older adults was 42.1%—nearly double the 21.3% observed in younger patients. These findings suggest that, when appropriately dosed and carefully monitored, lithium can be a highly effective treatment option even in the geriatric population.

Considerations for Treating Bipolar Disorder in Late Life

When treating older adults with bipolar disorder, several age-specific factors must be carefully considered, particularly comorbid medical conditions, altered pharmacokinetics, and increased brain vulnerability. Older patients often present with multiple medical comorbidities and are more likely to be on polypharmacy regimens. Therefore, a thorough evaluation of both comorbid conditions and current medications is essential to prevent adverse drug interactions and minimize iatrogenic complications.

For example, lithium may interact with angiotensin-converting enzyme (ACE) inhibitors, calcium channel blockers, thiazide and loop diuretics, and nonsteroidal anti-inflammatory drugs (NSAIDs)—all of which can elevate serum lithium levels [52]. Valproate, in contrast, can increase its free (active) concentration when co-administered with agents such as aspirin, warfarin, digoxin, or phenytoin, necessitating careful dose adjustments [53].

Pharmacokinetic changes associated with aging also warrant careful consideration. In older adults, renal clearance is reduced by approximately 50% compared to younger individuals, and the glomerular filtration rate (GFR) also declines [54]. Consequently, the half-life of lithium may be prolonged to 28–36 h in the elderly, making it advisable to initiate treatment at approximately half the standard adult dose.

Age-related decreases in muscle mass and total body water, along with increased body fat, further reduce the volume of distribution for hydrophilic drugs such as lithium, resulting in higher serum concentrations [55]. Additionally, serum albumin levels tend to decrease with age, which may increase the free (active) fraction of protein-bound medications like valproate [3]. Since valproate also inhibits hepatic enzyme activity, caution is warranted in patients with compromised liver function.

Another important consideration is the increased prevalence of structural brain abnormalities in older adults with bipolar disorder. In such cases, valproate may be preferred over lithium due to its more favorable tolerability in the presence of cerebrovascular pathology [56, 57]. Moreover, older patients are more susceptible to extrapyramidal symptoms (EPS), even when treated with atypical antipsychotics, which are generally associated with a lower risk of EPS [58]. Management of EPS in the elderly requires particular caution, as reduced brain reserve increases vulnerability to adverse effects. The use of anticholinergic agents or benzodiazepines in this population may precipitate delirium or exacerbate cognitive impairment. Additionally, atypical antipsychotics are linked to increased metabolic risks, including weight gain, dyslipidemia, and glucose dysregulation. Given the high prevalence of cerebrovascular disease among older adults with bipolar disorder, such metabolic side effects may be especially significant and could potentially aggravate preexisting medical conditions [59].

Treatment Course and Outcomes in Late-Life Bipolar Disorder

Overall, treatment outcomes for late-life bipolar disorder are relatively favorable and, in some respects, may even surpass those observed in younger populations. For instance, older adults tend to experience less manic exhaustion than younger patients [18]. In the STEP-BD (Systematic Treatment Enhancement Program for Bipolar Disorder) study, 66.8% of adult patients with bipolar disorder achieved recovery, whereas the recovery rate was even higher among older patients, at 78.5% [60]. Similarly, a six-year longitudinal study found that approximately 72% of elderly patients with bipolar disorder were able to maintain independent living without experiencing significant symptoms [40].

However, when compared specifically to older adults with unipolar depression, those with bipolar disorder—particularly individuals who experience manic episodes—tend to have a less favorable clinical course. Treatment response in geriatric mania is often poorer than in late-life depression, with some studies reporting recovery rates as low as 16% [61, 62]. Most patients do not achieve full remission but instead exhibit only partial symptom improvement. Additionally, cognitive impairment is more frequently observed in older adults with bipolar disorder than in those with unipolar depression [63]. The prevalence of general medical conditions, including cerebrovascular disease, is also higher in this population and contributes to increased mortality risk [18, 28, 40, 64]. Reported mortality rates among older adults with mania range from 11–16% over a two-year follow-up period, and up to 34% over five to seven years. These findings underscore the importance of managing medical comorbidities and ensuring careful monitoring throughout the course of treatment.

Conclusion

Although the prevalence and incidence of bipolar disorder in late life are lower than in younger populations, a relatively high proportion of older adults with bipolar disorder still receive psychiatric treatment. The diagnostic criteria for late-life bipolar disorder remain consistent with those for younger individuals; however, age-related factors increase the likelihood of diagnoses such as substance- or medication-induced bipolar disorder, or bipolar disorder secondary to a general medical condition. In some cases, individuals with a family history or genetic predisposition for bipolar disorder may initially present with depressive symptoms and later develop hypomania or mania—often triggered by antidepressant treatment—necessitating a re-evaluation of the initial diagnosis. Additionally, early manifestations of dementia can mimic bipolar symptoms, underscoring the importance of differential diagnosis in geriatric populations. Identifying secondary causes of bipolar-like symptoms is crucial for accurate diagnosis and appropriate management.

Compared to early-onset bipolar disorder, late-life presentations tend to involve milder, atypical symptom profiles, with cognitive impairment more frequently observed by age-related neurobiological changes. Sex differences further contribute to clinical heterogeneity: female patients are more likely to experience anxiety, somatic complaints, and severe mood symptoms, with higher rates of hospitalization, whereas male patients show a higher lifetime prevalence of comorbid substance use disorders.

The potential association between late-life bipolar disorder and dementia has garnered increasing attention. Recurrent mood episodes may accelerate cognitive decline and heighten the risk of dementia, particularly in individuals with diminished brain reserve. Notably, long-term lithium treatment appears to mitigate this risk, while other psychotropic medications have not shown comparable protective effects. Some researchers posit that, in certain cases, late-onset bipolar disorder may represent an early clinical manifestation of neurodegenerative disease.

Pharmacological treatment strategies for late-life bipolar disorder generally parallel those used in younger adults but require careful consideration of age-related changes in drug metabolism, medical comorbidities, and heightened sensitivity to side effects. Dose adjustments and close monitoring are especially important when prescribing lithium, valproate, or antipsychotics. Although treatment outcomes are generally favorable, they are often less robust than those seen in late-life depression. Furthermore, comorbid medical conditions are associated with increased mortality, highlighting the importance of an integrated treatment model. Accordingly, the management of bipolar disorder in the elderly should involve a multidisciplinary approach that brings together psychiatrists, neurologists, geriatricians, and caregivers to address the complex interplay of psychiatric, neurological, and medical factors that influence treatment outcomes.

While pharmacotherapy remains the cornerstone of management, individualized psychosocial interventions play a complementary and often decisive role in promoting recovery and preventing relapse. Such approaches include psychoeducation to enhance illness insight and medication adherence, sleep hygiene programs to stabilize circadian rhythms, and cognitive rehabilitation to mitigate neurocognitive deficits frequently observed in this population. A coordinated model of care—integrating medical optimization, psychosocial support, and caregiver education—offers the best prospect for maintaining functional independence and improving quality of life in elderly patients with bipolar disorder.

Declarations

Competing Interests The author(s) has no competing interests to declare that are relevant to the content of this manuscript.

Ethics Approval The author(s) declares that this manuscript does not include primary research with human participants.

The author(s) declares that this manuscript does not include primary studies involving animals.

References

1. Azorin JM, Kaladjian A, Adida M, Fakra E. Late-onset bipolar illness: the geriatric bipolar type VI. CNS Neurosci Ther. 2012;18(3):208–13. https://doi.org/10.1111/j.1755-5949.2011.00255.x.
2. Sami M, Khan H, Nilforooshan R. Late onset mania as an organic syndrome: a review of case reports in the literature. J Affect Disord. 2015;188:226–31. https://doi.org/10.1016/j.jad.2015.08.027.
3. Sajatovic M, Chen P. Geriatric bipolar disorder. Psychiatr Clin North Am. 2011;34(2):319–33, vii. https://doi.org/10.1016/j.psc.2011.02.007.
4. Chen ST, Altshuler LL, Spar JE. Bipolar disorder in late life: a review. J Geriatr Psychiatry Neurol. 1998;11(1):29–35. https://doi.org/10.1177/089198879801100107.
5. Almeida OP, Fenner S. Bipolar disorder: similarities and differences between patients with illness onset before and after 65 years of age. Int Psychogeriatr. 2002;14(3):311–22.
6. Aziz R, Lorberg B, Tampi RR. Treatments for late-life bipolar disorder. Am J Geriatr Pharmacother. 2006;4(4):347–64. https://doi.org/10.1016/j.amjopharm.2006.12.007.
7. Shobassy A. Elderly bipolar disorder. Curr Psychiatry Rep. 2021;23(2):5. https://doi.org/10.1007/s11920-020-01216-6.
8. Banga A, Gyurmey T, Matuskey D, Connor DF, Kaplan RF, Steffens DC. Late-life onset bipolar disorder presenting as a case of pseudo-dementia: a case discussion and review of literature. Yale J Biol Med. 2013;86(2):235–44.
9. Elefante C, Brancati GE, Beatino MF, Nerli BF, D'Alessandro G, Fustini C, et al. Clinical predictors of cognitive impairment in a cohort of patients with older age bipolar disorder. Brain Sci. 2025;15(4). https://doi.org/10.3390/brainsci15040349.
10. Depp CA, Jeste DV. Bipolar disorder in older adults: a critical review. Bipolar Disord. 2004;6(5):343–67. https://doi.org/10.1111/j.1399-5618.2004.00139.x.
11. Weissman MM, Leaf PJ, Tischler GL, Blazer DG, Karno M, Bruce ML, et al. Affective disorders in five United States communities. Psychol Med. 1988;18(1):141–53.
12. Hirschfeld RM, Calabrese JR, Weissman MM, Reed M, Davies MA, Frye MA, et al. Screening for bipolar disorder in the community. J Clin Psychiatry. 2003;64(1):53–9.
13. Kessler RC, Berglund P, Demler O, Jin R, Merikangas KR, Walters EE. Lifetime prevalence and age-of-onset distributions of DSM-IV disorders in the National Comorbidity Survey Replication. Arch Gen Psychiatry. 2005;62(6):593–602. https://doi.org/10.1001/archpsyc.62.6.593.
14. Yassa R, Nair V, Nastase C, Camille Y, Belzile L. Prevalence of bipolar disorder in a psychogeriatric population. J Affect Disord. 1988; 14(3):197–201.
15. Depp CA, Lindamer LA, Folsom DP, Gilmer T, Hough RL, Garcia P, et al. Differences in clinical features and mental health service use in bipolar disorder across the lifespan. Am J Geriatr Psychiatry. 2005;13(4):290–8. https://doi.org/10.1176/appi.ajgp.13.4.290.
16. Rasanen P, Tiihonen J, Hakko H. The incidence and onset-age of hospitalized bipolar affective disorder in Finland. J Affect Disord. 1998;48(1):63–8.
17. Akiskal HS, Pinto O. The evolving bipolar spectrum. Prototypes I, II, III, and IV. Psychiatr Clin North Am. 1999;22(3):517–34, vii. https://doi.org/10.1016/s0193-953x(05)70093-9.
18. Young RC. Bipolar mood disorders in the elderly. Psychiatr Clin North Am. 1997;20(1):121–36.
19. Besga A, Martinez-Cengotitabengoa M, Gonzalez-Ortega I, Gutierrez M, Barbeito S, Gonzalez-Pinto A. The role of white matter damage in late onset bipolar disorder. Maturitas. 2011;70(2):160–3. https://doi.org/10.1016/j.maturitas.2011.07.005.
20. de Asis JM, Greenwald BS, Alexopoulos GS, Kiosses DN, Ashtari M, Heo M, et al. Frontal signal hyperintensities in mania in old age. Am J Geriatr Psychiatry. 2006;14(7):598–604. https://doi.org/10.1097/01.JGP.0000200603.70504.d5.
21. Zanetti MV, Cordeiro Q, Busatto GF. Late onset bipolar disorder associated with white matter hyperintensities: a pathophysiological hypothesis. Prog Neuro-Psychopharmacol Biol Psychiatry. 2007;31(2):551–6. https://doi.org/10.1016/j.pnpbp.2006.10.004.
22. Satzer D, Bond DJ. Mania secondary to focal brain lesions: implications for understanding the functional neuroanatomy of bipolar disorder. Bipolar Disord. 2016;18(3):205–20. https://doi.org/10.1111/bdi.12387.
23. Fidan YS, Arman IH, Calli SY, Domac FM, Yeniceri EN, Tasdelen B, et al. Revisiting late-onset bipolar disorder associated with pituitary adenoma: a cross-sectional, multidisciplinary, case-based analysis. Brain Behav. 2025;15(6):e70611. https://doi.org/10.1002/brb3.70611.
24. Mittal T, Jalaja Haridas N. Late-onset bipolar disorder preceding the diagnosis of papillary thyroid carcinoma. Prim Care Companion CNS Disord. 2025;27(4). https://doi.org/10.4088/PCC.25cr03936.
25. Alexopoulos GS, Lieberman KW, Young RC, Shamoian CA. Platelet MAO activity and age at onset of depression in elderly depressed women. Am J Psychiatry. 1984;141(10):1276–8. https://doi.org/10.1176/ajp.141.10.1276.
26. Montejo L, Sole B, Fico G, Kalman JL, Budde M, Heilbronner U, et al. Contrasting genetic burden for bipolar disorder: early onset versus late onset in an older adult bipolar disorder sample. Eur Neuropsychopharmacol. 2025;92:29–37. https://doi.org/10.1016/j.euroneuro.2024.12.001.
27. Young RC, Schreiber MT, Nysewander RW. Psychotic mania. Biol Psychiatry. 1983;18(10):1167–73.
28. Stone K. Mania in the elderly. Br J Psychiatry. 1989;155:220–4.

29. Young RC, Kiosses D, Heo M, Schulberg HC, Murphy C, Klimstra S, et al. Age and ratings of manic psychopathology. Bipolar Disord. 2007;9(3):301–4. https://doi.org/10.1111/j.1399-5618.2007.00393.x.
30. Chen P, Sajatovic M, Briggs FBS, Mulsant B, Dols AA, Gildengers A, et al. Sociodemographic and clinical characteristics of people with oldest older age bipolar disorder in a global sample: results from the global aging and geriatric experiments in bipolar disorder project. Int J Geriatr Psychiatry. 2024;39(2):e6073. https://doi.org/10.1002/gps.6073.
31. Sajatovic M, Rej S, Almeida OP, Altinbas K, Balanza-Martinez V, Barbosa IG, et al. Bipolar symptoms, somatic burden and functioning in older-age bipolar disorder: a replication study from the global aging & geriatric experiments in bipolar disorder database (GAGE-BD) project. Int J Geriatr Psychiatry. 2024;39(3):e6057. https://doi.org/10.1002/gps.6057.
32. Orhan M, Montejo L, Sajatovic M, Eyler L, Dols A. Global Aging & Geriatric Experiments in Bipolar Disorder (GAGE-BD): building a global consortium benefiting people with bipolar disorder in later life. Curr Psychiatry Rep. 2025;27(5):231–8. https://doi.org/10.1007/s11920-025-01593-w.
33. Blanken M, Oudega ML, Almeida OP, Schouws S, Orhan M, Beunders AJM, et al. Sex differences among older adults with bipolar disorder: results from the Global Aging & Geriatric Experiments in Bipolar Disorder (GAGE-BD) project. Am J Geriatr Psychiatry. 2024;32(3):326–38. https://doi.org/10.1016/j.jagp.2023.10.008.
34. Klaus F, Ng HX, Barbosa IG, Beunders A, Briggs F, Burdick KE, et al. Cognition in older age bipolar disorder: an analysis of archival data across the globe. J Affect Disord. 2024;355:231–8. https://doi.org/10.1016/j.jad.2024.03.126.
35. Scaini G, Fries GR, Valvassori SS, Zeni CP, Zunta-Soares G, Berk M, et al. Perturbations in the apoptotic pathway and mitochondrial network dynamics in peripheral blood mononuclear cells from bipolar disorder patients. Transl Psychiatry. 2017;7(5):e1111. https://doi.org/10.1038/tp.2017.83.
36. Kim Y, Santos R, Gage FH, Marchetto MC. Molecular mechanisms of bipolar disorder: progress made and future challenges. Front Cell Neurosci. 2017;11:30. https://doi.org/10.3389/fncel.2017.00030.
37. Depp CA, Dev S, Eyler LT. Bipolar depression and cognitive impairment: shared mechanisms and new treatment avenues. Psychiatr Clin North Am. 2016;39(1):95–109. https://doi.org/10.1016/j.psc.2015.09.004.
38. Samalin L, Boyer L, Murru A, Pacchiarotti I, Reinares M, Bonnin CM, et al. Residual depressive symptoms, sleep disturbance and perceived cognitive impairment as determinants of functioning in patients with bipolar disorder. J Affect Disord. 2017;210:280–6. https://doi.org/10.1016/j.jad.2016.12.054.
39. Altshuler LL. Bipolar disorder: are repeated episodes associated with neuroanatomic and cognitive changes? Biol Psychiatry. 1993;33(8–9):563–5. https://doi.org/10.1016/0006-3223(93)90093-s.
40. Dhingra U, Rabins PV. Mania in the elderly: a 5-7 year follow-up. J Am Geriatr Soc. 1991;39(6):581–3.
41. Nunes PV, Forlenza OV, Gattaz WF. Lithium and risk for Alzheimer's disease in elderly patients with bipolar disorder. Br J Psychiatry. 2007;190:359–60. https://doi.org/10.1192/bjp.bp.106.029868.
42. Velosa J, Delgado A, Finger E, Berk M, Kapczinski F, de Azevedo CT. Risk of dementia in bipolar disorder and the interplay of lithium: a systematic review and meta-analyses. Acta Psychiatr Scand. 2020;141(6):510–21. https://doi.org/10.1111/acps.13153.
43. Kessing LV, Andersen PK. Does the risk of developing dementia increase with the number of episodes in patients with depressive disorder and in patients with bipolar disorder? J Neurol Neurosurg Psychiatry. 2004;75(12):1662–6. https://doi.org/10.1136/jnnp.2003.031773.
44. Chen MH, Li CT, Tsai CF, Lin WC, Chang WH, Chen TJ, et al. Risk of subsequent dementia among patients with bipolar disorder or major depression: a nationwide longitudinal study in Taiwan. J Am Med Dir Assoc. 2015;16(6):504–8. https://doi.org/10.1016/j.jamda.2015.01.084.
45. Nielsen JL, Kaltoft K, Wium-Andersen IK, Wium-Andersen MK, Osler M. Association of early- and late-life bipolar disorder with incident dementia. A Danish cohort study. J Affect Disord. 2024;367:367–73. https://doi.org/10.1016/j.jad.2024.09.015.
46. Alexander L, Beck K, Bocharova M, Young AH, Stewart R, Carter R, et al. Late-life affective disorders and risk of progression to dementia: retrospective cohort study of patients in secondary care. Br J Psychiatry. 2025:1–7. https://doi.org/10.1192/bjp.2025.45.
47. Kessing LV, Sondergard L, Forman JL, Andersen PK. Lithium treatment and risk of dementia. Arch Gen Psychiatry. 2008;65(11):1331–5. https://doi.org/10.1001/archpsyc.65.11.1331.
48. Dunn N, Holmes C, Mullee M. Does lithium therapy protect against the onset of dementia? Alzheimer Dis Assoc Disord. 2005;19(1):20–2.
49. Kessing LV, Forman JL, Andersen PK. Does lithium protect against dementia? Bipolar Disord. 2010;12(1):87–94. https://doi.org/10.1111/j.1399-5618.2009.00788.x.
50. Chang WH, Su CC, Chen KC, Hsiao YY, Chen PS, Yang YK. Which severe mental illnesses most increase the risk of developing dementia? Comparing the risk of dementia in patients with schizophrenia, major depressive disorder and bipolar disorder. Clin Psychopharmacol Neurosci. 2023;21(3):478–87. https://doi.org/10.9758/cpn.22.991.
51. Chancel R, Lopez-Castroman J, Baca-Garcia E, Mateos Alvarez R, Courtet P, Conejero I. Biomarkers of bipolar disorder in late life: an evidence-based systematic review.

Curr Psychiatry Rep. 2024;26(3):78–103. https://doi.org/10.1007/s11920-024-01483-7.
52. Eastham JH, Jeste DV, Young RC. Assessment and treatment of bipolar disorder in the elderly. Drugs Aging. 1998;12(3):205–24.
53. Sajatovic M. Treatment of bipolar disorder in older adults. Int J Geriatr Psychiatry. 2002;17(9):865–73. https://doi.org/10.1002/gps.719.
54. Shulman KI, Mackenzie S, Hardy B. The clinical use of lithium carbonate in old age: a review. Prog Neuro-Psychopharmacol Biol Psychiatry. 1987;11(2–3):159–64.
55. Sproule BA, Hardy BG, Shulman KI. Differential pharmacokinetics of lithium in elderly patients. Drugs Aging. 2000;16(3):165–77.
56. Mazure CM, Druss BG, Cellar JS. Valproate treatment of older psychotic patients with organic mental syndromes and behavioral dyscontrol. J Am Geriatr Soc. 1992;40(9):914–6.
57. Lott AD, McElroy SL, Keys MA. Valproate in the treatment of behavioral agitation in elderly patients with dementia. J Neuropsychiatry Clin Neurosci. 1995;7(3):314–9. https://doi.org/10.1176/jnp.7.3.314.
58. Crystal S, Olfson M, Huang C, Pincus H, Gerhard T. Broadened use of atypical antipsychotics: safety, effectiveness, and policy challenges. Health Aff (Millwood). 2009;28(5):w770–81. https://doi.org/10.1377/hlthaff.28.5.w770.
59. Schneider LS, Dagerman K, Insel PS. Efficacy and adverse effects of atypical antipsychotics for dementia: meta-analysis of randomized, placebo-controlled trials. Am J Geriatr Psychiatry. 2006;14(3):191–210. https://doi.org/10.1097/01.JGP.0000200589.01396.6d.
60. Al Jurdi RK, Marangell LB, Petersen NJ, Martinez M, Gyulai L, Sajatovic M. Prescription patterns of psychotropic medications in elderly compared with younger participants who achieved a "recovered" status in the systematic treatment enhancement program for bipolar disorder. Am J Geriatr Psychiatry. 2008;16(11):922–33. https://doi.org/10.1097/JGP.0b013e318187135f.
61. Angst J, Preisig M. Outcome of a clinical cohort of unipolar, bipolar and schizoaffective patients. Results of a prospective study from 1959 to 1985. Schweiz Arch Neurol Psychiatr (1985). 1995;146(1):17–23.
62. Gildengers AG, Mulsant BH, Begley AE, McShea M, Stack JA, Miller MD, et al. A pilot study of standardized treatment in geriatric bipolar disorder. Am J Geriatr Psychiatry. 2005;13(4):319–23. https://doi.org/10.1176/appi.ajgp.13.4.319.
63. Berrios GE, Bakshi N. Manic and depressive symptoms in the elderly: their relationships to treatment outcome, cognition and motor symptoms. Psychopathology. 1991;24(1):31–8. https://doi.org/10.1159/000284694.
64. Shulman KI, Tohen M, Satlin A, Mallya G, Kalunian D. Mania compared with unipolar depression in old age. Am J Psychiatry. 1992;149(3):341–5. https://doi.org/10.1176/ajp.149.3.341.

8 Child and Adolescent Bipolar Disorder

MoonSoo Lee and Se Hoon Shim

Introduction

Interest in bipolar disorder manifesting in childhood and adolescence has increased since the 1990s. One study reported that between 1994 and 2003, the rate of bipolar disorder diagnoses in youth outpatient visits in the United States increased approximately 40-fold [1]. Many clinicians now believe that bipolar disorder can indeed present in children and adolescents and that aside from developmental influences, it is essentially similar to the adult illness. There has been considerable debate, however, about the phenotype of bipolar disorder in younger children and early adolescents. Over the past few decades, some of these controversies have been partially resolved by research evidence, while others remain under discussion, similar to specific unresolved issues even in adult bipolar disorder, which will require future investigation. At this point, the concept of pediatric bipolar disorder has become more clearly established, and accordingly, the previously rising prevalence rates have now leveled off in epidemiological studies. Nevertheless, in terms of treatment, a strong evidence base from clinical trials is still lacking, underscoring the need for further research.

M. Lee (✉)
Department of Psychiatry, Korea University, College of Medicine, Seoul, Republic of Korea
e-mail: npboard@korea.ac.kr

S. H. Shim
Department of Psychiatry, Soonchunhyang University, College of Medicine, Cheonan, Republic of Korea

Epidemiology

Prevalence and incidence estimates of pediatric bipolar disorder vary widely across studies depending on methodological factors. In a 2011 meta-analysis, Van Meter and colleagues analyzed 12 studies (total $n = 16{,}222$) published between 1985 and 2007 examining bipolar disorder prevalence in individuals up to 21 years old. The pooled prevalence of bipolar spectrum disorder in youth was 1.8% [2]. About a decade later, the same group conducted an updated meta-analysis of epidemiological studies through 2019. During this interval, the diagnostic criteria evolved (notably with Diagnostic and Statistical Manual of Mental Disorder, fifth Edition [DSM-V] introducing disruptive mood dysregulation disorder, DMDD, as a new diagnosis that could affect bipolar diagnoses). In the updated analysis, there was significant heterogeneity among studies' prevalence estimates, but the pooled prevalence of pediatric bipolar spectrum disorder was 3.9%, with bipolar I specifically around 0.6% [3]. These findings suggest that the prevalence of pediatric bipolar disorder has not continued to increase and may have stabilized, likely reflecting more consistent diagnostic practices.

In clinical settings, bipolar disorder is less common in children and adolescents than disor-

W.-M. Bahk et al. (eds.), *Bipolar Disorder*, https://doi.org/10.1007/978-981-92-1323-8_8

ders such as depression [4] or attention-deficit/hyperactivity disorder (ADHD) [5]. Prevalence appears higher in post-pubertal adolescents than in pre-pubertal children [6].

Risk Factors

Relatively little is definitively known about risk factors for pediatric bipolar disorder, but research indicates a complex interplay of genetic, neurobiological, psychological, and environmental factors.

Genetic Factors

Bipolar disorder is one of the most heritable psychiatric illnesses, and earlier age of onset is associated with higher heritability. Heritability estimates for bipolar disorder exceed 80% in many studies [7]. Twin studies report concordance rates ranging from 60% to 90% in monozygotic twins (though results vary by study), which are among the highest concordance rates compared to other psychiatric conditions [8]. One landmark study addressing familial risk is the Pittsburgh Bipolar Offspring Study (BIOS). BIOS reported that when one biological parent has bipolar disorder, the offspring have about a 10.6% risk of developing bipolar disorder; if both parents have bipolar disorder, the risk rises to ~29%. In other words, having a biological parent with bipolar disorder was associated with a 14-fold increase in the odds of bipolar spectrum disorder in offspring. Moreover, over 75% of those offspring who developed bipolar disorder experienced their first mood episode before age 12. Among these youth, the most common initial diagnosis was bipolar disorder not otherwise specified (bipolar NOS), followed by major depressive disorder [9].

Neuroimaging Studies

Neuroimaging research in adolescents with bipolar disorder has identified several structural and functional brain abnormalities. Structural findings include reduced amygdala volumes, decreased gray matter in the orbitofrontal cortex (OFC) and anterior cingulate cortex (ACC), and abnormally reduced fractional anisotropy in white matter tracts connecting frontal lobe regions with subcortical areas [10]. Functional imaging studies (including meta-analyses) suggest that, unlike adults with bipolar disorder, youths with bipolar disorder exhibit hyperactivation in the amygdala, frontal lobes, and visual processing regions, along with hypoactivation in the ACC [11]. Synthesizing current findings, one conceptualization is that adolescent bipolar disorder involves dysfunction in neural circuits for emotion processing and regulation (involving bilateral frontal cortices—particularly the ventrolateral prefrontal cortex—plus the hippocampus and amygdala) alongside a parallel hyperactivation of reward-processing circuits (linking the left ventral striatum with the ventrolateral prefrontal and orbitofrontal cortices) [12]. These neural activation changes are thought to underlie emotion regulation difficulties, increased reward sensitivity, and the propensity toward manic symptoms. Emerging resting-state functional magnetic resonance imaging (fMRI) studies provide further support for these network-level abnormalities [13]. Concerning treatment effects on the brain, some pharmacological interventions appear to improve function in prefrontal cortical regions.

In contrast, subcortical hyperactivity (e.g., in the amygdala) may normalize only after long-term treatment [14]. Different medications target different neural circuit components, suggesting that combination therapy is necessary in severe cases to address the array of circuit dysfunctions adequately. It should be noted, however, that many neuroimaging studies to date have limitations such as small sample sizes and potential confounds (e.g., medication effects), so additional research—including long-term prospective studies—is needed to clarify how mood symptom trajectories and treatments impact neurodevelopment, and to determine the predictive value of early neuroimaging findings on long-term outcomes.

Clinical Presentation

Characteristics of Pediatric Bipolar Disorder

The clinical manifestations of bipolar disorder in children and adolescents have some distinctive features compared to adults. Psychotic symptoms and mixed mood states are relatively common in youth, and mood, energy, and behavior can be highly variable, lacking the sustained periods typical in adults. Irritable mood, belligerence, and mixed (dysphoric) mood states are more frequent in pediatric bipolar disorder than classic euphoric mood episodes [15]. Rapid cycling (frequent mood episode shifts) is also more prevalent in youths; some pediatric patients may even show ultrarapid cycling. Furthermore, full inter-episode recovery is less common in bipolar youth than in adults [16]. In the era of DSM-IV, many children and adolescents were diagnosed with "bipolar disorder not otherwise specified (NOS)" rather than bipolar I, because their mood episodes often did not meet the strict duration or symptom count criteria for bipolar I. Thus, bipolar NOS was a frequently used diagnosis in youth [17].

Neurocognitive profiles in pediatric bipolar disorder resemble those in adults, with deficits observed across multiple cognitive domains. Notably, impairments in verbal memory and working memory have been consistently found in a significant proportion of studies [15]. These cognitive deficits have implications for treatment planning—clinicians should consider neurocognitive functioning when designing a comprehensive treatment approach for children and adolescents with bipolar disorder.

Comorbid Conditions

Children and adolescents with bipolar disorder have high rates of comorbid psychiatric disorders. Common co-occurring diagnoses include ADHD, oppositional defiant disorder (ODD), conduct disorder, anxiety disorders, and substance use disorders. A recent systematic review of comorbidity in pediatric bipolar disorder found that the most frequent comorbid conditions were ADHD (in roughly 60% of cases) and ODD (about 47%) [18]. Pediatric bipolar disorder with comorbid ADHD tends to have an earlier onset of mood episodes (by about 5 years on average), a greater number of mood episodes, more suicide attempts, and a more chronic course than bipolar disorder without ADHD [19]. Bipolar disorder with comorbid conduct disorder is associated with more frequent hospitalizations and greater functional impairment. In contrast, comorbid anxiety disorders in bipolar youth correlate with earlier onset, longer duration of episodes in adulthood, and higher rates of suicide attempts. In general, the presence of comorbid conditions portends a poorer prognosis and a higher likelihood of functional impairment in pediatric bipolar disorder.

Diagnosis and Assessment

Diagnostic Criteria and DSM-V Changes

When evaluating a child or adolescent for possible bipolar disorder, standard diagnostic criteria and guidelines used for adults should be applied, with appropriate inclusion of parents or caregivers in the assessment and consideration of the youth's educational and social functioning. One major change in DSM-V aimed at reducing the overdiagnosis and overtreatment of pediatric bipolar disorder was the introduction of disruptive mood dysregulation disorder (DMDD) as a new depressive disorder category [20]. In earlier conceptualizations of pediatric bipolar disorder, chronic severe irritability was often considered a hallmark symptom. However, irritability is not specific to bipolar disorder—it can manifest in a range of other disorders—and using chronic, non-episodic irritability as a primary diagnostic criterion for bipolar disorder led to considerable confusion. Research tracking chronically irritable youth (those characterized as having severe mood dysregulation, SMD) found that these youths generally did not develop bipolar disorder over time, but instead were more likely to develop unipolar depressive disorders [21]. Accordingly, the SMD construct (with some modifications) was formalized as DMDD and incorporated into DSM-V under depressive disorders, defined by recurrent temper outbursts and persistent chronic irritability in youth up to 18 years of age. With the designation of prototypical chronic irritability as DMDD (a separate diagnosis to be ruled out before diagnosing bipolar disorder), much of the diagnostic ambiguity has been resolved. Essentially, pediatric bipolar disorder is now recognized as fundamentally the same illness as adult bipolar disorder, requiring the presence of distinct mood episodes (e.g., manic or hypomanic episodes) that meet standard criteria. The same diagnostic criteria apply across age groups, a principle that is increasingly acknowledged in clinical practice.

Diagnostic Process in Youth

Some authors have expressed concern about potential overdiagnosis and overtreatment of presumed bipolar disorder in children; however, it remains true that bipolar disorder in adolescents is often under-recognized and undertreated, contributing to poor outcomes such as elevated suicide rates and multiple comorbidities. While vigilance against overdiagnosis is important, clinicians must equally guard against the risk of underdiagnosing pediatric bipolar disorder, as delayed treatment can lead to worse adult outcomes [22].

Differentiating bipolar disorder from other childhood-onset psychiatric conditions can be challenging because of overlapping symptomatology and the influence of development on symptom expression. ADHD, ODD, DMDD, substance use disorders, personality disorders, and anxiety disorders can all share some symptoms with bipolar disorder. It is critical to evaluate the longitudinal course of symptoms and look for episodic changes to distinguish bipolar disorder. In particular, when ADHD coexists with suspected bipolar disorder, clinicians should consider a diagnosis of mania or hypomania only if symptoms such as distractibility, impulsivity, and hyperactivity markedly worsen exclusively during distinct periods of elevated or irritable mood. ADHD represents a chronic baseline neurodevelopmental condition, whereas bipolar disorder is episodic. Moreover, specific symptoms—such as decreased need for sleep, increased (inappropriate) goal-directed or pleasurable activities (e.g., age-inappropriate sexual behaviors), hallucinations or delusions, and homicidal or suicidal ideation or behaviors—can be seen in pediatric bipolar manic episodes but are rare in ADHD. Mainly, a positive family history of bipolar disorder provides a strong rationale to pursue a more detailed evaluation and can be very helpful in the diagnostic process [23].

Another critical differential diagnosis is between unipolar depression and bipolar depression in youth. Approximately 28% of children and adolescents initially diagnosed with major depressive disorder (MDD) will eventually be diagnosed with bipolar disorder, highlighting the importance of careful assessment for bipolar features in depressed youth. Clinical features that raise suspicion for bipolar depression (as opposed to unipolar depression) in youth include particularly severe depression or greater functional impairment associated with the depressive episode, poorer peer and family relationships, higher rates of school-related problems, and a greater number of days with impaired functioning during depression. Additionally, if a depressed child or adolescent has comorbid diagnoses such as ODD, conduct disorder, or anxiety disorders [24], or if there is a family history of mood disorders or disruptive behavior disorders [25], the likelihood of a later bipolar diagnosis is higher.

Assessment Tools

To aid in the diagnostic assessment, a variety of rating scales and structured instruments can be utilized. For broad screening of emotional and behavioral symptoms, one commonly used tool is the Child Behavior Checklist (CBCL)—particularly the CBCL dysregulation profile, which can indicate general behavioral dysregulation [26]. In addition, several instruments have been developed specifically to screen for or assess bipolar disorder symptoms in youth; these can be helpful adjuncts in evaluation. Notable tools include:

- *Mood Disorder Questionnaire–Adolescent version (MDQ-A)*—a self-report screening questionnaire for bipolar symptoms in adolescents [27].
- *Child Mania Rating Scale (CMRS)*—a parent-report measure assessing mania symptoms in children and adolescents [28].
- *Young Mania Rating Scale (YMRS)*—a clinician-administered scale for mania symptom severity [29].
- *Child Bipolar Questionnaire 2.0 (CBQ 2.0)*—a caregiver-report instrument for bipolar symptoms [30].
- *General Behavior Inventory (GBI)*—a questionnaire that measures depressive and hypomanic/biphasic symptoms over time [31].

Among these, the Young Mania Rating Scale (YMRS) is considered the gold standard clinician rating scale for assessing manic symptoms in pediatric bipolar disorder, as it is in adults [29]. However, because the YMRS focuses on manic symptoms and does not evaluate depressive symptoms, it should be supplemented with separate measures for depressive symptomatology when assessing bipolar youth. In clinical and research practice, a YMRS score of ≤ 12 is often interpreted as indicating remission of manic symptoms, whereas a score ≥ 20 is a commonly used cutoff for defining a significant manic state (e.g., as an inclusion threshold in clinical trials).

For a definitive diagnosis, a diagnostic interview is often employed. The Kiddie Schedule for Affective Disorders and Schizophrenia Present and Lifetime version (K-SADS-PL) is a semi-structured diagnostic interview that can be administered with the child and parent to systematically evaluate the presence of mood episodes (mania, hypomania, depression) and comorbid conditions, using developmentally appropriate criteria. The K-SADS-PL has demonstrated good reliability and validity in diagnosing pediatric bipolar disorder in clinical and research settings [32]. When conducting such an interview, clinicians should remain mindful that bipolar spectrum conditions—such as bipolar II disorder, cyclothymic disorder, and other specified (formerly "not otherwise specified") bipolar disorders—may be more common in youth than full bipolar I disorder. These diagnoses should be carefully considered in the evaluation of a child with mood dysregulation, rather than an all-or-nothing approach of only considering bipolar I.

Treatment

Pharmacotherapy

Pharmacological care for children and adolescents with bipolar disorder borrows core principles from adult practice but requires developmental tailoring and vigilant safety monitoring. The overarching aims are acute symptom control, restoration of age-appropriate functioning, and prevention of relapse, achieved through phase-specific treatment, systematic laboratory and metabolic surveillance, and shared decision-making with families. Youth are more vulnerable than adults to weight gain and cardiometabolic adverse effects—particularly with atypical antipsychotics—and they frequently present with mixed features and comorbid conditions such as ADHD, all of which should shape medication selection and monitoring plans. Psychosocial interventions are not optional adjuncts but integral elements initiated early and continued across phases [19, 22, 33–36].

Clinical decision-making should begin with illness phase and severity. In acute manic or mixed episodes, first-line pharmacotherapies are atypical antipsychotics—such as risperidone, aripiprazole, asenapine, or quetiapine—and lithium. Syntheses of pediatric trials indicate that atypical antipsychotics tend to produce stronger short-term antimanic effects than traditional mood stabilizers, but at the cost of greater metabolic liability; this necessitates anticipatory guidance on nutrition, sleep, and activity, along with close follow-up of weight, fasting lipids, and glucose. Valproate and ziprasidone are reasonable second-line choices or adjuncts in selected cases; clozapine is reserved for treatment-refractory mania under stringent safety protocols. In adolescent females who are or could become pregnant, valproate should be avoided because of teratogenic risk. Combination therapy is appropriate early when presentations are severe, psychotic, highly mixed or rapid-cycling, or when an optimized monotherapy yields only partial response. Age-stratified guidance in the 2022 Korean Medication Algorithm recommends, for children 12 years and younger with mania, either atypical antipsychotic monotherapy or an atypical antipsychotic plus a mood stabilizer as first-line; for adolescents 13–18 years, mood stabilizer plus atypical antipsychotic is generally preferred first, although either agent as monotherapy may be acceptable depending on clinical context [33–35, 37, 38].

Bipolar depression in youth remains challenging because of high placebo response rates and a comparatively thin pediatric evidence base. Current data and consensus support lurasidone as a first-line option given its pediatric trials and tolerability. Lithium and lamotrigine are reasonable second-line choices, drawing on adult efficacy and emerging youth data, whereas olanzapine–fluoxetine combination and quetiapine are typically deferred to later lines after careful risk–benefit discussions, especially in view of metabolic concerns. Antidepressants, if considered at all, should never be used as monotherapy; they must be paired with a mood stabilizer or atypical antipsychotic and monitored closely for affective switch or cycle acceleration. Psychotherapy—particularly family-focused and skills-based approaches—should be embedded from the outset and sustained throughout depressive phases. The Korean algorithm aligns with this approach, listing atypical antipsychotic monotherapy or mood stabilizer plus atypical antipsychotic as first-line for both children and adolescents, with lamotrigine-containing and antidepressant-containing combinations reserved for non-response [34–36].

Maintenance treatment should continue the acute-phase responder whenever feasible, emphasizing simplicity, tolerability, and adherence. Common anchors include lithium, divalproex, and aripiprazole; combinations such as risperidone with lithium or divalproex are reasonable for recurrence-prone courses. Lamotrigine becomes a useful option for adolescents—particularly when depressive polarity predominates. Long-acting injectable antipsychotics may improve adherence in selected older adolescents who struggle with daily dosing. Longer-term randomized data in youth support aripiprazole's efficacy and tolerability over a 30-week continuation phase following stabilization from acute mania, lending confidence to its role in relapse prevention [35, 36, 39].

Safety, monitoring, and special populations require explicit planning. At baseline and periodically thereafter, clinicians should assess weight or body mass index (BMI), waist circumference, and blood pressure, and obtain fasting lipids and glucose, increasing monitoring frequency during the first months of antipsychotic treatment and then spacing to every 3–6 months once stable. Agent-specific laboratory and safety checks are essential: for lithium, monitor thyroid and renal function and counsel on hydration and intercurrent illness; for valproate, monitor hepatic function and platelets and provide rigorous teratogenicity counseling to adolescent females; for ziprasidone, consider baseline and follow-up electrocardiography in at-risk patients; and for prolactin-elevating or high-metabolic-risk atypical antipsychotics such as risperidone or olanzapine, incorporate prolactin and intensified metabolic surveillance. Suicidality and activation should be reviewed at every visit, paired with interventions that stabilize sleep and circadian rhythms and with family supervision of medication administration and restriction of lethal means. Deprescribing should proceed gradually; abrupt discontinuation—especially of lithium and atypical antipsychotics—raises relapse risk and is best avoided [19, 33, 34].

Comorbidity should be addressed within, not after, mood treatment. The general rule is to stabilize mood first, then target residual impairment from comorbid conditions. In bipolar youth with ADHD, carefully introduced psychostimulants can improve attention and hyperactivity once a mood stabilizer or atypical antipsychotic has achieved mood control; controlled pediatric studies show ADHD benefits without destabilizing mania under these conditions, although close observation for irritability, sleep disruption, or mood shift remains prudent. In adolescents with comorbid substance use disorders, integrated care is indicated, and there is evidence that effective mood stabilization—for example with lithium—can also reduce substance-related symptoms. For anxiety disorders, psychotherapy should be first-line; when pharmacotherapy is needed, selective serotonin reuptake inhibitors should be co-prescribed with a mood-stabilizing agent and monitored carefully for switch phenomena [40–44].

In practical terms, the acute manic or mixed phase in youth is typically managed first with an atypical antipsychotic or with lithium, adding the other agent early when presentations are severe, psychotic, highly mixed, or only partially responsive to optimized monotherapy; valproate is avoided in adolescent females who are or could become pregnant, and metabolic risks are anticipated and monitored when atypical antipsychotics are used. Bipolar depression is approached conservatively with lurasidone as a preferred initial medication, psychotherapy as a constant foundation, and lithium or lamotrigine considered when depressive symptoms persist; antidepressant monotherapy is contraindicated, and combinations that include antidepressants are reserved for non-responders with vigilant monitoring. For maintenance, the agent or regimen that achieved remission is continued when tolerated, with lithium, divalproex, and aripiprazole serving as common anchors; combination strategies and, in select cases, long-acting injectables are reasonable for recurrence-prone illness or adherence challenges, and abrupt discontinuation is avoided in favor of slow tapers to mitigate relapse [19, 22, 33–36, 39].

Non-pharmacological Treatment

Psychosocial interventions are a critical component of managing pediatric bipolar disorder, in conjunction with medication. The American Academy of Child and Adolescent Psychiatry (AACAP) Practice Parameter on bipolar disorder in youth [19] outlines several key non-pharmacological strategies:

- *Psychoeducation*: Educating the patient and family about the illness's symptoms, course, causes, and treatments, as well as its impact on the child's social and family functioning. Improving understanding of bipolar disorder can enhance treatment adherence and empower families.
- *Relapse prevention*: Teaching patients and families to recognize early warning signs of mood episodes and to maintain routines that promote stability. Psychoeducation improves medication compliance and enables early detection of prodromal symptoms, which is crucial for preventing full relapses. Strategies include stress reduction, establishing healthy sleep patterns, and improving social and coping skills.
- *Individual psychotherapy*: Therapeutic modalities such as cognitive–behavioral therapy (CBT) or interpersonal therapy, adapted for youth, alongside supportive individual therapy, can help the child develop insight, learn coping strategies, regulate emotions, and address age-appropriate developmental issues. Psychotherapy provides a space to monitor symptoms and promote psychological growth and skill acquisition.
- *Social and family functioning*: Given the influence of bipolar disorder on family dynamics, peer relationships, academic performance, and overall development, it is important to involve the family and possibly peers/teachers in treatment. Family-focused therapy and social skills training aims to improve communication, problem-solving, and conflict resolution within the family, and to enhance the child's social functioning. Cultural factors should be considered to ensure interventions are appropriate and effective.
- *Educational and academic functioning*: Many children with bipolar disorder experience academic difficulties. Collaboration with schools

is often necessary—for example, developing individualized education programs (IEPs) or 504 plans to accommodate the child's needs, providing school-based counseling, or adjusting workloads. Teaching organizational and learning strategies can help the child keep up academically.

- *Community consultation*: Children and adolescents with bipolar disorder may benefit from community resources, such as after-school programs, mentorship, or support groups. Connecting families with community agencies and programs can provide additional support and respite. In some cases, especially if the home environment is very stressful or unsafe, therapeutic foster care or residential treatment programs may be considered to provide a structured environment for stabilization.

Among the various psychosocial intervention models, those with demonstrated efficacy in youth via randomized controlled trials include multifamily psychoeducational psychotherapy and family-focused therapy. These family-centric psychoeducational programs have been shown to reduce relapse rates and improve outcomes. It is recommended that, whenever possible, all youth with bipolar disorder and their families should be offered such psychoeducational interventions. Moreover, the National Institute for Health and Care Excellence (NICE) guidelines for bipolar disorder management suggest that for bipolar depression in youth, at least a three-month trial of psychotherapy (such as CBT or interpersonal therapy) should be undertaken before initiating medication for depression [34].

Course and Prognosis

Pediatric bipolar disorder often follows a chronic, relapsing course and frequently presents with mixed features. In longitudinal studies, the majority of children and adolescents with bipolar disorder exhibit a chronic course with mixed manic-depressive symptomatology [45]. Recovery rate from an index episode was 81.5–100%, and recurrence rate was reported to be about 35–67% [46]. Early-onset bipolar disorder tends to be at least as episodic as the adult form of the illness. However, studies indicate it can be more chronic and resistant to treatment than bipolar disorder with adult onset [6].

Conclusion

While bipolar disorder has long been recognized as a serious adult psychiatric illness, it is now understood that the disorder often has its onset in childhood or adolescence. Early-onset bipolar disorder tends to have a more chronic course, and if it manifests in youth, it can lead to a prolonged illness burden affecting the young person and their family over many years. Increasing awareness of pediatric bipolar disorder, along with improvements in screening and diagnostic tools, has helped the field differentiate chronic, non-episodic irritability that progresses to depressive disorders from true episodic bipolar disorder. From phenomenology and neurobiology to psychosocial interventions and pharmacotherapy, ongoing research efforts are gradually illuminating various aspects of pediatric bipolar disorder, and these advances are expected to improve outcomes over time.

From a clinical standpoint, it is crucial to focus not only on symptom reduction but also on restoring age-appropriate functioning in youth with bipolar disorder. As our understanding of the underlying causes and risk factors improves, we anticipate the development of preventative strategies and more targeted treatments for at-risk youth. Research into sustained acute-phase treatment and maintenance strategies will clarify how to achieve lasting stabilization and prevent relapse in this population. Providing timely and appropriate treatment is key to preventing early-onset bipolar disorder from becoming a lifelong, refractory illness. Currently, many effective treatment strategies in adults are being adapted for use in children and adolescents, but clinicians must account for developmental differences that influence treatment response. Recent evidence supports the acute efficacy of atypical antipsychotics for manic and mixed episodes in youths, but further studies are needed to establish their long-term safety and effectiveness in younger patients. Additionally, there remain substantial gaps in evidence regarding the treatment of bipolar depression in youth, management of common comorbidities in pediatric bipolar disorder, and interventions for asymptomatic youth at high genetic risk for bipolar illness. Addressing these gaps through future research will help resolve clinical uncertainties and guide improvements in diagnosis, treatment selection, long-term monitoring, and relapse prevention for children and adolescents with bipolar disorder.

Declarations

Competing Interests The author(s) has no competing interests to declare that are relevant to the content of this manuscript.

Ethics Approval The author(s) declares that this manuscript does not include primary research with human participants.

The author(s) declares that this manuscript does not include primary studies involving animals.

References

1. Moreno C, Laje G, Blanco C, Jiang H, Schmidt AB, Olfson M. National trends in the outpatient diagnosis and treatment of bipolar disorder in youth. Arch Gen Psychiatry. 2007;64(9):1032–9.
2. Van Meter AR, Moreira AL, Youngstrom EA. Meta-analysis of epidemiologic studies of pediatric bipolar disorder. J Clin Psychiatry. 2011;72(9):1250–6.
3. Van Meter A, Moreira ALR, Youngstrom E. Updated meta-analysis of epidemiologic studies of pediatric bipolar disorder. J Clin Psychiatry. 2019;80(3).
4. Thapar A, Collishaw S, Pine DS, Thapar AK. Depression in adolescence. Lancet. 2012;379(9820):1056–67.
5. Parry P, Allison S, Bastiampillai T. 'Pediatric bipolar disorder' rates are still lower than claimed: a re-examination of eight epidemiological surveys used by an updated meta-analysis. Int J Bipolar Disord. 2021;9(1):21.
6. Perlis RH, Miyahara S, Marangell LB, Wisniewski SR, Ostacher M, DelBello MP, et al. Long-term implications of early onset in bipolar disorder: data from the first 1000 participants in the systematic treatment enhancement program for bipolar disorder (STEP-BD). Biol Psychiatry. 2004;55(9):875–81.
7. McGuffin P, Rijsdijk F, Andrew M, Sham P, Katz R, Cardno A. The heritability of bipolar affective disorder and the genetic relationship to unipolar depression. Arch Gen Psychiatry. 2003;60(5):497–502.
8. O'Connell KS, Coombes BJ. Genetic contributions to bipolar disorder: current status and future directions. Psychol Med. 2021;51(13):2156–67.
9. Birmaher B, Axelson D, Monk K, Kalas C, Goldstein B, Hickey MB, et al. Lifetime psychiatric disorders in school-aged offspring of parents with bipolar disorder: the Pittsburgh Bipolar Offspring study. Arch Gen Psychiatry. 2009;66(3):287–96.
10. Pavuluri M. Neuroscience-based formulation and treatment for early-onset bipolar disorder: a paradigm shift. Curr Treat Options Psychiatry. 2015;2:229–51.
11. Wegbreit E, Cushman GK, Puzia ME, Weissman AB, Kim KL, Laird AR, et al. Developmental meta-analyses of the functional neural correlates of bipolar disorder. JAMA Psychiatry. 2014;71(8):926–35.
12. Phillips ML, Swartz HA. A critical appraisal of neuroimaging studies of bipolar disorder: toward a new conceptualization of underlying neural circuitry and a road map for future research. Am J Psychiatry. 2014;171(8):829–43.
13. Cattarinussi G, Bellani M, Maggioni E, Sambataro F, Brambilla P, Delvecchio G. Resting-state functional connectivity and spontaneous brain activity in early-onset bipolar disorder: a review of functional magnetic resonance imaging studies. J Affect Disord. 2022;311:463–71.
14. Yang H, Lu LH, Wu M, Stevens M, Wegbreit E, Fitzgerald J, et al. Time course of recovery showing initial prefrontal cortex changes at 16 weeks, extending to subcortical changes by 3 years in pediatric bipolar disorder. J Affect Disord. 2013;150(2):571–7.
15. DelBello MP, Carlson GA, Tohen M, Bromet EJ, Schwiers M, Strakowski SM. Rates and predictors of developing a manic or hypomanic episode 1 to 2 years following a first hospitalization for major depression with psychotic features. J Child Adolesc Psychopharmacol. 2003;13(2):173–85.
16. Findling RL, Gracious BL, NK MN, Youngstrom EA, Demeter CA, Branicky LA, et al. Rapid, continuous cycling and psychiatric co-morbidity in pediatric bipolar I disorder. Bipolar Disord. 2001;3(4):202–10.
17. Safer DJ, Rajakannan T, Burcu M, Zito JM. Trends in subthreshold psychiatric diagnoses for youth in community treatment. JAMA Psychiatry. 2015;72(1):75–83.
18. Fahrendorff AM, Pagsberg AK, Kessing LV, Maigaard K. Psychiatric comorbidity in patients with pediatric bipolar disorder – a systematic review. Acta Psychiatr Scand. 2023;148(2):110–32.
19. McClellan J, Kowatch R, Findling RL, Work Group on Quality I. Practice parameter for the assessment and treatment of children and adolescents with bipo-

lar disorder. J Am Acad Child Adolesc Psychiatry. 2007;46(1):107–25.
20. Tandon R. Bipolar and depressive disorders in diagnostic and statistical manual of mental Disorders-5: clinical implications of revisions from diagnostic and statistical manual of mental disorders-IV. Indian J Psychol Med. 2015;37(1):1–4.
21. Stringaris A, Baroni A, Haimm C, Brotman M, Lowe CH, Myers F, et al. Pediatric bipolar disorder versus severe mood dysregulation: risk for manic episodes on follow-up. J Am Acad Child Adolesc Psychiatry. 2010;49(4):397–405.
22. Yatham LN, Kennedy SH, Parikh SV, Schaffer A, Bond DJ, Frey BN, et al. Canadian Network for Mood and Anxiety Treatments (CANMAT) and International Society for Bipolar Disorders (ISBD) 2018 guidelines for the management of patients with bipolar disorder. Bipolar Disord. 2018;20(2):97–170.
23. Nierenberg AA, Miyahara S, Spencer T, Wisniewski SR, Otto MW, Simon N, et al. Clinical and diagnostic implications of lifetime attention-deficit/hyperactivity disorder comorbidity in adults with bipolar disorder: data from the first 1000 STEP-BD participants. Biol Psychiatry. 2005;57(11):1467–73.
24. Buckley V, Young AH, Smith P. Child and adolescent anxiety as a risk factor for bipolar disorder: a systematic review of longitudinal studies. Bipolar Disord. 2023;25(4):278–88.
25. Goldstein BI, Shamseddeen W, Axelson DA, Kalas C, Monk K, Brent DA, et al. Clinical, demographic, and familial correlates of bipolar spectrum disorders among offspring of parents with bipolar disorder. J Am Acad Child Adolesc Psychiatry. 2010;49(4):388–96.
26. Mbekou V, Gignac M, MacNeil S, Mackay P, Renaud J. The CBCL dysregulated profile: an indicator of pediatric bipolar disorder or of psychopathology severity? J Affect Disord. 2014;155:299–302.
27. Wagner KD, Hirschfeld RM, Emslie GJ, Findling RL, Gracious BL, Reed ML. Validation of the Mood Disorder Questionnaire for bipolar disorders in adolescents. J Clin Psychiatry. 2006;67(5):827–30.
28. Pavuluri MN, Henry DB, Devineni B, Carbray JA, Birmaher B. Child mania rating scale: development, reliability, and validity. J Am Acad Child Adolesc Psychiatry. 2006;45(5):550–60.
29. Youngstrom EA, Gracious BL, Danielson CK, Findling RL, Calabrese J. Toward an integration of parent and clinician report on the Young Mania Rating Scale. J Affect Disord. 2003;77(2):179–90.
30. Papolos D, Hennen J, Cockerham MS, Thode HC Jr, Youngstrom EA. The child bipolar questionnaire: a dimensional approach to screening for pediatric bipolar disorder. J Affect Disord. 2006;95(1–3):149–58.
31. Depue RA, Krauss S, Spoont MR, Arbisi P. General behavior inventory identification of unipolar and bipolar affective conditions in a nonclinical university population. J Abnorm Psychol. 1989;98(2):117–26.
32. Matuschek T, Jaeger S, Stadelmann S, Dolling K, Grunewald M, Weis S, et al. Implementing the K-SADS-PL as a standard diagnostic tool: effects on clinical diagnoses. Psychiatry Res. 2016;236:119–24.
33. Pillay J, Boylan K, Newton A, Hartling L, Vandermeer B, Nuspl M, et al. Harms of antipsychotics in children and Young adults: a systematic review update. Can J Psychiatr. 2018;63(10):661–78.
34. NICE. National Institute for Health and Care Excellence. Bipolar disorder: assessment and management (CG185). NICE; 2014 (amended 2020, 2023).
35. Woo YS, Bahk WM, Jeong JH, Lee JG, Kim W, Sohn I, et al. Korean medication algorithm project for bipolar disorder 2022, fifth revision: an executive summary. Clin Psychopharmacol Neurosci. 2022;20(4):747–61.
36. Goldstein BI, Birmaher B, Carlson GA, MP DB, Findling RL, Fristad M, et al. The International Society for Bipolar Disorders Task Force report on pediatric bipolar disorder: knowledge to date and directions for future research. Bipolar Disord. 2017;19(7):524–43.
37. Findling RL, Cavus I, Pappadopulos E, Vanderburg DG, Schwartz JH, Gundapaneni BK, et al. Efficacy, long-term safety, and tolerability of ziprasidone in children and adolescents with bipolar disorder. J Child Adolesc Psychopharmacol. 2013;23(8):545–57.
38. Masi G, Mucci M, Millepiedi S. Clozapine in adolescent inpatients with acute mania. J Child Adolesc Psychopharmacol. 2002;12(2):93–9.
39. Findling RL, Correll CU, Nyilas M, Forbes RA, McQuade RD, Jin N, et al. Aripiprazole for the treatment of pediatric bipolar I disorder: a 30-week, randomized, placebo-controlled study. Bipolar Disord. 2013;15(2):138–49.
40. Scheffer RE, Kowatch RA, Carmody T, Rush AJ. Randomized, placebo-controlled trial of mixed amphetamine salts for symptoms of comorbid ADHD in pediatric bipolar disorder after mood stabilization with divalproex sodium. Am J Psychiatry. 2005;162(1):58–64.
41. Findling RL, Short EJ, McNamara NK, Demeter CA, Stansbrey RJ, Gracious BL, et al. Methylphenidate in the treatment of children and adolescents with bipolar disorder and attention-deficit/hyperactivity disorder. J Am Acad Child Adolesc Psychiatry. 2007;46(11):1445–53.
42. Goldsmith M, Singh M, Chang K. Antidepressants and psychostimulants in pediatric populations: is there an association with mania? Paediatr Drugs. 2011;13(4):225–43.
43. Chiorean A, Jones BDM, Murong M, Gonzalez-Torres C, Kloiber S, Ortiz A, et al. Prescribed psychostimulants and other pro-cognitive medications in bipolar disorder: a systematic review and meta-analysis of recurrence of manic symptoms. Bipolar Disord. 2024;26(5):418–30.
44. Geller B, Cooper TB, Sun K, Zimerman B, Frazier J, Williams M, et al. Double-blind and placebo-controlled study of lithium for adolescent bipolar

disorders with secondary substance dependency. J Am Acad Child Adolesc Psychiatry. 1998;37(2):171–8.
45. Wozniak J, DiSalvo M, Farrell A, Joshi G, Uchida M, Faraone SV, et al. Long term outcomes of pediatric Bipolar-I disorder: a prospective follow-up analysis attending to full syndomatic, subsyndromal and functional types of remission. J Psychiatr Res. 2022;151:667–75.
46. Cirone C, Secci I, Favole I, Ricci F, Amianto F, Davico C, et al. What do we know about the long-term course of early onset bipolar disorder? A review of the current evidence. Brain Sci. 2021;11(3).

9 Bipolar Disorder and Attention-Deficit/Hyperactivity Disorder (ADHD): Importance and Differential Diagnosis

Hyun-Ju Yang and Young-Eun Jung

Introduction

The clinical features of bipolar disorder and attention-deficit/hyperactivity disorder (ADHD) are quite similar, and the two disorders also show high rates of comorbidity, making accurate diagnosis challenging [1]. In childhood and adolescent bipolar disorder, ADHD is diagnosed in 50–90% of cases, while 10–25% of children with ADHD are found to have bipolar disorder [2]. Among adults, approximately one in six patients with bipolar disorder is currently diagnosed with ADHD or has a history of the condition [3, 4]. When bipolar disorder co-occurs with ADHD, the onset of mood symptoms tends to occur earlier, the illness course becomes more chronic, mood episodes—particularly depressive episodes—are more frequent, and suicide risk is higher. Even after mood symptoms improve, deficits in social and occupational functioning often persist due to the impact of ADHD symptoms [4–6].

Despite this clinical significance, many patients do not receive an appropriate diagnosis or treatment in practice. For example, a patient presenting with increased energy, distractibility, irritability, talkativeness, impulsivity, and hyperactivity may, if a child, often be presumed to have only ADHD; in adults, given the perception that ADHD is mainly a childhood disorder, clinicians may focus more on mood symptoms. Even when both bipolar disorder and ADHD are considered, and a comprehensive evaluation is conducted, it remains difficult to distinguish between the two disorders or diagnose their comorbidity. In pediatric and adolescent populations, several developmental factors further complicate the differential diagnosis. Unlike adults, the most common mood symptoms of childhood and adolescent bipolar disorder are irritability with unstable affect or persistent and aggressive anger outbursts. Furthermore, nonspecific mixed features can make it difficult to distinguish between episodes, and the younger the patient, the more atypical the clinical presentation becomes, further complicating diagnosis [7]. These atypical and mixed features in youth constitute important diagnostic pitfalls when differentiating bipolar disorder from ADHD and related conditions. In adults, the pattern of symptom expression changes again, creating a different set of diagnostic pitfalls. Diagnosing ADHD in adults is also challenging. When ADHD persists into adulthood, attention-deficit symptoms usually predominate, while hyperactivity and impulsivity tend to diminish. Instead, emotional dysregulation—manifested as irritability, mood swings, and rapid shifts in emotional state—becomes

H.-J. Yang · Y.-E. Jung (✉)
Department of Psychiatry, Jeju National University Hospital, School of Medicine, Jeju National University, Jeju, Republic of Korea
e-mail: jyejye77@daum.net

W.-M. Bahk et al. (eds.), *Bipolar Disorder*, https://doi.org/10.1007/978-981-92-1323-8_9

more prominent, features that are easily confused with bipolar spectrum conditions such as hypomania, mixed mania, or agitated depression [1]. Such changes in symptom profile over the lifespan create specific diagnostic pitfalls in adult patients, particularly when relying on cross-sectional assessment alone.

Therefore, clinicians must recognize the distinguishing features of bipolar disorder and ADHD, as well as understand the clinical course and prognosis when both disorders coexist, in order to make an accurate diagnosis and develop an appropriate treatment plan.

Symptoms That Help Differentiate Bipolar Disorder and ADHD

To facilitate clinical decision-making, the differential features between bipolar disorder and ADHD can be conceptually organized into three levels: core differentiators, supportive features, and misleading overlaps. This section briefly introduces this framework and then describes the clinical characteristics in more detail. Generally, the distinct characteristic symptoms of bipolar disorder and ADHD are summarized in Table 9.1 [1]. Among these, episodicity versus chronicity represents a core differentiator. The most significant differential point between the two is that bipolar disorder presents episodic features. In contrast, ADHD is a chronic condition that typically begins in childhood before the age of 12 and shows no symptom-free intervals or functional recovery between episodes, distinguishing it from bipolar disorder. Therefore, it is crucial to differentiate whether symptoms occur episodically and apply this distinction appropriately within each diagnostic criterion.

Table 9.1 Comparison of clinical features between bipolar disorder and ADHD

Features	ADHD	Bipolar disorder
Age of onset	Childhood	Early adulthood
Course	Persistent, chronic	Distinct episodes
Symptoms	Emotional dysregulation Low self-esteem Difficulty sustaining attention, restless	Persistently elevated, irritable mood Grandiosity, inflated self-esteem Goal-directed activity
Sleep	Usually not a core diagnostic feature	Decreased need for sleep
Libido	Not affected	Increased sexual drive (during mania)
Psychotic symptoms	None	May be present

By contrast, several overlapping symptoms may be misleading and should be interpreted with caution. Manic episodes can resemble ADHD symptoms, such as inattention, hyperactivity, and impulsivity, complicating diagnosis. According to Geller et al., both disorders can exhibit increased energy and distractibility, but elated mood, grandiosity, racing thoughts, and decreased need for sleep are more characteristic of manic episodes [8]. However, in childhood and adolescent bipolar disorder, grandiosity and elated mood are less common, making differentiation difficult. A meta-analysis found that the most frequent manic symptoms in children included increased energy (89%), inattention (84%), pressured speech (82%), irritability (81%), grandiose ideas (78%), and elevated mood (70%) [9].

There is also substantial overlap in depressive symptoms between bipolar disorder and ADHD. This overlap often leads to frustration, low achievement, and low self-esteem, which can mimic persistent depressive feelings and warrant careful evaluation for depression or comorbidity. By contrast, psychomotor retardation, fatigue, hypersomnia, anhedonia, and suicidal ideation are more typical of bipolar depression and are not features of ADHD [10]. Compared to ADHD, childhood and adolescent bipolar disorder tends to involve more severe negative emotional reactions and verbal aggression after minor stressors [11]. While untreated ADHD may cause irritability or depressed mood, these symptoms usually do not meet the criteria for a major depressive episode [12].

These findings can be regarded as supportive features that strengthen the diagnosis of bipolar disorder over ADHD. Another distinguishing factor is the higher prevalence of psychotic symptoms in bipolar disorder [9], such as mood-incongruent hallucinations and delusions. Recurrent mood episodes also increase suicide risk [2]; in childhood bipolar disorder, serious suicidal behaviors occur in about 25% of cases. Such suicidality helps differentiate bipolar disorder from ADHD, conduct disorder, or anxiety disorders [12]. Family history also provides diagnostic clues; children with a parental history of bipolar disorder have an elevated risk themselves [13].

Irritability and temper outbursts require special consideration. Irritability is common in children and occurs in both ADHD and bipolar disorder. According to Diagnostic and Statistical Manual of Mental Disorder, Fifth edition (DSM-V), irritability with mood instability or persistent, aggressive outbursts—even in the absence of elated mood or grandiosity—can justify a bipolar disorder diagnosis. These outbursts can be severe, lasting over an hour, and often triggered by minor stressors. DSM-V also introduced disruptive mood dysregulation disorder (DMDD), classified under depressive disorders because longitudinal data suggest a trajectory toward unipolar depression rather than bipolar disorder [14, 15]. DMDD is defined by frequent (≥3 per week), intense temper outbursts and persistently irritable or negative mood between outbursts, lasting for at least 12 months. The diagnosis applies to children aged 6 or older, with onset before age 10. Up to 25% of childhood and adolescent bipolar patients may also meet DMDD criteria. The key difference is that DMDD is persistent, whereas bipolar disorder involves distinct episodes. If (hypo)manic episodes last more than one day, a diagnosis of bipolar disorder—not DMDD—is warranted. Notably, approximately 65% of children with DMDD also have ADHD. Clinicians must be aware of these distinctions and comorbidities to ensure accurate diagnosis of bipolar disorder, ADHD, and DMDD.

Comorbidity of Bipolar Disorder and ADHD

As described above, bipolar disorder and ADHD show high comorbidity. In children, comorbidity is associated with poorer adaptation, greater risk of academic failure, more psychiatric and cognitive comorbidities, and worse overall prognosis. In adults, the coexistence of the two disorders is linked to more frequent mood episodes, more severe symptoms, mixed features, interpersonal aggression, impulsivity, legal problems, suicide attempts, substance use, personality disorders, lower quality of life, and social difficulties [4–6].

Comorbidity rates vary across age groups and study designs. In childhood and adolescent bipolar disorder, comorbidity with ADHD has been reported in 50–90% of cases, depending on sample characteristics, age group, and bipolar subtype. Wozniak et al. reported ADHD in up to 98% of bipolar disorder cases under the age of 12 [16]. Other studies have found rates of approximately 49–58.6% in adolescents with bipolar disorder [17]. In the Course and Outcome of Bipolar Youth (COBY) study, ADHD comorbidity was 58.6% overall: 62.1% in type I, 43.3% in type II, and 59.8% in bipolar disorder not otherwise specified [7, 13]. Conversely, among children diagnosed with ADHD, the comorbidity rate of bipolar disorder is approximately 10% [18]. In adults, a meta-analysis of 71 studies found that 17.11% of bipolar disorder patients have comorbid ADHD, whereas 7.95% of adults with ADHD are diagnosed with bipolar disorder [3].

Several hypotheses have been proposed to explain this comorbidity. First, several studies suggest that ADHD may serve as an early warning sign or a developmental marker of bipolar disorder. Notably, it has been reported that individuals with both ADHD and bipolar disorder have a significantly higher frequency of prepubertal onset and an earlier average age of onset compared to those with bipolar disorder alone [9, 19]. According to the large-scale U.S. study Systematic Treatment Enhancement Program for Bipolar Disorder (STEP-BD), adult patients with bipolar disorder who had prepubertal onset (20.4%) showed a significantly higher rate of comorbid ADHD than those with adolescent-onset (7.6%) or adult-onset (5.7%). Moreover, those with both bipolar disorder and ADHD had an average bipolar onset age approximately five years younger than those without ADHD (13.9 vs. 18 years) [20]. On the other hand, findings from studies indicate that even after ADHD symptoms improve through treatment, symptoms consistent with bipolar disorder persist, or attention and behavioral control problems associated with ADHD appear independently of the course of bipolar disorder. This has led to the simultaneous proposal that the two disorders coexist independently. A recent analysis of prospective cohort studies on bipolar disorder high-risk groups (patients and their offspring) showed that the diagnosis of ADHD in childhood is not a reliable predictor of later bipolar onset. However, preliminary results suggest that for bipolar disorder high-risk groups, ADHD symptoms may represent a neurodevelopmental phenotype of specific bipolar subtypes [21, 22].

In conclusion, there is still a lack of research clarifying the clinical, developmental, and biological relationships distinguishing ADHD and bipolar disorder and their comorbidity. It remains unclear whether the frequent coexistence of the two disorders arises from mere overlap of diagnostic criteria symptoms, the characteristic clinical features of childhood and adolescent bipolar disorder reflecting developmental differences, or the independent coexistence of two disorders due to dual genetic susceptibilities. Although hypotheses propose shared genetic and neurobiological risk factors commonly observed in both disorders, current evidence remains insufficient [23]. To clarify comorbidity and characteristics of childhood and adolescent bipolar disorder and ADHD, further longitudinal and neurobiological research is necessary.

Treatment Strategies and Precautions

Accurate diagnosis of bipolar disorder and ADHD is both challenging and essential, as misdiagnosis can delay appropriate treatment and lead to unnecessary side effects or severe functional impairment, including academic failure or job loss. In children, misdiagnosis may further disrupt development and family functioning. Clinicians are understandably cautious about initiating lifelong medication without diagnostic certainty, particularly in childhood and adolescent populations. Nevertheless, in children presenting with complex symptomatology such as ADHD, irritability, or aggression, timely recognition of possible bipolar disorder is crucial to avoid missing the appropriate treatment window. While misdiagnosing ADHD as bipolar disorder is relatively uncommon, bipolar disorder is frequently misdiagnosed as ADHD, conduct disorder, or DMDD. Such diagnostic errors may result in inappropriate use of stimulants or antidepressants, potentially exacerbating mood symptoms and worsening the overall course of illness [17, 24]. Careful differentiation of bipolar disorder from ADHD, DMDD, oppositional defiant disorder, and conduct disorder is therefore critical to prevent both over- and under-diagnosis and to ensure appropriate intervention.

Various medications can be used to treat bipolar disorder and ADHD (see Table 9.2). Generally, mood stabilizers (lithium, valproate/divalproex, carbamazepine) administered alone or in combination with atypical antipsychotics (e.g., aripiprazole), are effective for managing manic episodes but do not improve ADHD symptoms. Use of psychostimulants in bipolar disorder remains unclear in terms of efficacy and risk, as these medications may exacerbate manic symptoms. Some studies report that patients with prior stimulant use have more severe manic episodes and poorer treatment outcomes [25]. However, these data primarily come from child and adolescent populations, and evidence supporting pharmacological treatment efficacy for adult ADHD is limited. Methylphenidate and atomoxetine have demonstrated efficacy in adult ADHD, and lithium—well-known for its antimanic properties—has shown effectiveness comparable to methylphenidate in treating irritability and aggression associated with adult ADHD [26]. Importantly, careful consideration should be given to the time course for treatment effects (e.g., psychostimulants for ADHD show rapid

Table 9.2 Expected effects of pharmacological treatments in bipolar disorder and ADHD

	Treatment effect	
Medication	Bipolar disorder	ADHD
Psychostimulants (e.g., methylphenidate, amphetamine mixed salts)	May induce of exacerbate manic or psychotic symptoms [25] May be helpful for bipolar depression but requires careful monitoring [26] In children with comorbid bipolar disorder and ADHD, adjunctive use of amphetamine mixed salts to valproate may improve ADHD symptoms [27] Adjunctive methylphenidate to aripiprazole shows no effect on ADHD symptoms [28]	Known to be effective on core symptoms (inattention, hyperactivity, impulsivity); relatively rapid effect
Alpha-2 adrenergic agonists (e.g., guanfacine, clonidine)	Case reports suggest effects for secondary mania due to ADHD treatment; no established effects in primary bipolar disorder	May be effective for impulsivity, hyperactivity [38]
Noradrenergic agents (e.g., atomoxetine, nortriptyline, desipramine)	Theoretical risk of inducing mania Open-label studies with atomoxetine in combination with antimanic medications show significant improvement of ADHD symptoms without worsening manic episode [29]	May be effective for inattention, hyperactivity Especially effective with comorbid tic disorders or anxiety disorders [30]
Other antidepressants	Unclear efficacy and risk	In adults, bupropion is more than 2.5 times as effective as placebo [31]
Dopamine agonists (e.g., bromocriptine, pramipexole, ropinirole)	May be helpful as augmentation for treatment-resistant bipolar depression [32] Pramipexole may improve cognitive function in bipolar disorder patients [33]	Theoretically may help attention, but no evidence exists
Lithium	Proven antimanic efficacy Anti-suicidal effect reported May impair cognitive functions such as verbal memory, short- and long-term memory, motor speed [34]	Reported to improve irritability and aggression in adults [35]
Valproate/divalproex	Proven antimanic efficacy May impair attention and verbal memory [34]	Combination with stimulants is more effective for ADHD-related aggression than stimulants plus placebo [36]
Carbamazepine	Proven antimanic efficacy May impair learning and visuomotor speed [34]	Less effective for impulsivity and hyperactivity compared to clonidine [37]
Lamotrigine	Reported efficacy for bipolar depression More effective for preventions of depressive episodes than for acute treatment No reported cognitive adverse effects	No studies report efficacy for ADHD
Atypical antipsychotics	In case of comorbidity, aripiprazole is effective for manic episodes but not for ADHD symptoms [38]	Some agents may improve impulsivity and aggression; no efficacy for inattentive symptoms has been reported

effects within hours to days), differential efficacy across core symptom domains (inattention vs. impulsivity-hyperactivity), and the cognitive adverse effects associated with mood stabilizers and antipsychotics. The balance of therapeutic benefits and potential adverse effects of these medications must be thoroughly evaluated.

When bipolar disorder and ADHD truly coexist, clinical care requires heightened caution in developing treatment strategies. As shown in

Table 9.2, the two disorders respond to entirely different classes of medications, so clinicians must carefully understand the constellation of symptoms that respond individually to each drug class. First and foremost, in patients with confirmed or suspected bipolar disorder—especially those with a family history of the disorder—it is advisable to avoid first-line use of antidepressants or psychostimulants. However, if ADHD symptoms persistently cause functional impairment even after mood symptoms have stabilized sufficiently with mood stabilizers (monotherapy or combinations) or atypical antipsychotics, augmentation treatment with low-dose psychostimulants may be considered. Some researchers have suggested that once mood symptoms improve with one or more mood stabilizers, low-dose psychostimulant augmentation could be used as adjunctive therapy when ADHD symptoms persist [26, 27]. Additionally, bupropion can be considered to address depressive symptoms and improve attention in patients with bipolar depression comorbid with ADHD [31].

Conclusion

This chapter reviewed comorbidity, differential diagnosis, and treatment strategies for ADHD and bipolar disorder. Although diagnosis is complex, it remains essential. A thorough understanding of the clinical features, course, illness trajectory, and treatment response of each disorder is critical. In comorbid cases, mood stabilization should be given priority, with ADHD symptoms addressed subsequently through the cautious use of stimulant medications at low doses.

Declarations

Competing Interests The author(s) has no competing interests to declare that are relevant to the content of this manuscript.

Ethics Approval The author(s) declares that this manuscript does not include primary research with human participants.

The author(s) declares that this manuscript does not include primary studies involving animals.

References

1. Brus MJ, Solanto MV, Goldberg JF. Adult ADHD vs. bipolar disorder in the DSM-5 era: a challenging differentiation for clinicians. J Psychiatr Pract. 2014;20:428–37.
2. Pavuluri MN, Birmaher B, Naylor M. Pediatric bipolar disorder: a review of the past 10 years. J Am Acad Child Adolesc Psychiatry. 2005;44:846–71.
3. Schiweck C, Arteaga-Henriquez G, Aichholzer M, Edwin Thanarajah S, Vargas-Cáceres S, Matura S, et al. Comorbidity of ADHD and adult bipolar disorder: a systematic review and meta-analysis. Neurosci Biobehav Rev. 2021;124:100–23.
4. Karaahmet E, Konuk N, Dalkilic A, Saracli O, Atasoy N, Kurçer MA, et al. The comorbidity of adult attention-deficit/hyperactivity disorder in bipolar disorder patients. Compr Psychiatry. 2013;54:549–55.
5. McIntyre RS, Kennedy SH, Soczynska JK, Nguyen HT, Bilkey TS, Woldeyohannes HO, et al. Attention deficit/hyperactivity disorder in adults with bipolar disorder or major depressive disorder: results from the international mood disorders collaborative project. Prim Care Companion J Clin Psychiatry. 2010:12.
6. Perugi G, Ceraudo G, Vannucchi G, Rizzato S, Toni C, Dell'Osso L. Attention deficit/hyperactivity disorder symptoms in Italian bipolar adult patients: a preliminary report. J Affect Disord. 2013;149:430–4.
7. Axelson D, Birmaher B, Strober M, Gill MK, Valeri S, Chiappetta L, et al. Phenomenology of children and adolescents with bipolar spectrum disorders. Arch Gen Psychiatry. 2006;63:1139–48.
8. Geller B, Zimerman B, Williams M, Delbello MP, Bolhofner K, Craney JL, et al. DSM-IV mania symptoms in a prepubertal and early adolescent bipolar disorder phenotype compared to attention-deficit hyperactive and normal controls. J Child Adolesc Psychopharmacol. 2002;12:11–25.
9. Kowatch RA, Youngstrom EA, Danielyan A, Findling RL. Review and meta-analysis of the phenomenology and clinical characteristics of mania in children and adolescents. Bipolar Disord. 2005;7:483–96.
10. Torrente F, López P, Lischinsky A, Cetkovich-Bakmas M, Manes F. Depressive symptoms and the role of affective temperament in adults with attention-deficit/hyperactivity disorder (ADHD): a comparison with bipolar disorder. J Affect Disord. 2017;221:304–11.
11. Doerfler LA, Connor DF, Toscano PF Jr. Aggression, ADHD symptoms, and dysphoria in children and adolescents diagnosed with bipolar disorder and ADHD. J Affect Disord. 2011;131:312–9.
12. Geller B, Warner K, Williams M, Zimerman B. Prepubertal and young adolescent bipolarity versus ADHD: assessment and validity using the WASH-U-KSADS, CBCL and TRF. J Affect Disord. 1998;51:93–100.
13. Birmaher B, Axelson D, Strober M, Gill MK, Valeri S, Chiappetta L, et al. Clinical course of children and

adolescents with bipolar spectrum disorders. Arch Gen Psychiatry. 2006;63:175–83.
14. Axelson DA, Birmaher B, Findling RL, Fristad MA, Kowatch RA, Youngstrom EA, et al. Concerns regarding the inclusion of temper dysregulation disorder with dysphoria in the diagnostic and statistical manual of mental disorders, Fifth Edition. J Clin Psychiatry. 2011;72:1257–62.
15. Leibenluft E, Charney DS, Towbin KE, Bhangoo RK, Pine DS. Defining clinical phenotypes of juvenile mania. Am J Psychiatry. 2003;160:430–7.
16. Wozniak J, Biederman J, Kiely K, Ablon JS, Faraone SV, Mundy E, et al. Mania-like symptoms suggestive of childhood-onset bipolar disorder in clinically referred children. J Am Acad Child Adolesc Psychiatry. 1995;34:867–76.
17. Soutullo CA, DelBello MP, Ochsner JE, McElroy SL, Taylor SA, Strakowski SM, et al. Severity of bipolarity in hospitalized manic adolescents with a history of stimulant or antidepressant treatment. J Affect Disord. 2002;70:323–7.
18. Brancati GE, Perugi G, Milone A, Masi G, Sesso G. Development of bipolar disorder in patients with attention-deficit/hyperactivity disorder: a systematic review and meta-analysis of prospective studies. J Affect Disord. 2021;293:186–96.
19. Faraone SV, Biederman J, Wozniak J, Mundy E, Mennin D, O'Donnell D. Is comorbidity with ADHD a marker for juvenile-onset mania? J Am Acad Child Adolesc Psychiatry. 1997;36:1046–55.
20. Kessler RC, Adler L, Barkley R, Biederman J, Conners CK, Demler O, et al. The prevalence and correlates of adult ADHD in the United States: results from the National Comorbidity Survey Replication. Am J Psychiatry. 2006;163:716–23.
21. Duffy A. The nature of the association between childhood ADHD and the development of bipolar disorder: a review of prospective high-risk studies. Am J Psychiatry. 2012;169:1247–55.
22. Biederman J, Faraone SV, Petty C, Martelon MK, Woodworth KY, Wozniak J. Further evidence that pediatric-onset bipolar disorder comorbid with ADHD represents a distinct subtype: results from a large controlled family study. J Psychiatr Res. 2013;47:15.
23. van Hulzen KJE, Scholz CJ, Franke B, Ripke S, Klein M, McQuillin A, et al. Genetic overlap between attention-deficit/hyperactivity disorder and bipolar disorder: evidence from genome-wide association study meta analysis. Biol Psychiatry. 2017;82:634–41.
24. Biederman J, Mick E, Bostic JQ. The naturalistic course of pharmacologic treatment of children with manic-like symptoms: a systematic chart review. J Clin Psychiatry. 1998;59:628–37.
25. DelBello MP, Soutullo CA, Hendricks W, Niemeier RT, McElroy SL, Strakowski SM. Prior stimulant treatment in adolescents with bipolar disorder: association with age at onset. Bipolar Disord. 2001;3:53–7.
26. Dell'Osso B, Ketter TA. Use of adjunctive stimulants in adult bipolar depression. Int J Neuropsychopharmacol. 2013;16:55–68.
27. Scheffer RE, Kowatch RA, Carmody T, Rush AJ. Randomized, placebo-controlled trial of mixed amphetamine salts for symptoms of comorbid ADHD in pediatric bipolar disorder after mood stabilization with divalproex sodium. Am J Psychiatry. 2005;162:58–64.
28. Zeni CP, Tramontina S, Ketzer CR, Pheula GF, Rohde LA. Methylphenidate combined with aripiprazole in children and adolescents with bipolar disorder and attention-deficit/hyperactivity disorder: a randomized crossover trial. J Child Adolesc Psychopharmacol. 2009;19:553–61.
29. Chang K, Nayar D, Howe M, Rana M. Atomoxetine as an adjunct therapy in the treatment of co-morbid attention deficit/ hyperactivity disorder in children and adolescents with bipolar I or II disorder. J Child Adolesc Psychopharmacol. 2009;19:547–51.
30. Kratochvil CJ, Milton DR, Vaughan BS, Greenhill LL. Acute atomoxetine treatment of younger and older children with ADHD: a meta-analysis of tolerability and efficacy. Child Adolesc Psychiatry Ment Health. 2008;2:25.
31. Verbeeck W, Tuinier S, Bekkering GE. Antidepressants in the treatment of adult attention-deficit hyperactivity disorder: a systematic review. Adv Ther. 2009;26:170–84.
32. Perugi G, Toni C, Ruffolo G, Frare F, Akiskal H. Adjunctive dopamine agonists in treatment-resistant bipolar II depression: an open case series. Pharmacopsychiatry. 2001;34:137–41.
33. Burdick KE, Braga RJ, Nnadi CU, Shaya Y, Stearns WH, Malhotra AK. Placebo-controlled adjunctive trial of pramipexole in patients with bipolar disorder: targeting cognitive dysfunction. J Clin Psychiatry. 2012;73:103–12.
34. Goldberg JF. Adverse cognitive effects of psychotropic medications. In: Burdick KE, Goldberg JF, editors. Cognitive dysfunction in bipolar disorder: a guide for clinicians. Arlington: American Psychiatric Publishing; 2008. p. 137–58.
35. Dorrego MF, Canevaro L, Kuzis G, Sabe L, Starkstein SE. A randomized, double-blind, crossover study of methylphenidate and lithium in adults with attention-deficit/hyperactivity disorder: preliminary findings. J Neuropsychiatry Clin Neurosci. 2002;14:289–95.
36. Blader JC, Schooler NR, Jensen PS, Pliszka SR, Kafantaris V. Adjunctive divalproex versus placebo for children with ADHD and aggression refractory to stimulant monotherapy. Am J Psychiatry. 2009;166:1392–401.
37. Nair V, Mahadevan S. Randomised controlled study: efficacy of clonidine versus carbamazepine in children with ADHD. J Trop Pediatr. 2009;55:116–21.
38. Tramontina S, Zeni CP, Ketzer CR, Pheula GF, Narvaez J, Rohde LA. Aripiprazole in children and adolescents with bipolar disorder comorbid with attention-deficit/hyperactivity disorder: a pilot randomized clinical trial. J Clin Psychiatry. 2009;70:756–64.

Obesity and Metabolic Syndrome in Bipolar Disorder

10

Sung Hoon Yoon and Young Sup Woo

Introduction

Over the past two decades, numerous studies have investigated the relationship between various metabolic disorders, including obesity, insulin resistance, dyslipidemia, and bipolar disorder. These studies have consistently demonstrated a clear link between the two, suggesting substantial overlap in their underlying pathophysiological mechanisms. Epidemiologically, the prevalence of metabolic syndrome, which encompasses abdominal obesity, insulin resistance or glucose intolerance, hypertension, and dyslipidemia, among patients with bipolar disorder has been reported to range from 20 to 65%, with a meta-analysis estimating an average prevalence of approximately 37 [1]. This is nearly twice the prevalence observed in the general population.

Metabolic syndrome and related metabolic disorders not only increase the risk of cardiovascular disease and type 2 diabetes but are also associated with greater medical risks like premature mortality. Additionally, they are known to negatively affect the course and prognosis of bipolar disorder [2–4]. Of particular importance is the fact that bipolar disorder and metabolic disorders share overlapping pathogenic mechanisms, and that medications commonly used to treat bipolar disorder may themselves contribute to the development of metabolic disturbances [5, 6].

This chapter aims to review the evidence regarding the comorbidity of obesity, metabolic disorders, and metabolic syndrome in individuals with bipolar disorder, and to summarize the key pathophysiological features that may underlie these associations.

Obesity

Obesity is commonly observed among individuals with psychiatric disorders, including those with bipolar disorder. While it remains unclear whether obesity represents a more serious issue in patients with mental illness or bipolar disorder specifically compared to the general population, several findings suggest that it may be particularly relevant in this group. For example, studies have reported that up to 90% of individuals undergoing surgical treatment for severe obesity fall within the bipolar spectrum, with bipolar II disorder being the most prevalent subtype [7]. These findings highlight the clinical importance of addressing obesity in bipolar disorder.

The prevalence of obesity among individuals with bipolar disorder varies depending on the characteristics of the study population and the diagnostic criteria used, with rates reported as

S. H. Yoon
Department of Psychiatry, Wonkwang University Hospital, School of Medicine, Iksan, Republic of Korea

Y. S. Woo (✉)
Woo and Bahk Psychiatry Clinic, Seoul, Republic of Korea
e-mail: woo.youngsup@hotmail.com

W.-M. Bahk et al. (eds.), *Bipolar Disorder*, https://doi.org/10.1007/978-981-92-1323-8_10

high as 55.4%. A recent meta-analysis found that the prevalence of obesity, defined as a body mass index (BMI) ≥ 30, was 29.0%, approximately twice that observed in the general population. Abdominal obesity, in particular, was found in 51% of individuals with bipolar disorder [8]. Conversely, the prevalence of bipolar disorder among individuals with obesity has been reported to range from 3 to 11%. A recent meta-analysis reported a significantly increased odds ratio of 1.32, indicating that bipolar disorder is more common in obese individuals than in the general population [9]. An umbrella review of 12 meta-analyses including approximately 60 million participants found that individuals with bipolar disorder have a 1.6 -fold increased likelihood of obesity compared with the general population [10]. Moreover, the association appears bidirectional: bipolar disorder confers a 1.68-fold higher odds of subsequent obesity, whereas obesity is linked to a 1.32-fold greater odds of developing bipolar disorder [9].

One of the most prominent factors contributing to obesity in patients with bipolar disorder is the effect of medications. Commonly prescribed pharmacological agents such as lithium, valproate, and antipsychotics are well known to promote weight gain. In addition, individuals with bipolar disorder often engage in unhealthy lifestyle behaviors, including irregular eating patterns, poor dietary quality, and physical inactivity. The risk of being overweight or obese increases with a chronic course and longer illness duration [11], particularly in the presence of depressive episodes [12]. While overall obesity is not strongly associated with sex, abdominal obesity is more frequently observed in women, and obese women have a heightened risk of experiencing atypical major depressive episodes [8, 13].

Eating disorders, which frequently co-occur with bipolar disorder, are also associated with increased carbohydrate intake and decreased physical activity, both of which contribute to overweight and obesity. However, eating disorders alone cannot fully account for the observed weight gain [12]. When bipolar disorder is accompanied by obesity, the clinical course tends to be more severe and chronic, with greater functional impairment, increased suicide risk, and more frequently accompanied by comorbid anxiety disorders compared to those without obesity [5]. Furthermore, overweight or obese individuals with bipolar disorder exhibit more pronounced cognitive impairment than their normal-weight counterparts [14].

Dyslipidemia

Dyslipidemia is typically defined as hypertriglyceridemia (serum triglycerides ≥150 mg/dL) and/or low levels of high-density lipoprotein cholesterol (HDL-C), defined as <40 mg/dL in men and <50 mg/dL in women. Increased serum lipid levels in patients with bipolar disorder have been reported since the 1960s [15]. Since then, the reported prevalence of dyslipidemia in bipolar disorder has varied widely across studies, ranging from 1 to 57%, depending on the definitions applied. In a Korean study, dyslipidemia was observed in 21% of hospitalized patients with bipolar I disorder [16]. When data from international studies are aggregated, the prevalence is estimated at approximately 17%, which is comparable to that seen in individuals with schizophrenia and nearly ten times higher than in the general population [17]. Indeed, one study reported that 16% of individuals with bipolar disorder or schizophrenia were prescribed lipid-lowering medications, compared to only 10% in the general population [18]. The high comorbidity of dyslipidemia in bipolar disorder is likely influenced by the use of atypical antipsychotics [19].

Diabetes Mellitus

The high comorbidity of diabetes mellitus among individuals with bipolar disorder has been recognized since the early twentieth century [20]. International studies have reported comorbidity rates of up to 44% in patients with bipolar disorder, and one Korean study found a comparable rate of 43.5% [16]. While some studies have suggested that the prevalence of diabetes in patients with bipolar disorder is not significantly higher than that in the general population, other research has shown that 10% of individuals with bipolar disorder or schizophrenia were taking antidiabetic medications, compared to only 6% in the general population [18]. This difference suggests that diabetes comorbidity is indeed more common in bipolar disorder.

A recent meta-analysis estimated the prevalence of type 2 diabetes among patients with bipolar disorder is approximately 9.6%, which is about 1.6 times higher than that in age- and sex-matched controls. Furthermore, impaired fasting glucose (IFG), defined as fasting blood glucose levels ≥100 mg/dL, was observed in 22.4% of bipolar patients; when IFG was defined using a threshold of ≥110 mg/dL, the prevalence was 14.8%. For comparison, the prevalence of IFG based on the 110 mg/dL threshold in the general European population is reported to be 10.1% in men and 5.9% in women [8]. Further reinforcing these findings, a comprehensive umbrella review of 12 meta-analyses ($N \approx 60$ million) reported an equivalent odds ratio of 1.98 for type 2 diabetes in individuals with bipolar disorder relative to controls [10].

The age at first hospitalization for bipolar disorder and the overall illness duration do not appear to be associated with the development of diabetes [21]. However, glucose intolerance, insulin resistance, and diabetes mellitus may all be linked to pharmacologic treatments commonly used in bipolar disorder, including lithium, valproate, and atypical antipsychotics.

Hypertension

Hypertension is generally defined as a systolic blood pressure ≥130 mm Hg or a diastolic blood pressure ≥85 mm Hg. Among patients with bipolar disorder, the reported prevalence of hypertension varies from 2.5 to 67.5%. Although several studies have suggested that the prevalence of hypertension is higher in individuals with bipolar disorder compared to the general population, other studies have not found a significant difference. When data from multiple studies are combined, the estimated prevalence is approximately 15%, which is comparable to that observed in patients with major depressive disorder and in the general population [17]. A large-scale meta-analysis, encompassing data from around 60 million individuals, underscored this link showing that bipolar disorder is associated with a 1.28-fold increased likelihood of hypertension compared with controls [10].

Metabolic Syndrome

Metabolic syndrome is a cluster of metabolic abnormalities including abdominal obesity, glucose intolerance, hypertension, and dyslipidemia that is strongly associated with an increased risk of cardiovascular disease. The World Health Organization (WHO) first proposed diagnostic criteria for metabolic syndrome. Subsequently, modified definitions were introduced by several organizations to improve ease of use and enhance predictive accuracy for cardiovascular risk. These include the European Group for the Study of Insulin Resistance (EGIR), the National Cholesterol Education Program—Third Adult Treatment Panel (NCEP ATP III), the American College of Endocrinology (ACE)/American Association of Clinical Endocrinologists (AACE), and the International Diabetes Federation (IDF). In addition, the American Heart Association and the National Heart, Lung, and Blood Institute (AHA/NHLBI) published a revised version based on the NCEP ATP III criteria. Most recently, in 2009, a joint statement from the ATP III and IDF harmonized the existing diagnostic criteria [22].

The major diagnostic criteria for metabolic syndrome are summarized in Table 10.1 [23]. The variety of definitions reflects ongoing efforts to develop criteria that can accurately predict cardiovascular disease and diabetes mellitus. In fact, the distribution of adipose tissue may be a more important predictor than overall obesity. Measurements such as waist-to-hip ratio (WHR) and waist circumference may predict the risk of hypertension, coronary artery disease, and diabetes more effectively than body mass index (BMI).

Table 10.1 Diagnostic criteria for metabolic syndrome

Criterion	WHO (1998)	NCEP ATP III (2001)	IDF (2005)	AHA/NHLBI (2005)	ATP III / IDF Harmonized (2009)
Definition of metabolic syndrome	Insulin resistance +2 or more components	3 or more of 5 components	Central obesity +2 or more components	3 or more of 5 components	3 or more of 5 components
Insulin resistance / hyperglycemia	Impaired glucose tolerance, impaired fasting glucose, or reduced insulin sensitivity	Fasting glucose >110 mg/dL (revised to >100 mg/dL in 2004), or diabetes	Fasting glucose ≥100 mg/dL, or diabetes	Fasting glucose ≥100 mg/dL or under treatment	Fasting glucose ≥100 mg/dL or under treatment
Obesity / body weight	WHR >0.90 (M), >0.85 (F) and/or BMI >30 kg/m^2	WC ≥102 cm (M), ≥88 cm (F)	WC above population-specific threshold	WC ≥102 cm (M), ≥88 cm (F)	WC above population-specific threshold
Dyslipidemia	TG ≥150 mg/dL and/or HDL-C < 35 mg/dL (M), <39 mg/dL (F)	TG ≥150 mg/dL; HDL-C < 40 mg/dL (M), <50 mg/dL (F)	TG ≥150 mg/dL or under treatment; HDL-C < 40 mg/dL (M), <50 mg/dL (F) or under treatment	Same as IDF	Same as IDF
Blood pressure	≥140/90 mmHg	≥130/85 mmHg	Systolic ≥130 mmHg or diastolic ≥85 mmHg or under treatment	Same as IDF	Same as IDF
Other criteria	Microalbuminuria	–	–	–	–

WHO World Health Organization, *NCEP ATP III* National Cholesterol Education Program-Third Adult Treatment Panel, *IDF* International Diabetes Federation, *AHA* American Heart Association, *NHLBI* National Heart Lung and Blood Institute; *BMI* body mass index, *TG* triglyceride, *HDL-C* high-density lipoprotein-cholesterol, *WC* waist circumference, *WHR* waist-hip ratio, *M* male, *F* female

In patients with bipolar disorder, excess fat tends to accumulate centrally, making it particularly useful to assess waist circumference in addition to BMI. For Korean populations, the diagnostic thresholds include abdominal obesity defined as a waist circumference ≥ 90 cm in men or ≥ 85 cm in women; elevated blood pressure defined as systolic ≥130 mmHg and/or diastolic ≥85 mmHg or current use of antihypertensive medication; elevated fasting glucose ≥100 mg/dL or ongoing treatment for hyperglycemia; low HDL-C (<40 mg/dL in men, <50 mg/dL in women) or treatment for low HDL-C; and elevated triglycerides ≥150 mg/dL or treatment for hypertriglyceridemia [24].

The prevalence of metabolic syndrome in Western populations is estimated to range from approximately 15–25%, while in Korea, it has been reported to be around 30% [24]. The prevalence increases with age and is more common in women. As previously mentioned, the comorbidity of metabolic syndrome in individuals with bipolar disorder is significantly higher ranging from 20 to 65% in international studies and approximately 37% according to a meta-analysis [1]. This elevated rate, roughly two to three times higher than that in the general population, appears to be consistent across different regions of the world [25].

The prevalence of metabolic syndrome increases with the duration of bipolar illness, which may reflect either illness-specific mechanism or, more likely, age-related physiological changes [26]. As noted earlier, not only is metabolic syndrome more common in individuals with bipolar disorder, but its constituent components are also frequently observed. Notably, hypertriglyceridemia and hypertension are the most prevalent, with hypertriglyceridemia and abdominal obesity identified as the most robust predictors of metabolic syndrome in this population [27].

The presence of metabolic syndrome adversely affects the overall course of bipolar disorder. One study found that patients with rapid-cycling bipolar disorder and co-occurring metabolic abnormalities, including obesity, experienced more severe depressive symptoms and responded poorly to treatment [28]. Another study reported that abdominal obesity negatively influenced the severity of bipolar symptoms and overall functional outcomes [29]. In individuals with both bipolar disorder and metabolic syndrome, recovery rates were reduced, episode frequency increased, and suicide attempts were more common [30].

Furthermore, metabolic syndrome has been associated with greater cognitive impairment in patients with bipolar disorder, which may negatively impact treatment response and illness trajectory [31]. Even in euthymic bipolar patients, higher BMI was negatively correlated with cognitive domains such as attention and psychomotor speed, and overweight or obese individuals exhibited significantly lower verbal fluency than their normal-weight counterparts [14].

Taken together, the metabolic comorbidities reviewed above, obesity, dyslipidemia, impaired glucose regulation, diabetes, and hypertension, frequently co-occur in bipolar disorder and can amplify one another over time. Metabolic syndrome is common in bipolar disorder, and its relevance becomes especially clear in routine practice where weight and metabolic change often intersect with the illness course and treatment exposure [1, 30]. Viewed together, the preceding sections describe a coherent clinical pattern in bipolar disorder: weight gain and metabolic change often unfold alongside illness course and treatment exposure, with downstream abnormalities spanning lipids, glycemic regulation, and blood pressure—an observation consistent with the possibility that shared biological pathways may contribute to this pattern.

Beyond comorbidity, metabolic dysregulation in bipolar disorder has been associated in some studies with a greater overall burden of illness and less favorable outcomes and may also be linked to cognitive vulnerabilities such as reduced executive function [14, 30, 31].

With this clinical framework in mind, the next section shifts from describing the individual components to examining shared biological pathways that have been proposed to link bipolar disorder with metabolic syndrome, while noting that much of the evidence remains observational.

The Association Between Metabolic Syndrome and Bipolar Disorder

The association between bipolar disorder and metabolic syndrome, or broader metabolic abnormalities including obesity, is well established. Various factors, such as limited access to healthcare, behavioral characteristics, shared neurobiological alterations, and genetic vulnerability, have been proposed as contributing factors to this comorbidity. However, the precise pathophysiological mechanisms underlying this comorbidity remain unclear (Fig. 10.1).

Pharmacological factors are among the primary considerations when explaining the high prevalence of metabolic syndrome and related metabolic disorders in individuals with bipolar disorder. One study found that the prevalence of metabolic syndrome was 2.3 times higher in bipolar patients treated with antipsychotics compared to the general population, highlighting the potential risk posed by atypical antipsychotics used in the treatment of bipolar disorder [32]. A meta-analysis reported a significantly higher prevalence of metabolic syndrome among patients taking antipsychotic medications (45.3%) compared to those not taking antipsychotics (32.4%) [1]. Recent studies have suggested that psychotropic medications may influence metabolic risk, *potentially* through changes in gene expression [9].

However, it is important to note that the relationship between obesity and bipolar depression was reported as early as the Kraepelin era—prior

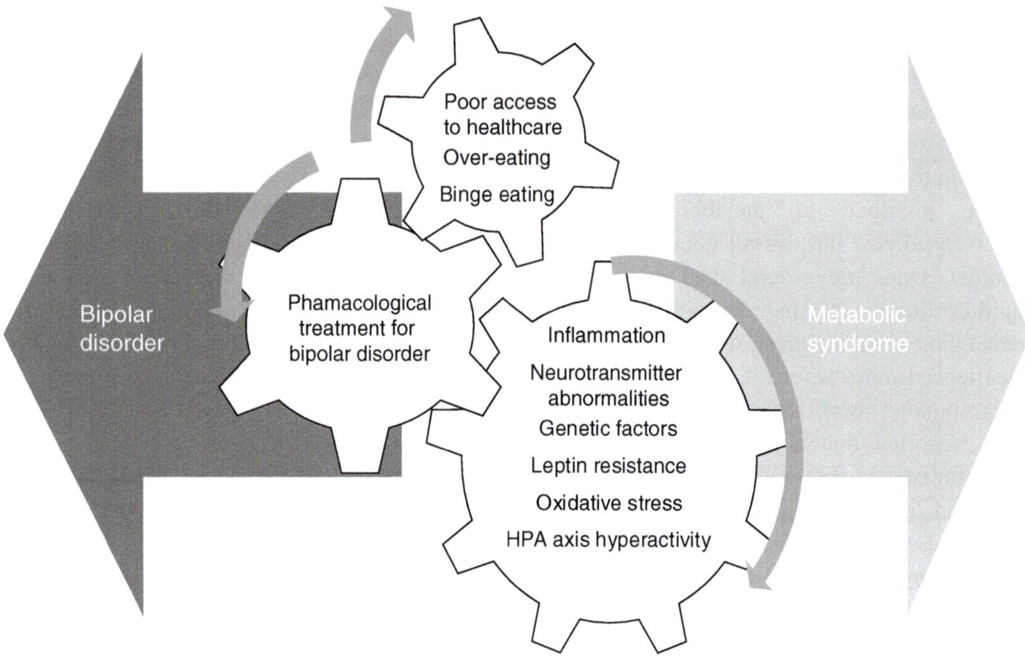

Fig. 10.1 Pathophysiological link between bipolar disorder and metabolic syndrome

to the introduction of pharmacological treatment. Additionally, several studies have shown elevated rates of metabolic abnormalities, such as dyslipidemia and insulin resistance, even in drug-naïve patients with bipolar disorder [12, 33]. These findings suggest that the development of metabolic syndrome in bipolar disorder may not be due solely to pharmacotherapy, but rather to an interaction between medication effects and an inherent metabolic vulnerability in this population.

From a behavioral perspective, individuals with bipolar disorder often experience functional impairment, unemployment, and financial difficulties. These factors are associated with unhealthy lifestyle habits and difficulties in weight management, thereby increasing the risk of metabolic disturbances. Moreover, limited access to healthcare may delay preventive or early interventions [34]. Symptoms of bipolar depression, such as overeating, fatigue, lethargy, and sleep disturbances, further reduce physical activity levels and contribute to overeating and obesity [35]. Binge eating, a common comorbidity in bipolar disorder, is strongly associated with depressive symptoms and obesity. While metabolic syndrome is frequently observed in patients with binge eating disorder, this relationship appears to extend beyond the effects of obesity alone [36, 37].

Recent research suggests that metabolic network dysregulation—including alterations in insulin-glucose homeostasis, inflammatory responses, and adipokine synthesis—may play a critical role in mood disorders [38]. A growing body of evidence has identified inflammation as a mediator linking metabolic abnormalities with depressive and bipolar disorders [39, 40]. Chronic, subclinical inflammation is known to impair insulin sensitivity and promote metabolic syndrome, particularly in mechanistic and experimental studies. In animal models, pro-inflammatory cytokines have been shown to induce insulin resistance. In humans, levels of inflammatory markers such as C-reactive protein (CRP) are elevated during acute episodes of bipolar disorder and decrease during remission, although they may not return fully to baseline [41, 42]. Elevated CRP has also been associated with the presence of comorbid metabolic syndrome in bipolar patients [43].

Genetic predispositions related to inflammation have also been observed in bipolar disorder. Compared to the general population, individuals with bipolar disorder are more likely to exhibit variants in inflammation-related genes such as CASP1 and STAT. CASP1 is involved in the production of interleukin-1β, while STAT encodes transcription factors that regulate the inflammatory response [44, 45]. Variants in genes associated with innate immunity have also been identified in bipolar disorder, including homozygosity for the TLR4 rs1927914 A and rs11536891 T alleles, which are more frequently found in early-onset bipolar disorder [46]. In contrast, the NOC2 rs2066482 polymorphism is rarely seen in bipolar patients. This finding may help explain the increased incidence and earlier onset of inflammatory bowel disease (IBD) in individuals with bipolar disorder compared to those without it [47, 48].

In addition, the adipocyte-derived hormone leptin has been proposed as a potential link between obesity and depression [49]. Leptin regulates appetite and energy expenditure, and animal studies have demonstrated its antidepressant effects. However, in individuals with obesity, leptin resistance may attenuate these beneficial effects [49]. Other proposed mechanisms that may contribute to the relationship between bipolar disorder and metabolic abnormalities include oxidative stress, sympathetic nervous system activation, platelet activation, endothelial dysfunction, and dysregulation of the hypothalamic–pituitary–adrenal (HPA) axis [50]. In parallel, insulin levels have also been shown to be elevated in euthymic bipolar patients compared with healthy controls, further implicating dysregulated appetite-regulating hormones in the shared neurobiology of mood and metabolic disturbances [51]. Interestingly, adiponectin, which is a hormone with anti-inflammatory and vasoprotective properties, did not differ overall between bipolar and control groups, but was positively correlated with both longer illness duration and a higher proportion of bipolar I disorder [51]. Given adiponectin's role in enhancing endothelial function and improving insulin sensitivity [52], reductions in its activity over the course of illness may be associated with a progressively less favorable cardiometabolic risk profile in bipolar disorder. In other words, while leptin and insulin dysregulation may be linked to early metabolic disturbance, diminished adiponectin-related protective effects with chronic illness may contribute to blood pressure and vascular risk in this population. Patients with mood disorders, including bipolar disorder, frequently experience chronic stress due to both environmental factors such as early-life adversity and persistent illness-related stressors. These chronic stress exposures may be associated with biological changes that affect both mood symptoms and metabolic risk factors. In individuals with bipolar disorder, cortisol levels are elevated across all mood states—including euthymia, depression, and mania [53]. Notably, cortisol levels are even higher in those with rapid cycling, a history of suicide attempts, or frequent relapses [54, 55].

Chronic HPA axis hyperactivation in bipolar disorder has been associated with impaired glucocorticoid signaling and a blunted response to cortisol [56, 57]. Under normal conditions, glucocorticoid receptor activation exerts anti-inflammatory effects. However, glucocorticoid receptor resistance in the context of chronic stress may disrupt this negative feedback mechanism and may result in sustained immune activation [58]. Chronically elevated cortisol levels have been linked to weight gain and insulin resistance in bipolar disorder [59–61].

Childhood trauma and adverse early-life experiences are also associated with bipolar disorder and elevated levels of inflammatory cytokines. More than half of adult patients with bipolar disorder report a history of childhood abuse, and such individuals are more likely to experience early onset of illness, increased suicide risk, rapid cycling, and psychotic symptoms [62, 63]. Because the brain and immune system are still developing during childhood, early stress may have long-lasting effects and has been proposed to involve epigenetic modifications that may affect neuroplasticity and may contribute to chronic inflammation, glucocorticoid receptor dysfunction, and HPA-axis hyperactivation [64].

Dopamine dysregulation may also play an important role. In bipolar disorder, dopamine transporter function in the striatum is reduced [65], and dopaminergic agents have shown efficacy in treating bipolar depression. Dysfunction of the dopaminergic system is also observed in obesity and binge eating disorder. Furthermore, dopamine D2 receptor agonists have been shown to improve metabolic parameters in patients with obesity and diabetes, including blood glucose levels, resting energy expenditure, systolic blood pressure, lipid profiles, and overall glycemic control [66].

Collectively, these findings underscore the complexity of the relationship between bipolar disorder and metabolic syndrome, which appears to arise from the convergence of multiple pathophysiological pathways.

Management of Metabolic Syndrome and Metabolic Disorders in Patients with Bipolar Disorder

In clinical practice, management of metabolic syndrome and related metabolic disorders in bipolar disorder is best approached in a stepwise manner, beginning with systematic screening and monitoring and early implementation of lifestyle interventions. When clinically feasible, clinicians should also consider optimizing the psychotropic regimen—through dose adjustment, simplification, or switching to lower metabolic-risk agents—while adjunctive pharmacotherapy and specialist referral can be guided by established cardiometabolic recommendations. Where available, evidence from bipolar disorder populations is highlighted, while management of dyslipidemia, hypertension, and diabetes often draws on broader population-based guidance. Accordingly, the discussion below first addresses bipolar disorder–specific strategies—particularly lifestyle interventions and psychotropic optimization/weight-mitigation—and then summarizes management of dyslipidemia, hypertension, and diabetes, which generally follows population-based cardiometabolic guidelines.

According to international studies, over 60% of patients with comorbid bipolar disorder and metabolic syndrome or related metabolic disorders remained untreated [27]. Even among those receiving treatment, the proportion achieving adequate metabolic control remains low. In general populations with metabolic syndrome, effective management of blood pressure and lipid parameters has been shown to reduce the incidence of cardiovascular disease by nearly 50%, underscoring the importance of actively addressing these conditions in patients with bipolar disorder.

Despite this clinical need, research on the treatment of metabolic disorders specifically in bipolar populations remains limited. Because bipolar disorder–specific evidence for treating dyslipidemia, hypertension, and diabetes remains limited, treatment targets and pharmacologic strategies are commonly adapted from general population guidelines, with attention to bipolar-specific considerations such as relapse risk, cumulative treatment exposure, and drug–drug interactions. For patients with bipolar disorder who are at risk for metabolic disorders, careful monitoring of body mass index (BMI), waist circumference, serum lipid levels, and fasting glucose is warranted—especially in those receiving antipsychotic medications. Importantly, dyslipidemia can occur independently of BMI, necessitating regular screening even in patients who are of normal weight or not taking medications associated with weight gain.

When treating individuals with bipolar disorder, it is advisable to select medications that are both effective in managing mood symptoms and associated with a lower risk of weight gain or metabolic abnormalities. Clinicians should weigh the severity of mood symptoms, the patient's physical health history (including baseline metabolic risk factors), prior medication use, and the potential side effects of treatment when conducting a risk–benefit analysis to guide pharmacologic decisions. Alongside pharmacologic decision-making, lifestyle modification should be initiated early, particularly when depressive symptoms, sleep disturbance, or treatment exposure increases metabolic risk. Lifestyle interventions and adherence to a Mediterranean-style dietary pattern have been associated with reduced cardiometabolic risk and improvements in depressive symptoms in some studies [67, 68]. Although smoking cessation is known to increase the risk of weight gain [69], subsequent research has demonstrated that it nonetheless lowers cardiovascular risk despite modest weight increases [70].

Weight management in bipolar disorder relies heavily on lifestyle changes, including the promotion of sleep hygiene. In the Korean Medication Algorithm Project for Bipolar Disorder (KMAP-BP 2022), lifestyle interventions such as exercise and dietary control are strongly recommended as first-line strategies for patients with weight-related concerns [71]. Reductions in body weight and abdominal obesity also contribute positively to other components of metabolic syndrome. In line with international practice, the Canadian Network for Mood and Anxiety Treatments together with the International Society for Bipolar Disorders (CANMAT & ISBD 2018) guidelines, the Royal Australian and New Zealand College of Psychiatrists' Mood Disorders Clinical Practice Guideline (RANZCP 2020), and the UK's National Institute for Health and Care Excellence (NICE) Guideline (2020 update) all concur that lifestyle modification must serve as the first-line intervention for metabolic syndrome in patients receiving bipolar disorder treatments [72–74]. Specifically, they recommend initiating structured programs of dietary counseling (emphasizing a Mediterranean-style or heart-healthy diet), regular physical activity, sleep hygiene, and smoking cessation at the earliest signs of metabolic disturbance. Only if these measures prove insufficient after a defined trial period (typically 3–6 months) should clinicians consider optimizing the psychotropic regimen (e.g., switching to a lower–metabolic–risk agent when clinically feasible) and/or adding adjunctive weight-mitigation pharmacotherapy (e.g., metformin, topiramate, or GLP-1 receptor agonists) [72–74].

If the patient is in a stable phase of bipolar disorder, a medication switch may be considered, provided that relapse risk is carefully evaluated and the alternative agent has a lower propensity for weight gain. If switching is not feasible, adjunctive pharmacologic interventions aimed at weight reduction may be considered. Evidence for bupropion as a weight-mitigation strategy in bipolar depression is limited; however, it may indirectly support weight management by reducing fatigue and overeating in some patients.

Recent meta-analyses suggest that medications such as topiramate, zonisamide, metformin, glucagon-like peptide-1 receptor agonists (GLP-1RAs), and nizatidine are effective in mitigating antipsychotic-induced weight gain [75]. Furthermore, bariatric surgery can be highly effective in cases of severe obesity and may be considered for patients with bipolar disorder following a thorough psychiatric and medical evaluation. For the remaining components of metabolic syndrome, evidence specific to bipolar disorder is limited; therefore, management typically follows general cardiometabolic guidelines, with attention to psychotropic interactions and illness-related factors.

Even in cases where dyslipidemia, hypertension, and hyperglycemia are present, lifestyle modification should be the first-line intervention. The importance of healthy eating, regular physical activity, and adequate sleep cannot be overstated. When necessary, pharmacologic interventions such as lipid-lowering agents, antihypertensive medications, or antidiabetic drugs may be considered, typically following cardiometabolic guidelines used in the general population.

For dyslipidemia, commonly used agents include statins (inhibitors of beta-hydroxymethylglutaryl-coenzyme A [HMG-CoA] reductase), fibric acid derivatives, nicotinic acid, and bile acid sequestrants. Concerns have been raised about potential increases in depression and suicide risk associated with statin use. However, a large-scale study involving over 20,000 patients reported no significant difference in suicide risk between statin-treated and placebo groups [76]. Another study even suggested that statin therapy may reduce the risk of depression [77]. When selecting lipid-lowering therapy, clinicians should also consider the overall medication burden and potential drug–drug interactions in patients receiving long-term psychotropic treatment.

Nutritional supplements such as omega-3 fatty acids have been shown to lower triglyceride (TG) levels, increase high-density lipoprotein cholesterol (HDL-C), and improve depressive symptoms. A meta-analysis found that adjunctive treatment with omega-3 fatty acids improved depressive symptoms in patients with bipolar disorder [78]. In patients receiving antipsychotic treatment, switching to agents with a lower metabolic risk may help reduce TG and BMI while improving HDL-C. Additionally, combining lipid-lowering agents or omega-3 fatty acids may further improve metabolic profiles.

For hypertension, dietary modifications are essential and should include increased intake of fruits and vegetables, low-fat dairy products, and reduced consumption of salt and saturated fats. Various antihypertensive agents may also be considered. However, caution is required when using certain antihypertensives in patients taking lithium, as thiazide diuretics, loop diuretics, angiotensin-converting enzyme (ACE) inhibitors, and angiotensin receptor blockers (ARBs) can increase the risk of lithium toxicity. Despite initial concerns, more recent studies have shown that beta-blockers do not significantly worsen depressive symptoms [79]. In cases of comorbid hyperglycemia, metformin is the preferred first-line agent, especially in patients treated with atypical antipsychotics, as it improves weight, waist circumference, and insulin resistance. Thiazolidinediones have also been shown to delay the progression to diabetes in insulin-resistant individuals [50].

Glucagon-like peptide-1 receptor agonists (GLP-1RAs)—a class of antidiabetic medications that has gained attention for their weight-reducing properties—have also demonstrated cognitive benefits and antidepressant effects in patients with mood disorders [80, 81]. These findings suggest a potential link between insulin signaling, obesity, and cognitive function and may contribute to a better understanding of the shared pathophysiology underlying the frequent co-occurrence of mood disorders, including bipolar disorder, and metabolic diseases.

Conclusion

Metabolic syndrome and related metabolic disorders are highly prevalent among individuals with bipolar disorder, yet they are often overlooked in clinical practice. Given the nature of bipolar disorder—where depressive episodes tend to be more prolonged than manic or hypomanic episodes—metabolic conditions may exert an even greater impact when co-occurring with depressive symptoms.

Although recent treatment guidelines, including the Korean Medication Algorithm Project for Bipolar Disorder (KMAP-BP 2022), have begun to address the management of metabolic syndrome and metabolic disorders in patients with bipolar disorder, clinical research specifically targeting this population remains limited. Consequently, existing guidelines are largely based on evidence from studies conducted in the general population.

Psychiatrists should be vigilant in assessing the risk of metabolic syndrome and related conditions when treating patients with bipolar disorder. Routine screening and monitoring should be implemented when appropriate. In selecting pharmacologic treatments, clinicians must consider the potential metabolic side effects and weigh them accordingly, particularly in patients at elevated risk for metabolic complications.

For at-risk individuals, lifestyle interventions—such as dietary changes, increased physical activity, and sleep hygiene—are essential. In addition, adjunctive pharmacologic therapies that target metabolic risk factors may also be necessary. Proper identification and management of metabolic syndrome and related disorders can help prevent further comorbidities such as cardiovascular disease and diabetes, while also improving the overall course and prognosis of bipolar disorder.

Declarations

Competing Interests The author(s) has no competing interests to declare that are relevant to the content of this manuscript.

Ethics Approval The author(s) declares that this manuscript does not include primary research with human participants.

The author(s) declares that this manuscript does not include primary studies involving animals.

References

1. Vancampfort D, et al. Metabolic syndrome and metabolic abnormalities in bipolar disorder: a meta-analysis of prevalence rates and moderators. Am J Psychiatry. 2013;170(3):265–74.
2. Gans RO. The metabolic syndrome, depression, and cardiovascular disease: interrelated conditions that share pathophysiologic mechanisms. Med Clin North Am. 2006;90(4):573–91.
3. Taylor V, MacQueen G. Associations between bipolar disorder and metabolic syndrome: a review. J Clin Psychiatry. 2006;67(7):1034–41.
4. Gimenez-Palomo A, et al. Does metabolic syndrome or its component factors alter the course of bipolar disorder? A systematic review. Neurosci Biobehav Rev. 2022;132:142–53.
5. Mansur RB, Brietzke E, McIntyre RS. Is there a "metabolic-mood syndrome"? A review of the relationship between obesity and mood disorders. Neurosci Biobehav Rev. 2015;52:89–104.
6. Kapczinski F, et al. Allostatic load in bipolar disorder: implications for pathophysiology and treatment. Neurosci Biobehav Rev. 2008;32(4):675–92.
7. Alciati A, et al. Bipolar spectrum disorders in severely obese patients seeking surgical treatment. J Affect Disord. 2007;101(1–3):131–8.
8. Liu YK, et al. Prevalence of type 2 diabetes mellitus, impaired fasting glucose, general obesity, and abdominal obesity in patients with bipolar disorder: a systematic review and meta-analysis. J Affect Disord. 2022;300:449–61.
9. Kambey PA, et al. The bi-directional association between bipolar disorder and obesity: evidence from meta and bioinformatics analysis. Int J Obes. 2023;47(6):443–52.
10. Kang J, et al. Comorbid physical health outcomes in patients with bipolar disorder: an umbrella review of systematic reviews and meta-analyses. Asian J Psychiatr. 2024;99:104138.
11. Calkin C, et al. Can body mass index help predict outcome in patients with bipolar disorder? Bipolar Disord. 2009;11(6):650–6.
12. Maina G, et al. Prevalence and correlates of overweight in drug-naive patients with bipolar disorder. J Affect Disord. 2008;110(1–2):149–55.
13. Pickering RP, et al. Are overweight, obesity, and extreme obesity associated with psychopathology? Results from the national epidemiologic survey on alcohol and related conditions. J Clin Psychiatry. 2007;68(7):998–1009.
14. Yim CY, et al. The effect of overweight/obesity on cognitive function in euthymic individuals with bipolar disorder. Eur Psychiatry. 2012;27(3):223–8.
15. Brandrup E, Randrup A. A controlled investigation of plasma lipids in manic-depressives. Br J Psychiatry. 1967;113(502):987–92.
16. Kim B, et al. Correlates of metabolic abnormalities in bipolar I disorder at initiation of acute phase treatment. Psychiatry Investig. 2009;6(2):78–84.
17. Fountoulakis KN. Bipolar Disorder: An Evidence-Based Guide to Manic Depression. Heidelberg: Springer-Verlag; 2015.
18. Bai YM, et al. Risk of developing diabetes mellitus and hyperlipidemia among patients with bipolar disorder, major depressive disorder, and schizophrenia: a 10-year nationwide population-based prospective cohort study. J Affect Disord. 2013;150(1):57–62.
19. Huang TL, Chen JF. Serum lipid profiles and schizophrenia: effects of conventional or atypical antipsychotic drugs in Taiwan. Schizophr Res. 2005;80(1):55–9.
20. Raphael T, Parsons J. Blood sugar studies in dementia praecox and manic-depressive insanity. Arch Neurol Psychiatr. 1921;5(6):687–709.
21. Cassidy F, Ahearn E, Carroll BJ. Elevated frequency of diabetes mellitus in hospitalized manic-depressive patients. Am J Psychiatry. 1999;156(9):1417–20.
22. Alberti KG, et al. Harmonizing the metabolic syndrome: a joint interim statement of the International Diabetes Federation Task Force on Epidemiology and Prevention; National Heart, Lung, and Blood Institute; American Heart Association; World Heart Federation; International Atherosclerosis Society; and International Association for the Study of Obesity. Circulation. 2009;120(16):1640–5.
23. Dommermuth R, Ewing K. Metabolic syndrome: systems thinking in heart disease. Prim Care. 2018;45(1):109–29.
24. Kang H, et al. Clinical practice guideline of prevention and treatment for metabolic syndrome. Korean J Fam Pract. 2015;5(3):375–420.
25. McIntyre RS, et al. Bipolar disorder and metabolic syndrome: an international perspective. J Affect Disord. 2010;126(3):366–87.
26. Salvi V, et al. Age-specific prevalence of metabolic syndrome in Italian patients with bipolar disorder. Psychiatry Clin Neurosci. 2011;65(1):47–54.
27. Correll CU, et al. Findings of a U.S. national cardiometabolic screening program among 10,084 psychiatric outpatients. Psychiatr Serv. 2010;61(9):892–8.

28. Kemp DE, et al. Medical comorbidity in bipolar disorder: relationship between illnesses of the endocrine/metabolic system and treatment outcome. Bipolar Disord. 2010;12(4):404–13.
29. Fagiolini A, et al. Metabolic syndrome in patients with bipolar disorder. J Clin Psychiatry. 2008;69(4):678–9.
30. de Almeida KM, Moreira CL, Lafer B. Metabolic syndrome and bipolar disorder: what should psychiatrists know? CNS Neurosci Ther. 2012;18(2):160–6.
31. Leboyer M, Kupfer DJ. Bipolar disorder: new perspectives in health care and prevention. J Clin Psychiatry. 2010;71(12):1689–95.
32. Godin O, et al. Metabolic syndrome in a French cohort of patients with bipolar disorder: results from the FACE-BD cohort. J Clin Psychiatry. 2014;75(10):1078–85. quiz 1085
33. Stemmle PG, et al. Insulin resistance and hyperlipidemia in women with bipolar disorder. J Psychiatr Res. 2009;43(3):341–3.
34. Keck PE, McElroy SL. Bipolar disorder, obesity, and pharmacotherapy-associated weight gain. J Clin Psychiatry. 2003;64(12):1426–35.
35. Markwald RR, et al. Impact of insufficient sleep on total daily energy expenditure, food intake, and weight gain. Proc Natl Acad Sci USA. 2013;110(14):5695–700.
36. Hudson JI, et al. Longitudinal study of the diagnosis of components of the metabolic syndrome in individuals with binge-eating disorder. Am J Clin Nutr. 2010;91(6):1568–73.
37. Tanofsky-Kraff M, et al. Children's binge eating and development of metabolic syndrome. Int J Obes. 2012;36(7):956–62.
38. McIntyre RS, et al. Should depressive syndromes be reclassified as "metabolic syndrome type II"? Ann Clin Psychiatry. 2007;19(4):257–64.
39. Leboyer M, et al. Can bipolar disorder be viewed as a multi-system inflammatory disease? J Affect Disord. 2012;141(1):1–10.
40. Soczynska JK, et al. Mood disorders and obesity: understanding inflammation as a pathophysiological nexus. NeuroMolecular Med. 2011;13(2):93–116.
41. Goldstein BI, et al. Inflammation and the phenomenology, pathophysiology, comorbidity, and treatment of bipolar disorder: a systematic review of the literature. J Clin Psychiatry. 2009;70(8):1078–90.
42. Tsai SY, et al. Inflammatory markers and their relationships with leptin and insulin from acute mania to full remission in bipolar disorder. J Affect Disord. 2012;136(1–2):110–6.
43. Vuksan-Cusa B, Sagud M, Jakovljevic M. C-reactive protein and metabolic syndrome in patients with bipolar disorder compared to patients with schizophrenia. Psychiatr Danub. 2010;22(2):275–7.
44. Vasilakos J, Shivers B. Watch for ICE in neurodegeneration. Mol Psychiatry. 1996;1(1):72–6.
45. Brierley MM, Fish EN. Stats: multifaceted regulators of transcription. J Interf Cytokine Res. 2005;25(12):733–44.
46. Oliveira J, et al. Polymorphism of toll-like receptor 4 gene in bipolar disorder. J Affect Disord. 2014;152-154:395–402.
47. Oliveira J, et al. Genetic association between a 'standing' variant of NOD2 and bipolar disorder. Immunobiology. 2014;219(10):766–71.
48. Walker JR, et al. The Manitoba IBD cohort study: a population-based study of the prevalence of lifetime and 12-month anxiety and mood disorders. Am J Gastroenterol. 2008;103(8):1989–97.
49. Lu XY. The leptin hypothesis of depression: a potential link between mood disorders and obesity? Curr Opin Pharmacol. 2007;7(6):648–52.
50. McElroy SL, Keck PE Jr. Metabolic syndrome in bipolar disorder: a review with a focus on bipolar depression. J Clin Psychiatry. 2014;75(1):46–61.
51. Misiak B, et al. Appetite-regulating hormones in bipolar disorder: a systematic review and meta-analysis. Front Neuroendocrinol. 2022;67:101013.
52. Khoramipour K, et al. Adiponectin: structure, physiological functions, role in diseases, and effects of nutrition. Nutrients. 2021;13(4):1180.
53. Cervantes P, et al. Circadian secretion of cortisol in bipolar disorder. J Psychiatry Neurosci. 2001;26(5):411–6.
54. Havermans R, et al. Patterns of salivary cortisol secretion and responses to daily events in patients with remitted bipolar disorder. Psychoneuroendocrinology. 2011;36(2):258–65.
55. Kamali M, et al. Associations between suicide attempts and elevated bedtime salivary cortisol levels in bipolar disorder. J Affect Disord. 2012;136(3):350–8.
56. Spiliotaki M, et al. Altered glucocorticoid receptor signaling cascade in lymphocytes of bipolar disorder patients. Psychoneuroendocrinology. 2006;31(6):748–60.
57. Daban C, et al. Hypothalamic-pituitary-adrenal axis and bipolar disorder. Psychiatr Clin North Am. 2005;28(2):469–80.
58. Cohen S, et al. Chronic stress, glucocorticoid receptor resistance, inflammation, and disease risk. Proc Natl Acad Sci USA. 2012;109(16):5995–9.
59. Cole DP, et al. Slower treatment response in bipolar depression predicted by lower pretreatment thyroid function. Am J Psychiatry. 2002;159(1):116–21.
60. Berrettini WH, et al. Cerebrospinal fluid and plasma monoamines and their metabolites in euthymic bipolar patients. Biol Psychiatry. 1985;20(3):257–69.
61. Gregoire F, et al. Glucocorticoids induce a drastic inhibition of proliferation and stimulate differentiation of adult rat fat cell precursors. Exp Cell Res. 1991;196(2):270–8.
62. Garno JL, et al. Impact of childhood abuse on the clinical course of bipolar disorder. Br J Psychiatry. 2005;186:121–5.
63. Hammersley P, et al. Childhood trauma and hallucinations in bipolar affective disorder: preliminary investigation. Br J Psychiatry. 2003;182:543–7.

64. SayuriYamagata A, et al. Medical comorbidity in bipolar disorder: the link with metabolic-inflammatory systems. J Affect Disord. 2017;211:99–106.
65. Anand A, et al. Striatal dopamine transporter availability in unmedicated bipolar disorder. Bipolar Disord. 2011;13(4):406–13.
66. Kok P, et al. Activation of dopamine D2 receptors simultaneously ameliorates various metabolic features of obese women. Am J Physiol Endocrinol Metab. 2006;291(5):E1038–43.
67. Thompson PD, et al. Exercise and physical activity in the prevention and treatment of atherosclerotic cardiovascular disease: a statement from the Council on Clinical Cardiology (Subcommittee on Exercise, Rehabilitation, and Prevention) and the Council on Nutrition, Physical Activity, and Metabolism (Subcommittee on Physical Activity). Circulation. 2003;107(24):3109–16.
68. Sanchez-Villegas A, et al. Association of the Mediterranean dietary pattern with the incidence of depression: the Seguimiento Universidad de Navarra/University of Navarra follow-up (SUN) cohort. Arch Gen Psychiatry. 2009;66(10):1090–8.
69. Berlin I. Smoking-induced metabolic disorders: a review. Diabetes Metab. 2008;34(4 Pt 1):307–14.
70. Clair C, et al. Association of smoking cessation and weight change with cardiovascular disease among adults with and without diabetes. JAMA. 2013;309(10):1014–21.
71. Woo YS, et al. Korean medication algorithm project for bipolar disorder 2022, fifth revision: an executive summary. Clin Psychopharmacol Neurosci. 2022;20(4):747–61.
72. Health NIf, Excellence C. Bipolar disorder: assessment and management. NICE, National Institute for Health and Care Excellence; 2019.
73. Malhi GS, et al. The 2020 Royal Australian and New Zealand College of Psychiatrists clinical practice guidelines for mood disorders. Aust N Z J Psychiatry. 2021;55(1):7–117.
74. Yatham LN, et al. Canadian Network for Mood and Anxiety Treatments (CANMAT) and International Society for Bipolar Disorders (ISBD) 2018 guidelines for the management of patients with bipolar disorder. Bipolar Disord. 2018;20(2):97–170.
75. Wang Y, et al. Efficacy and tolerability of pharmacological interventions on metabolic disturbance induced by atypical antipsychotics in adults: a systematic review and network meta-analysis. J Psychopharmacol. 2021;35(9):1111–9.
76. Heart Protection Study Collaborative G. MRC/BHF Heart Protection Study of cholesterol lowering with simvastatin in 20,536 high-risk individuals: a randomised placebo-controlled trial. Lancet. 2002;360(9326):7–22.
77. Yang CC, Jick SS, Jick H. Lipid-lowering drugs and the risk of depression and suicidal behavior. Arch Intern Med. 2003;163(16):1926–32.
78. Sarris J, Mischoulon D, Schweitzer I. Omega-3 for bipolar disorder: meta-analyses of use in mania and bipolar depression. J Clin Psychiatry. 2012;73(1):81–6.
79. van Melle JP, et al. Beta-blockers and depression after myocardial infarction: a multicenter prospective study. J Am Coll Cardiol. 2006;48(11):2209–14.
80. Mansur RB, et al. Liraglutide promotes improvements in objective measures of cognitive dysfunction in individuals with mood disorders: a pilot, open-label study. J Affect Disord. 2017;207:114–20.
81. Pozzi M, et al. A systematic review of the antidepressant effects of glucagon-like peptide 1 (GLP-1) functional agonists: Further link between metabolism and psychopathology: Special Section on "Translational and Neuroscience Studies in Affective Disorders". Section Editor, Maria Nobile MD, PhD. This Section of JAD focuses on the relevance of translational and neuroscience studies in providing a better understanding of the neural basis of affective disorders. The main aim is to briefly summaries relevant research findings in clinical neuroscience with particular regards to specific innovative topics in mood and anxiety disorders. J Affect Disord. 2019;257:774–8.

Bipolar Disorder and Addiction

11

Eunsung Lim and Inki Sohn

Introduction

Bipolar disorder (BD) affects approximately 1–4% of the global population and is recognized as one of the psychiatric disorders with the highest comorbidity rates across multiple meta-analyses [1]. The most common comorbid psychiatric disorders in BD include substance use disorders (SUDs), encompassing both alcohol and behavioral addictions [2]. Given the reciprocal and detrimental relationship between BD and SUDs, a comprehensive treatment approach targeting both conditions is essential. This chapter aims to elucidate the relationship between BD and comorbid addictive disorders.

BD and AUD

Issues in Comorbidity of AUD

> Alcoholism occurs among male patients in about a quarter of the cases, but it is to be regarded as the consequence of debaucheries committed in excitement, not as a cause. —Kraepelin [3]

Alcohol use disorder (AUD) co-occurs with over 50% of other psychiatric disorders [1]. As Kraepelin noted, it is particularly prevalent among individuals with BD, often leading to significant social and legal complications. The lifetime prevalence of AUD in South Korea is reported at 11.6% (17.6% in males, 5.4% in females), showing a gradual decreasing trend. However, it remains higher than that of major depressive disorder (MDD; 7.7%) and anxiety disorders (9.3%) and represents one of the most common psychiatric disorders requiring clinical intervention [4]. The comorbidity rate of alcohol abuse in patients with BD ranges from 6% to 69% (average 48.5%) [5]. Notably, Grant et al. reported that BD exhibits the highest comorbidity rate with AUD among all psychiatric disorders (Table 11.1).

Several genetic associations have been proposed to explain this high comorbidity rate, [6–8] although the exact mechanisms remain unclear. Recent studies have highlighted a significant association between both disorders and suicidality, with a markedly increased risk of suicide when both conditions coexist [9, 10]. Furthermore, alcohol use in BD patients can exacerbate the clinical course and impede treatment efficacy [11]. Despite these issues, research on the comorbidity of these two disorders remains limited.

E. Lim (✉)
Department of Psychiatry, Shinsegae Hyo Hospital, Gimje, Republic of Korea
e-mail: calvaria0416@naver.com

I. Sohn
Department of Psychiatry, Keyo Hospital, Uiwang, Republic of Korea

W.-M. Bahk et al. (eds.), *Bipolar Disorder*, https://doi.org/10.1007/978-981-92-1323-8_11

Table 11.1 Association between alcohol use disorder and selected psychiatric conditions [3]

Psychiatric condition	Population prevalence (12 months, %)	Proportion with AUD (%)	Relative risk (odds ratio)
Bipolar spectrum disorder	2.82	30.97–43.6	3.5
Depressive disorder	7.06	13.70	1.8
Anxiety-related disorders	11.08	17.05	1.7
Personality pathology	14.8	28.6	2.6

Comorbidity Rates

Several studies examining the association between AUD and mood disorders have indicated that BD comorbid with AUD is more prevalent than major depressive disorder (MDD) comorbid with AUD [6]. Specifically, nearly half of individuals with bipolar I disorder experience lifetime alcohol dependence, which is more than twice the rate observed in MDD. Furthermore, patients with BD are more likely to exhibit alcohol dependence rather than alcohol abuse [6].

Cassidy et al., [4] in a cohort study of 392 patients with substance abuse, including AUD, and comorbid BD, reported a higher comorbidity rate in men compared to women. They also observed that individuals with comorbid AUD and BD had a higher frequency of psychiatric hospitalizations, although the prevalence of AUD decreased with age.

Hypotheses for High Comorbidity

Despite the strong association between BD and AUD, the underlying mechanisms remain unclear. Strakowski et al. [11] proposed several hypotheses to explain the co-occurrence of SUDs, including AUD, and BD:

1. *Substance use as a risk factor*: Substance abuse may act as a risk factor for specific psychiatric disorders. For example, alcohol withdrawal symptoms may trigger the onset or recurrence of BD.
2. *Self-medication hypothesis*: Patients in a manic state may consume alcohol to maintain a state of euphoria, while those in a depressive state may use alcohol to alleviate agitation.
3. *Shared neurobiological mechanisms*: The neurotransmitters involved in alcohol consumption or withdrawal may overlap with those implicated in BD, such that changes in one disorder affect the clinical course of the other. For example, dopamine, a neurotransmitter involved in the reward system of AUD, is associated with dopamine excess in manic states, whereas decreased serotonin and norepinephrine during alcohol withdrawal may contribute to depressive symptoms [12]. Thus, AUD and BD interact bidirectionally, where cause and effect influence each other, making elucidation of the underlying causes of comorbidity particularly complex.

Genetic factors have also been highlighted. Family studies of BD and AUD report that shared genetic factors play a significant role [6, 7]. Other studies show that the association between BD and AUD (odds ratio 14.5) is substantially higher than that between unipolar depression and AUD (odds ratio 1.7) [8]. Neves et al. [13] reported that two BDNF haplotypes are frequently observed in patients with both BD and AUD. Lydall et al. [14] identified genes such as CDH11, COL11A2, NMUR2, XP07, and SEMA5A as being associated with both disorders. Le-Niculescu et al. [15] reported that the clock gene D-box binding protein(Dbp) is involved in the development of both disorders. Recently, several genetic markers have been discovered using genome-wide association study (GWAS) technology. For example, the ADH1B gene is associated with alcohol consumption, while the ALDH2 gene correlates with alcohol-related characteristics, [16] including alcohol dependence and flushing response in East Asian populations [17]. Polymorphisms in the dopamine D2 receptor, glucokinase regulator (GCKR) gene, and Klotho Beta (KLB) gene have also been linked to AUD [18, 19]. Bortolasci et al. [20] analyzed the PON1 Q192R polymorphism and found that the probability of BD increased depending on the QQ genotype of smokers, suggesting that this polymorphism modulates the effect of smoking on BD through pathways involving inflammation, oxidative stress, and nitration. Nevertheless, these findings cannot be considered direct causes of the comorbidity, and further research is warranted.

According to a review by Tohen et al., [21] covering literature published from 1980 to 1997, risk factors for coexisting SUDs, including AUD, and BD include (1) early onset of BD, (2) male sex, (3) mixed BD patterns, and (4) family history of SUD. Therefore, the close relationship between these two disorders necessitates consideration of their high comorbidity rate when implementing prevention or early treatment strategies.

Differential Diagnosis

Although AUD and mania can coexist, their symptoms—such as impulsivity and severe mood changes—can be similar, making accurate diagnosis challenging. Alcohol withdrawal symptoms often include decreased motivation, depression, anxiety, agitation, and insomnia, complicating differentiation from depressive disorders. Thus, longitudinal observation is critical, rather than relying on point-in-time assessments. Mood changes during intoxication should be reassessed after sobriety, and withdrawal symptoms should be evaluated after approximately two to four weeks of abstinence to allow for symptom resolution [22].

Type II BD and cyclothymic disorder are frequently overlooked due to milder symptoms than type I BD. If only AUD is diagnosed, treatment may be delayed, the clinical course may worsen, and prognosis may be poor; careful assessment is, therefore, essential.

Clinical Presentation

A synthesis of three studies by Deykin et al., [23] Tohen et al., [24] and Strakowski et al. [25] indicates that patients with comorbid AUD and BD experience earlier BD onset, more frequent relapses, and a higher likelihood of rapid-cycling or mixed episodes compared to BD patients without AUD. They also have more than twice as many hospitalizations due to psychotic symptoms and approximately four times as many comorbid psychiatric disorders. BD patients with AUD are often non-adherent to medication, exhibit residual symptoms after treatment, and experience more adverse drug effects [26]. Failure to treat these conditions can perpetuate alcohol addiction, creating a vicious cycle and resulting in functional decline and poor prognosis. According to Fabiano et al. [27], impulsivity is a core symptom shared between AUD and BD, and lifetime suicide attempts occur 1.8 times more frequently than in BD alone.

Treatment

Despite the high comorbidity rate, a clear therapeutic framework has not yet been established. Mood stabilizers such as lithium, valproate, carbamazepine, and lamotrigine are commonly used, [28, 29] with selection guided by side effects and tolerability rather than efficacy alone [29]. Recent reports indicate that atypical antipsychotics, such as quetiapine and aripiprazole, [30, 31] may be effective, although results are inconsistent and require further investigation [32].

Lithium has been shown to improve mania in younger BD patients and may reduce alcohol dependence, [28] but valproate is often preferred for mixed or rapid-cycling BD with comorbid AUD [33]. Multiple studies have confirmed valproate's efficacy, [34, 35] and the American Psychiatric Association guidelines recommend it as first-line treatment [36]. Although both valproate and alcohol are hepatotoxic, recent studies suggest valproate does not significantly elevate liver enzyme levels in patients with AUD [37]. Spijker et al. [38] reported optimal outcomes when lithium and valproate were used in combination. Periodic monitoring of liver and thyroid function is advised.

Naltrexone has been shown to reduce alcohol consumption in BD patients, [39] though its efficacy for acute BD remains uncertain [32]. Cognitive-behavioral therapy (CBT) is an important treatment modality, particularly when focused on relapse prevention and addressing real-life challenges rather than solely improving disease symptoms (Weiss et al.) [40].

Azolin et al. [41] summarized treatment recommendations for BD with comorbid AUD:

- Reduce alcohol consumption to normal levels or achieve abstinence in dependent patients.
- Initiate simultaneous treatment for BD and AUD after abstinence, preferably using valproate.
- Educate patients regarding the interaction between AUD and BD, highlighting the risks of depression.
- Emphasize that alcohol should not be used as self-medication for mood symptoms.
- Provide psychoeducation on environmental factors negatively affecting AUD or BD.
- Monitor treatment adherence and ensure appropriate interventions are administered.

BD and SUD

Illicit substances are considered major risk factors for inducing BD, as defined in the Diagnostic and Statistical Manual of Mental Disorders, Fifth Edition (DSM-V) diagnostic category of substance-induced bipolar and related disorders. Beyond alcohol, BD is frequently comorbid with other SUDs, with a prevalence of approximately 20% for cannabis and 17% for other substances, showing a strong statistical association (odds ratio: 4.96) [42]. Notably, increased frequency of cannabis use is associated with a higher risk of developing (hypo)mania in BD, making it a significant risk factor for disease onset [43, 44].

Patients with BD may use illicit drugs for various reasons, including self-medication, mood enhancement, tension relief, alleviating boredom, escaping reality, changing mood, and increasing energy [45]. Genetic factors, such as alcohol and acetaldehyde metabolizing enzymes and 5HT2C polymorphisms, as well as socioeconomic and environmental factors—including access to illicit drugs and community poverty—also contribute [42, 46, 47]. Comorbid conditions, such as suicide attempts, conduct disorder, borderline personality disorder, antisocial personality disorder, and post-traumatic stress disorder, further exacerbate the risk of SUD.

The comorbidity of BD and SUD worsens clinical outcomes, including earlier onset, rapid cycling, frequent relapse, higher suicide rates, and cognitive and negative symptom deterioration (Table 11.2). Misdiagnosis is more likely, leading to treatment delays, decreased adherence, reduced pharmacologic response (e.g., to lithium), and increased medical comorbidities such as hepatitis C and HIV. Poly-substance use is particularly associated with BD [48]. The relationship between BD and SUD is bidirectional: illicit drugs may precipitate BD, while BD may predispose patients to substance use due to disinhibition, elevated mood in mania, or escape from negative affect in depressive episodes.

Treatment of comorbid BD and SUD often requires more complex pharmacological approaches than standard BD treatment [49]. While polypharmacy has shown some efficacy for cannabis and cocaine use, there is limited

Table 11.2 Adverse effects of SUD on BD [45]

Clinical course
Early onset of disease
Accelerated progression of BD
Increased disease severity
Rapid cycling and frequent relapse
Increased risk of conversion to (hypo)mania
Treatment
Diagnostic difficulty
Poor treatment adherence
Decreased treatment response (e.g., to lithium)
Discontinuation or delay of treatment
Complications
Increased psychosocial problems (e.g., occupation, debt)
Impaired social support
Cognitive impairment
Elevated suicide risk
Physical comorbidities (e.g., hepatitis C, HIV)

evidence for heroin, amphetamine, or methamphetamine [50]. Mood stabilizers are generally more effective than atypical antipsychotics in treating BD with SUD [51]. Other medications, including benzodiazepines, gabapentin, pregabalin, and oxcarbazepine, are often employed to reduce craving, [52] alleviate substance-induced psychotic symptoms, manage withdrawal-related sleep or anxiety disturbances, and improve mood symptoms. The therapeutic effects of benzodiazepines remain unclear and warrant further investigation. Clinicians must carefully monitor for psychotic symptoms, ensure treatment aims for full remission, frequently assess for SUD relapse during maintenance, and evaluate suicide risk.

BD and Gambling Disorder

BD and behavioral addictions, particularly gambling disorder, are presumed to be clinically associated, though research remains limited [2]. Co-occurrence of BD and gambling disorder often leads to significant social problems and poor prognosis [53, 54]. McIntyre et al. [55] reported a 6.3% prevalence of gambling disorder among BD patients, significantly higher than in the general population (2%) or in MDD patients (2.5%). BD with gambling disorder is more common in men, frequently accompanied by anxiety and depression [54].

Brain imaging studies indicate volume reductions in the prefrontal cortex for both BD and gambling disorder, which may influence behavioral responses [56]. While genetic and biological studies are limited, shared core symptoms—including impulsivity, anxiety, emotional instability, pleasure-seeking, and impaired judgment—likely contribute to the high comorbidity rate [57, 58]. Clinically, treatment should prioritize emotional regulation to improve instability, with lithium reported as the most effective pharmacological option [59]. Future studies are needed to elucidate genetic, biological, and psychosocial factors underlying this comorbidity and to identify optimal treatment strategies [60].

BD and Other Behavioral Addictions

Bipolar disorder (BD) is frequently comorbid with a wide range of behavioral addictions beyond gambling, including problematic Internet use, gaming disorder, compulsive shopping, and hypersexual behaviors. These behavioral addictions share several core psychopathological features with BD, such as impulsivity, emotional dysregulation, and reward sensitivity, which are particularly pronounced during manic and hypomanic episodes [61]. The coexistence of BD and behavioral addictions not only complicates diagnostic processes but also negatively impacts clinical outcomes, often leading to poorer treatment response and increased functional impairment [62].

The relationship between BD and behavioral addictions appears to be bidirectional, where mood instability exacerbates addictive behaviors, and the presence of these addictions can, in turn, trigger mood episodes, creating a challenging cycle to manage [63]. During manic and hypomanic phases, heightened impulsivity and diminished impulse control tend to escalate behaviors such as excessive Internet use, gaming, shopping, and sexual activities, which serve as maladaptive coping mechanisms or reinforcing stimuli. Additionally, neurobiological studies suggest overlapping dysfunctions in frontolimbic circuits involved in impulse control and emotional regulation, further underpinning the comorbidity.

Effective treatment of BD with comorbid behavioral addictions necessitates an integrated approach that addresses both mood regulation and behavioral modification. Pharmacological interventions—including mood stabilizers like lithium, valproate, and atypical antipsychotics—have demonstrated efficacy in stabilizing mood symptoms and reducing impulsivity [50]. Lithium, in particular, has been noted for its anti-suicidal properties and potential benefits in preventing relapses in bipolar patients with impulsive behaviors [64]. Psychosocial interventions such as cognitive-behavioral therapy (CBT) are also crucial, targeting maladaptive thought patterns and reinforcing coping strategies to manage addictive impulses and stabilize mood. Furthermore, approaches like motivational interviewing and family psychoeducation can enhance treatment adherence and support recovery.

Despite these advances, there remains a significant need for further research focused on developing tailored therapeutic strategies that specifically address the complex interplay between BD and behavioral addictions. Longitudinal studies exploring neurobiological, psychological, and social factors will be instrumental in refining intervention models. Overall, a comprehensive, multidisciplinary approach integrating pharmacological, psychotherapeutic, and social support mechanisms is essential for improving outcomes in this population and reducing the burden associated with comorbid BD and behavioral addictions.

Psychodynamic Perspectives on the Coexistence of BD and SUDs

Evidence consistently shows a high comorbidity rate between BD and SUD, exceeding that observed with other mood or anxiety disorders. Factors contributing to this comorbidity include:

1. Attempts to self-treat BD mood symptoms with substance use.
2. Drug-induced changes in brain function leading to mood symptoms.
3. Shared vulnerabilities or risk factors, such as impulsivity and goal orientation.

These vulnerabilities can be explained from a psychodynamic perspective.

Goal Orientation in BD and SUD

Long-term personality traits significantly influence vulnerability to mental illness [65]. Goal-oriented behavior activates the reward system when an external goal is attractive or internal expectations for achievement are high. This increases cognitive and motor activity toward goal attainment and generates hope or planning. The mesolimbic dopamine system, including the ventral tegmental area to nucleus accumbens circuit and associated prefrontal areas, underlies positive reinforcement in drug use. BD patients are particularly sensitive to goal-oriented stimuli, including those derived from drug-induced rewards, which may contribute to excessive goal pursuit, decreased need for sleep, distractibility, irritability, and heightened self-confidence or optimism during (hypo)mania [66, 67]. In contrast, depressive episodes, characterized by sadness, anhedonia, low energy, psychomotor retardation, despair, and low self-confidence, reflect deactivation of goal-oriented behavior, often associated with perfectionistic personality traits [66].

Personality Vulnerability: Impulsivity

Impulsivity, defined as a tendency to act without planning or consideration of consequences, is a core trait in both SUD and BD [68]. It contributes to urgent, unplanned behaviors and is linked to prefrontal executive dysfunction [61]. Integrated addiction models suggest that goal orientation and impulsivity interact to promote substance use. High impulsivity prevents suppression of drug-seeking behavior once rewards are available, while high goal orientation amplifies pursuit of substance-induced rewards. Impulsivity is consistently elevated in BD patients and is further increased in BD with SUD, representing a shared vulnerability underlying comorbidity.

Summary

SUDs and AUDs in individuals with severe and chronic mental illnesses, such as BD, represent major challenges for public mental health systems and social functioning. AUD is the most common comorbidity, though other SUDs, including cannabis and cocaine use, are gradually increasing in South Korea. Comorbidity is associated with poor disease courses, including early onset, diagnostic difficulty, functional deterioration, frequent relapse, and increased risk of suicide and violence. Treatment adherence is typically low, resulting in suboptimal outcomes. Therefore, an intensive, integrated treatment program addressing both BD and SUD is essential, alongside close monitoring for relapse. Continued research is necessary to develop more effective treatment strategies for this high-risk population.

Declarations

Competing Interests The author(s) has no competing interests to declare that are relevant to the content of this manuscript.

Ethics Approval The author(s) declares that this manuscript does not include primary research with human participants.

The author(s) declares that this manuscript does not include primary studies involving animals.

References

1. Grant B, Dawson DA, Stinson FS, Chou SP, Dufour MC, Pickering RP. The 12-month prevalence and trends in DSM–IV alcohol abuse and dependence: United States, 1991–1992 and 2001–2002. Drug Alcohol Depend. 2004a;74:223–34.
2. Di Nicola M, Tedeschi D, Mazza M, Martinotti G, Harnic D, Catalano V, et al. Behavioural addictions in bipolar disorder patients: role of impulsivity and personality dimensions. J Affect Disord. 2010a;125:82–8.
3. Kraepelin E. Manic-depressive insanity and paranoia (1921). Translated by Barclay RM. Salem: Ayer; 1976.
4. Korean Ministry of Health and Welfare Mental Disorder Survey, 2021.
5. Cassidy F, Ahearn EP, Carroll BJ. Substance abuse in bipolar disorder. Bipolar Disord. 2001;3:181–8.
6. Regier DA, Farmer ME, Rae DS, Locke BZ, Keith SJ, Judd LL, et al. Comorbidity of mental disorders with alcohol and other drug abuse: results from the epidemiologic catchment area (ECA) study. JAMA. 1990;264:2511–8.
7. Berrettini WH, Ferraro TN, Goldin LR, Detera-Wadleigh SD, Choi H, et al. A linkage study of bipolar illness. Arch Gen Psychiatry. 1997;54:27–35.
8. Preisig M, Fenton BT, Stevens DS, Merikangas KR. Familial relationship between mood disorders and alcoholism. Compr Psychiatry. 2001;42:87–95.
9. Feinman JA, Dunner DL. The effect of alcohol and substance abuse on the course of bipolar affective disorder. J Affect Disord. 1996;37:43–9.
10. Tondo L, Baldessarini RJ, Hennen J, Minnai GP, Salis P, Scamonatti L, et al. Suicide attempts in major affective disorder patients with comorbid substance use disorders. J Clin Psychiatry. 1999;60:63–9.
11. Strakowski SM, DelBello MP. The co-occurrence of bipolar and substance use disorders. Clin Psychol Rev. 2000;20:191–206.
12. Markou A, Kosten TR, Koob GF. Neurobiological similarities in depression and drug dependence: a self-medication hypothesis. Neuropsychopharmacology. 1998;18:135–74.
13. Neves FS, Malloy-Diniz L, Romano-Silva MA, Campos SB, Miranda DM, De Marco L, et al. The role of BDNF genetic polymorphisms in bipolar disorder with psychiatric comorbidities. J Affect Disord. 2011;131:307–11.
14. Lydall GJ, Bass NJ, McQuillin A, Lawrence J, Anjorin A, Kandaswamy R, et al. Confirmation of prior evidence of genetic susceptibility to alcoholism in a genome-wide association study of comorbid alcoholism and bipolar disorder. Psychiatr Genet. 2011;21:294–306.
15. Le-Niculescu H, McFarland MJ, Ogden CA, Balaraman Y, Patel S, Tan J, et al. Phenomic, convergent functional genomic, and biomarker studies in a stress-reactive genetic animal model of bipolar disorder and co-morbid alcoholism. Am J Med Genet B Neuropsychiatr Genet. 2008;147B:134–66.
16. Joseph DD, Alex PM, Ian RG. Genetics of alcohol use disorder: a review. Curr Opin Psychol. 2019;27:56–61.
17. Jorgenson E, Thai KK. Genetic contributors to variation in alcohol consumption vary by race/ethnicity in a large multi-ethnic genome-wide association study. Mol Psychiatry. 2017;22:1359–67.
18. kranzler HR, Zhou H, et al. Genome-wide association study of alcohol consumption and use disorder in 274,424 individuals from multiple populations. Nat Commun. 2019;10:1499.
19. Zhou H, Sealock JM, et al. Genome-wide meta-analysis of problematic alcohol use in 435,563 individuals yields insights into biology and relationships with other traits. Nat Neurosci. 2020;23:809–18.
20. Bortolasci C, Vargas HO, et al. Lowered plasma paraoxonase (PON)1 activity is a trait marker of major depression and PON1 Q192R gene polymorphism-smoking interactions differentially predict the odds of major depression and bipolar disorder. J Affect Disord. 2014;159:23–30.
21. Tohen M, Freenfield SF, Weiss RD, Zarate CA Jr, Vagge LM. The effect of comorbid substance use disorders on the course of bipolar disorder. A review. Harv Rev Psychiatry. 1998;6:133–41.
22. Brown SE, Schuckit M. Changes in depression among abstinent alcoholics. J Stud Alcohol. 1988;49:412–7.
23. Deykin EY, Levy JC, Wells V. Adolescent depression, alcohol and drug abuse. Am J Public Health. 1987;77:178–82.
24. Tohen M, Waternaux CM, Tsuang MT. Outcome in mania: a 4-year prospective follow-up of 75 patients utilizing survival analysis. Arch Gen Psychiatry. 1990;47:1106–11.

25. Strakowski SM, Keck PE Jr, McElroy SL, West SA, Sax KW, Hawkins JM, et al. Twelve-month outcome after a first hospitalization for affective psychosis. Arch Gen Psychiatry. 1998;55:49–55.
26. Baldessarini RJ, Perry R, Pike J. Factors associated with treatment nonadherence among US bipolar disorder patients. Hum Psychopharmacol. 2008;23:95–105.
27. Fabiano GN, Angela MS, Fabiana NF, Fkavio F, Beny L. Prevalence and clinical correlates of alcohol use disorders among bipolar disorder patients: results from the Brazilian Bipolar Research Network. Compr Psychiatry. 2014;55:1116–21.
28. Geller B, Cooper TB, Sun K, Zimerman B, Frazier J, Williams M, et al. Double-blind and placebo-controlled study of lithium for adolescent bipolar disorders with secondary substance dependency. J Am Acad Child Adolesc Psychiatry. 1998;37:171–8.
29. Hirschfeld RM, Calabrese JR, Weissman MM, Reed M, Davies MA, Frye MA, et al. Screening for bipolar disorder in the community. J Clin Psychiatry. 2003;64:53–9.
30. Brown ES, Garza M, Carmody TJ. A randomized, double-blind, placebo-controlled add-on trial of quetiapine in outpatients with bipolar disorder and alcohol use disorders. J Clin Psychiatry. 2008;69:701–5.
31. Moallem N, Ray LA. Quetiapine improves response inhibition in alcohol dependent patients: a placebo-controlled pilot study. Pharmacol Biochem Behav. 2012;100:490–3.
32. Naqlich A, Adinoff B, Brown ES. Pharmacological treatment of bipolar disorder with comorbid alcohol use disorder. CNS Drugs. 2017;31:665–74.
33. Bowden CL. Predictors of response to divalproex and lithium. J Clin Psychiatry. 1995;56:25–30.
34. Brady KT, Sonne SC, Anton R, Ballenger JC. Valporate in the treatment of acute bipolar affective episodes complicated by substance abuse: a pilot study. J Clin Psychiatry. 1995;56:118–21.
35. Albanese MJ, Clodfelter RC, Khantzian EJ. Divalproex sodium in substance abusers with mood disorder. J Clin Psychiatry. 2000;61:916–21.
36. American Psychiatric Association. Practice guideline for the treatment of patients with substance use disorders, 2nd edition. 2006. Accessed on 10 Aug 2009.
37. Sonne SC, Brady KT. Safety of depakote in bipolar patients with comorbid alcohol abuse/dependence. Am J Psychiatry. 1999a;156:1122.
38. Spijker AT, van Zaane J, Koenders MA, Hoekstra R, Kupka RW. Bipolar disorder and alcohol use disorder: practical recommendations for treatment, based on a literature review. Tijdschr Psychiatr. 2018;60:87–95.
39. Brown ES, Beard L, Dobbs L, Rush AJ. Naltrexone in patients with bipolar disorder and alcohol dependence. Depress Anxiety. 2006;23:492–5.
40. Weiss RD, Kolodziej ME, Najavits LM, Greenfield SF, Fucito LM. Utilization of psychosocial treatments by patients diagnosed with bipolar disorder and substance abuse. Am J Addict. 2000;9:314–20.
41. Azorin JM, Bowden CL, Garay RP, Perugi G, Vieta E, Young AH. Possible new ways in the pharmacological treatment of bipolar disorder and comorbid alcoholism. Neuropsychiatr Dis Treat. 2010;6:37–46.
42. Hunt GE, Malhi GS, et al. Comorbidity of bipolar and substance use disorders in national surveys of general populations, 1990-2015: systematic review and meta-analysis. J Affect Disord. 2016;206:321–30.
43. Lalli M, Brouillette K, et al. Substance use as a risk factor for bipolar disorder: a systematic review. J Psychiatr Res. 2021;144:285–95.
44. Ratheesh SM, Cotton JK, et al. Prospective progression from high-prevalence disorders to bipolar disorder: exploring characteristics of pre-illness stages. J Affect Disord. 2015;10:1016.
45. Preuss UW, Schaefer M, et al. Bipolar disorder and comorbid use of illicit substances. Medicina (Kaunas). 2021;17; 57:1256.
46. Messer T, Lammers G, et al. Substance abuse in patients with bipolar disorder: a systematic review and meta-analysis. Psychiatry Res. 2017;253:338–50.
47. Grunze H, Schaefer M, et al. Comorbid bipolar and alcohol use disorder-a therapeutic challenge. Front Psych. 2021;12:660432.
48. Zamora-Rodriguez FJ. Uso de sustancias y curso del trastorno bipolar en una muestra de pacientes hospitalizados. Actas Esp Psiquiatr. 2018;46:183–91.
49. Kim AM, Salstein L. A systematic review of complex polypharmacy in bipolar disorder: prevalence, clinical features, adherence, and preliminary recommendations for practitioners. J Clin Psychiatry. 2021;82:20r13263.
50. Yatham LN, Kennedy SH. Canadian network for mood and anxiety treatments (CANMAT) and International Society for Bipolar Disorders (ISBD) 2018 guidelines for the management of patients with bipolar disorder. Bipolar Disord. 2018;20:97–170.
51. Brown ES, Sunderajan P, et al. A randomized, double-blind, placebo-controlled, trial of lamotrigine therapy in bipolar disorder, depressed or mixed phase and cocaine dependence. Neuropsychopharmacology. 2012;37:2347–54.
52. Maust DT, Lin LA, Blow FC. Benzodiazepine use and misuse among adults in the United States. Psychiatr Serv. 2019;70:97–106.
53. Mazza M, Mandelli L, Di Nicola M, Harnic D, Catalano V, Tedeschi D, et al. Clinical features, response to treatment and functional outcome of bipolar disorder patients with and without co-occurring substance use disorder: 1-year follow-up. J Affect Disord. 2009;115:27–35.
54. Kennedy SH, Welsh BR, Fulton K, Soczynska JK, McIntyre RS, O'Donovan C, et al. Frequency and correlates of gambling problems in outpatients with major depressive disorder and bipolar disorder. Can J Psychiatr. 2010;55:568–76.
55. McIntyre RS, McElroy SL, Konarski JZ, Soczynska JK, Wilkins K, Kennedy SH. Problem gambling in

bipolar disorder: results from the Canadian community health survey. J Affect Disord. 2007;102:27–34.
56. Wallis JD, Miller EK. Neuronal activity in primate dorsolateral and orbital prefrontal cortex during performance of a reward preference task. Eur J Neurosci. 2003;18:2069–81.
57. Olsen CM. Natural rewards, neuroplasticity, and non-drug addictions. Neuropharmacology. 2011;61:1109–22.
58. George O, Le Moal M, Koob GF. Allostasis and addiction: role of the dopamine and corticotropin-releasing factor systems. Physiol Behav. 2012;106:58–64.
59. Hollander E, Pallanti S, Allen A, Sood E, Baldini Rossi N. Does sustained-release lithium reduce impulsive gambling and affective instability versus placebo in pathological gamblers with bipolar spectrum disorders? Am J Psychiatry. 2005;162:137–45.
60. Di Nicola M, De Risio L, Pettorruso M, Caselli G, De Crescenzo F, Swierkosz-Lenart K, et al. Bipolar disorder and gambling disorder comorbidity: current evidence and implications for pharmacological treatment. J Affect Disord. 2014;167:285–98.
61. Swann AC, Dougherty DM, Pazzaglia P, Pham M, Moeller FG. Impulsivity: a link between bipolar disorder and substance abuse. Bipolar Disord. 2004;6:204–12.
62. Yen S, Fann JR, Kuo C. Behavioral addictions in bipolar disorder: a review of clinical evidence and neurobiological insights. J Affect Disord. 2019;259:330–6.
63. Billieux J, Van der Linden M, Rochat L. The role of impulsivity in externalizing and internalizing behaviors: implications for clinical practice. Revue Medico-Psychologique. 2015;16(3):290–7.
64. Cipriani A, Hawton K, Hetrick S, et al. Lithium in the prevention of suicide in mood disorders: updated systematic review and meta-analysis. Eur J Clin Pharmacol. 2013;69(5):523–31.
65. Gray JA. The neuropsychology of anxiety: an enquiry into the functions of the septo-hippocampal system. New York: Oxford University Press; 1982.
66. Depue RA, Iacono WG. Neurobehavioral aspects of affective disorders. Annu Rev Psychol. 1989;40:457–92.
67. Urosevic S, Abramson LY, Harmon-Jones E, Alloy LB. Dysregulation of the behavioral approach system (BAS) in bipolar spectrum disorders: review of theory and evidence. Clin Psychol Rev. 2008;28:1188–205.
68. Dawe S, Loxton NJ. The role of impulsivity in the development of substance use and eating disorders. Neurosci Biobehav Rev. 2004;28:343–51.

Suicide in Bipolar Disorder

12

Won-Seok Choi and Kyung Joon Min

Introduction

Individuals with bipolar disorder (BD) are known to have a shorter life expectancy than the general population, at approximately 10–20 years [1–3]. The causes of premature death can be divided into natural and unnatural causes. Natural causes include chronic diseases such as cardiovascular disease and chronic obstructive pulmonary disease, while unnatural causes include suicide. BD patients had a standardized mortality ratio (SMR) of 2.05 for all causes of death, which is approximately twice the mortality rate of the general population. In particular, suicide was the highest among various factors (14.14) [4]. In the same context, 15–20% of BD patients die by suicide; some of the reasons include that 30–60% of patients with BD attempt suicide at least once [3, 5], and they attempt more lethal methods of suicide than the general population [6].

Pharmacotherapy reduces the risk of suicide in BD to a certain extent [7–9]. However, individuals diagnosed with BD frequently remain undiagnosed or misdiagnosed [10], consequently missing out on appropriate treatment opportunities. In this chapter, we will examine the characteristics of suicide in patients with BD. In addition, we will review risk factors and protective factors for suicide and ultimately suggest effective suicide prevention strategies for patients with BD.

W.-S. Choi (✉)
Department of Psychiatry, Korea University Guro Hospital, Seoul, Republic of Korea
e-mail: sutak17@naver.com

K. J. Min
Department of Psychiatry, College of Medicine, Chung-Ang University, Seoul, Republic of Korea

Suicidal Behavior in Mood Disorders

Suicidal behavior is a common phenomenon in patients with mood disorders. According to early data, suicide occurs in 15–19% of individuals with mood disorders across their lifetime [11]. Nonetheless, later studies have identified substantial flaws in the data and methods used, noting that the elevated suicide risk estimates do not align with the widespread prevalence of depression in the general population [12]. In cross-sectional studies, the prevalence of suicide attempters is higher among patients with BD type I or II compared to those with unipolar depression [13, 14]. Prospective studies have shown that the incidence of suicide is either higher in individuals with BD compared to those with major depressive disorder or generally similar [15–17]. Longer-term prospective study shows twice as many suicide attempts in BD than in major depressive disorder over the same follow-up period [18]. Nevertheless, a recent meta-analysis found that the odds of suicide death from a mood disorder were 8.62 times higher for major depressive disorder and 8.66 times higher for

W.-M. Bahk et al. (eds.), *Bipolar Disorder*, https://doi.org/10.1007/978-981-92-1323-8_12

BD. Notably, for both disorders, these events were more common in women, and for major depressive disorder, there was a higher risk of suicidal behavior within the first year after discharge [19]. To summarize, suicide rates in BD are generally thought to be higher than in major depressive disorder, but this varies by environment and is likely due to patients with BD remaining in a high-risk state longer rather than the disorder itself [20].

Focusing on BD only, patients with BD choose a high lethality method of suicide, resulting in a rate of suicide attempts that is 10 times higher than that of the general population [21]. Among bipolar patients who received inpatient treatment, the suicide mortality rate for bipolar II patients was 4.2% compared to 2.8% for bipolar I patients [22]. In a study of people with BD on medication, over an 18-month period, people with bipolar II disorder (34.34%) had twice as many suicide deaths as people with bipolar I disorder (14.14%) [23]. In particular, the risk of suicidal behavior was higher for patients with mixed features (odds ratio [OR] = 3.39) or many previous depressive episodes (OR = 1.62) [24]. According to a recent national survey study conducted in China, suicidal behavior and non-suicidal self-injury (NSSI) in BD are strongly associated with depressive and mixed episodes, with mixed episodes exhibiting the highest prevalence of NSSI and the most prominent addictive characteristics [25].

Risk Factors for Suicide in BD

Key suicide risk factors in BD include a history of prior suicide attempts, current major depressive or mixed episodes, early illness onset with rapid cycling, comorbid substance use or anxiety disorders, family history of suicide, and prolonged untreated illness [26, 27].

Several recent studies have systematically investigated suicide risk factors in individuals with BD, using large-scale and longitudinal data. Baldessarini et al. [27] conducted a comparative analysis of 3284 patients with major affective disorders and found significantly higher rates of suicidal ideation, attempts, and completions among BD patients compared to those with major depressive disorder. Their multivariate analysis identified five independent risk factors: BD diagnosis, early onset (≤25 years), mixed features, hospitalization history, and greater depressive severity at intake. Hansson et al. [28], using registry data from 12,850 Swedish patients with BD, demonstrated that male sex, living alone, previous suicide attempts, comorbid psychiatric diagnoses, recent affective episodes, criminal conviction, psychiatric hospitalization, and involuntary commitment were all significant predictors of suicide death, with risk profiles varying between men and women. Miola et al. [29] expanded on prior findings through an eight-year prospective cohort study of 4307 BD and major depressive disorder patients. They recognized that bipolar patients were more likely to engage in suicidal behavior than those with major depressive disorder and highlighted five independent risk factors: bipolar diagnosis, longer duration of depressive morbidity, younger age at illness onset, lower functional status, and female sex in BD specifically.

Episode–Related Risk Factors

Suicidal behavior (suicide deaths, suicide attempts) and suicidal ideation in patients with BD occur mainly in severe depressive episodes, and rarely in euphoric mania/hypomania/euthymia [26]. These characteristics show that suicidal behavior in BD patients is influenced by the polarity or severity of the mood episode, but it is not just the nature of the mood episode that influences suicidality. For example, although it has been known that patients with mixed episodes have higher rates of suicide [3, 24, 30], the highest ORs for suicidal ideation have been found among those with manic/hypomanic symptoms (OR = 29.43) [31]. In this study, manic/hypomanic symptoms were also associated with higher ORs compared to depressive symptoms (OR = 21.98). As such, it is not simply the polarity of the mood episode or the predominant symptom that determines risk factors for suicide. Factors extrinsic to the disease itself include specific clinical characteristics such as comorbid psychiatric disorders, premorbid personality, family composition and characteristics, psychosocial factors, and genetic factors [21]. These clinical history and personality-related factors are also important in the care of bipolar patients because they can help identify patients at high risk for suicide.

Personality and Characteristics of Past Suicide Attempts

The underlying personality traits of patients with BD can also have a significant impact on suicide risk. Typical personality traits that increase suicide risk include aggression, impulsivity, and severe pessimism [20]. Among personality disorder cluster types, the presence of B or C cluster personality disorders increased the risk of suicide attempts in bipolar I disorder [32]. Considering these points, impulsivity and irritability are thought to have a significant impact on suicide in patients with BD, highlighting the importance of recognizing the patient's premorbid personality. Characteristics of previous suicide attempts are also predictors of suicide risk, and in particular, the use of aggressive and lethal suicidal methods is the strongest single predictor of suicide attempts or lethal suicide [20, 28, 33]. Previous suicide attempts increase the risk of suicide death by 37 times [34], and more than half of suicides occur among previous suicide attempters [23].

Psychosocial, Genetic, and Biological Risk Factors

Also, suicide risk in BD is influenced by social, genetic, and biological factors [35]. Social risk factors include social isolation, lack of family or peer support, unmarried or divorced status, unemployment, and low socioeconomic status. Adverse early life experiences—such as childhood abuse, neglect, and other forms of trauma—have also been strongly linked to increased suicide vulnerability [36, 37]. From a genetic perspective, a family history of suicide or mood disorders is considered a significant risk factor, suggesting a heritable component to suicidal behavior in BD [38, 39]. Biologically, emerging evidence points to dysregulation in the serotonergic system, hyperactivity of the hypothalamic-pituitary-adrenal axis, and increased inflammatory markers as potential contributors. These biological alterations may impair emotional regulation and stress response, thereby heightening susceptibility to suicidal behavior [40, 41]. While these findings are not yet fully conclusive, they underscore the importance of an integrative biopsychosocial approach to suicide risk assessment and prevention in individuals with BD [26, 42].

Diagnostic Delay and Treatment-Related Risk Factors

Delays in diagnosis or treatment of BD can also be risk factors for suicidal behavior [43, 44]. BD patients with a first episode of depression and a history of multiple depressive episodes also increase the risk of suicide [45]. Generally, patients with mood disorders experience a sharp increase in suicide risk immediately after discharge [19]. After discharge, suicide risk is highest in the order of depressive episodes, mixed episodes, and manic episodes. In particular, the suicide risk is highest after discharge in cases where the patient was hospitalized for a suicide attempt [46]. Not only during hospitalization but also immediately after discharge, suicide risk increases, so careful assessment of the patient's suicide risk is necessary [47].

Controversy continues to arise over whether antidepressant use in BD affects suicide risk. Previously, several researchers have argued for the risks of antidepressant use in BD [48]. The arguments were that antidepressants increase the risk of mania and long-term worsening of bipolar illness, that antidepressants have no suicide prevention and mortality reduction effect in BD, and that they should not generally be used in mild or moderate depressive episodes except in severe acute depressive episodes [48]. While some have suggested that the use of antidepressants may increase suicide rates, there are also reports that using them in combination with mood stabilizers may reduce this risk [49]. A number of large-scale studies have shown that antidepressant use is associated with a risk of switching from BD to mania [50–52]. Along the same lines, a study [53] has argued that the use of selective serotonin reuptake inhibitors in childhood and adolescence is a suicide risk because it increases the risk of suicide in undiagnosed bipolar depression. Many current treatment guidelines do not recommend the use of antidepressants alone [54, 55], question their effectiveness in BD, and argue that their traditional role in the past should be reconsidered [56]. However, there are also reports that antidepressant use in bipolar II disorder has been associated with significant depressive symptom improvement without mood switching [57–59], suggesting that the suicide risk of antidepressants may be variable depending on the type of BD and concomitant medications, requiring individualized treatment.

Table 12.1 summarizes the clinically identifiable risk factors for suicide in BD that are currently known. Suicide in patients with BD usually

Table 12.1 Clinically identifiable risk factors for suicide in bipolar disorder

Demographic risk factors
Male sex (associated with higher suicide mortality rate)
Female sex (associated with higher suicide attempt rate)
Marital status (single, widowed, divorced)
Living alone
No children
Young age (<35 years) or older age (>75 years)
Unemployed
Episode–related risk factors
Depressive episodes
in bipolar II disorder
with hopelessness, guilt, lack of reason for living
with mixed features
with psychotic features
with atypical features
Manic or hypomanic episode with mixed features
Personality traits
Aggressive or impulsive behavioral traits
Cyclothymic, irritable, depressive temperaments
Personal and medical history
History of suicide attempts, plans, ideations (especially using violent or highly lethal methods)
Early onset of disorder
Depressive polarity in the first mood episode
Rapid–cycling course
First or most recent episode being depressive
High number of depressive episodes
Early adverse life events and developmental trauma (such as loss or separation from parents, or emotional, physical, sexual abuse)
Acute psychosocial stress
Comorbid conditions
Anxiety disorders
Substance use disorders
Cluster B and C personality disorders
Serious physical illnesses
Treatment-related risk factors
Inadequate treatment
Delayed diagnosis or treatment
Early phase of treatment
Shortly after hospital admission
Early after discharge (following hospitalization for depressive or mixed episode)
High frequency of hospitalizations

occurs during clinically significant mood episodes, so the more suicide risk factors listed in Table 12.1 that are present in a patient, the higher the risk of suicidal behavior.

Protective Factors for Suicide in BD

There are many well-known risk factors for suicide, but protective factors are still not well understood. Generally known protective factors for suicide among patients with mood disorders include social connectedness, access to care, cultural/religious beliefs, reasons for living, self-efficacy, self-esteem, optimism, impulse control, and problem-solving skills [26, 29, 60, 61]. Particularly in BD, sustained and rapid treatment maintenance, prescription of mood stabilizers such as lithium, and medication adherence are closely associated with a reduction in suicide risk [35]. Also, problem-solving skills, resilience, and effective stress management skills also play a role in reducing the risk of repeated suicide attempts in BD [35, 62, 63]. According to recent findings, sleep and circadian rhythm disorders are also associated with an increased risk of suicide, so clinical management to normalize regular sleep and circadian rhythms is important for suicide prevention in BD [64]. Given these considerations, careful assessment of suicide risk and protective factors in patients with BD is important from an initial diagnosis.

Assessing Suicide Risk in BD Patients

Although many individuals with suicide attempts and suicide deaths have a history of mood disorders, not all individuals with mood disorders show suicidal behavior [16]. A leading cognitive model [65] suggests that suicidal thoughts emerge when a suicide-related schema is activated, triggering hopelessness and a narrowed focus on suicide-related cues that are difficult to disengage from. While past suicide attempts and the nature of the illness are important in assessing suicide risk, the timing and triggers for an individual's actual suicide attempt are also important [66]. Therefore, it is important to ask authentic and nonformulaic questions about suicide-related thoughts and behaviors in BD as well as other common cases of suicide prevention and assessment, and to convey curiosity and warmth to the patient during the assessment process [67]. In particular, while the assessment of risk factors is generally common and familiar to clinicians, the assessment of protective factors can be challenging, requiring a collaborative conversation with the patient to uncover and recognize them [68]. As well as the patient, additional information should be obtained from family, friends, or other health care colleagues to support the patient's assessment. Obviously, this process must be done with the patient's consent and with respect for confidentiality. By organizing information from the patient's report, additional information, and clinical observations, a comprehensive understanding of suicidal ideation and behavior can be formulated in one individual with BD [67].

Suicide Prevention in BD

To date, pharmacotherapy with lithium is strongly associated with a lower risk of suicide in both bipolar I and II disorder, even when mood stabilization is not fully achieved [66, 69]. In the same vein, abrupt discontinuation of lithium increases the risk of suicide [9]. Mood stabilizers such as valproic acid, lamotrigine, and carbamazepine have also reported some reductions in suicide risk, but these are lower and less consistent than lithium [66]. Recently reported multinational meta-analyses have even suggested that valproate may not reduce the risk of suicide [70].

Antipsychotic medications are increasingly being used in the treatment of patients with BD, and more recently for maintenance treatment [71, 72]. Clozapine has been recommended as a medication to reduce the risk of suicide, but it is currently limited to schizophrenia or schizoaffective disorder [73]. Among non-clozapine second-generation antipsychotics (SGA), olanzapine, quetiapine, ziprasidone, asenapine, and aripiprazole have been reported to reduce the risk of suicide, but this is not specific to BD [74]. Quetiapine as monotherapy or in combination with lithium/valproate has been shown to reduce suicide scale scores among bipolar patients in two randomized controlled trials [75, 76], but results are limited. Even, one retrospective study of veterans with BD found that SGA use is associated with higher rates of suicide attempts than lithium or valproate treatment in BD [77].

Intravenous ketamine and intranasal esketamine treatment are novel pharmacologic interventions in suicide prevention [66, 78]. However, the effectiveness of intranasal esketamine in preventing suicide in bipolar depression is limited [79]. Rather, intravenous ketamine has been shown to be effective in patients with severe suicidal ideation including those with BD, and to be more effective than in patients with major depressive disorder for reducing suicidal ideation (OR = 14.1 vs. OR = 1.3) [80]. In an observational study including only patients with bipolar I and II disorder, intravenous ketamine significantly reduced self-report measures of suicidal ideation [81].

Electroconvulsive therapy (ECT) or repetitive transcranial magnetic stimulation (rTMS) may also help reduce suicidal ideation in people with BD [82]. However, for both ECT and rTMS, the evidence is incomplete, due to a lack of studies that have focused exclusively on individuals with BD [66]. A number of broad psychosocial interventions can be also helpful, including public education, limiting means of suicide, and peer support, which can help prevent suicide by averting triggers or increasing treatment interventions through improved disease awareness [66, 83].

Conclusion

Suicide is an essential component in the management of BD and should be considered in all types of episodes. Although it is not easy to predict and prevent, recognizing the risk factors and protective factors of suicide can help ensure patient safety during clinical practice. Importantly, a multi-dimensional approach is needed to determine a patient's suicide risk, considering not only the patient's personal and disease characteristics but also psychosocial factors such as the surrounding environment of the patient. It is also recommended that therapists should evaluate the features of BD in patients with mood disorders, as early therapeutic and diagnostic access can help prevent suicide.

Declarations

Competing Interests The author(s) has no competing interests to declare that are relevant to the content of this manuscript.

Ethics Approval The author(s) declares that this manuscript does not include primary research with human participants.

The author(s) declares that this manuscript does not include primary studies involving animals.

References

1. Kessing LV, Vradi E, McIntyre RS, Andersen PK. Causes of decreased life expectancy over the life span in bipolar disorder. J Affect Disord. 2015;180:142–7. https://doi.org/10.1016/j.jad.2015.03.027.
2. Chang CK, Hayes RD, Perera G, Broadbent MT, Fernandes AC, Lee WE, et al. Life expectancy at birth for people with serious mental illness and other major disorders from a secondary mental health care case register in London. PLoS One. 2011;6(5):e19590. https://doi.org/10.1371/journal.pone.0019590.
3. McIntyre RS, Berk M, Brietzke E, Goldstein BI, López-Jaramillo C, Kessing LV, et al. Bipolar disorders. Lancet. 2020;396(10265):1841–56. https://doi.org/10.1016/S0140-6736(20)31544-0.
4. Hayes JF, Miles J, Walters K, King M, Osborn DP. A systematic review and meta-analysis of premature mortality in bipolar affective disorder. Acta Psychiatr Scand. 2015;131(6):417–25. https://doi.org/10.1111/acps.12408.
5. Gergel T, Adiukwu F, McInnis M. Suicide and bipolar disorder: opportunities to change the agenda. Lancet Psychiatry. 2024;11(10):781–4. https://doi.org/10.1016/S2215-0366(24)00172-X.
6. Gonda X, Pompili M, Serafini G, Montebovi F, Campi S, Dome P, et al. Suicidal behavior in bipolar disorder: epidemiology, characteristics and major risk factors. J Affect Disord. 2012;143(1–3):16–26. https://doi.org/10.1016/j.jad.2012.04.041.
7. Rihmer Z, Gonda X. The effect of pharmacotherapy on suicide rates in bipolar patients.

CNS Neurosci Ther. 2012;18(3):238–42. https://doi.org/10.1111/j.1755-5949.2011.00261.x.
8. Tondo L, Baldessarini RJ. History of suicide prevention with lithium treatment. Pharmaceuticals. 2025;18(2):258.
9. Tondo L, Vázquez GH, Baldessarini RJ. Prevention of suicidal behavior in bipolar disorder. Bipolar Disord. 2021;23(1):14–23. https://doi.org/10.1111/bdi.13017.
10. Shen H, Zhang L, Xu C, Zhu J, Chen M, Fang Y. Analysis of misdiagnosis of bipolar disorder in an outpatient setting. Shanghai Arch Psychiatry. 2018;30(2):93–101. https://doi.org/10.11919/j.issn.1002-0829.217080.
11. Miles CP. Conditions predisposing to suicide: a review. J Nerv Ment Dis. 1977;164(4):231–46. https://doi.org/10.1097/00005053-197704000-00002.
12. Blair-West GW, Cantor CH, Mellsop GW, Eyeson-Annan ML. Lifetime suicide risk in major depression: sex and age determinants. J Affect Disord. 1999;55(2–3):171–8. https://doi.org/10.1016/s0165-0327(99)00004-x.
13. Sokero TP, Melartin TK, Rytsälä HJ, Leskelä US, Lestelä-Mielonen PS, Isometsä ET. Suicidal ideation and attempts among psychiatric patients with major depressive disorder. J Clin Psychiatry. 2003;64(9):1094–100. https://doi.org/10.4088/jcp.v64n0916.
14. Valtonen H, Suominen K, Mantere O, Leppämäki S, Arvilommi P, Isometsä ET. Suicidal ideation and attempts in bipolar I and II disorders. J Clin Psychiatry. 2005;66(11):1456–62. https://doi.org/10.4088/jcp.v66n1116.
15. Fiedorowicz JG, Leon AC, Keller MB, Solomon DA, Rice JP, Coryell WH. Do risk factors for suicidal behavior differ by affective disorder polarity? Psychol Med. 2009;39(5):763–71. https://doi.org/10.1017/s0033291708004078.
16. Isometsä E. Suicidal behaviour in mood disorders--who, when, and why? Can J Psychiatr. 2014;59(3):120–30. https://doi.org/10.1177/070674371405900303.
17. Valtonen HM, Suominen K, Mantere O, Leppämäki S, Arvilommi P, Isometsä ET. Prospective study of risk factors for attempted suicide among patients with bipolar disorder. Bipolar Disord. 2006;8(5 Pt 2):576–85. https://doi.org/10.1111/j.1399-5618.2006.00341.x.
18. Tondo L, Lepri B, Baldessarini RJ. Suicidal risks among 2826 Sardinian major affective disorder patients. Acta Psychiatr Scand. 2007;116(6):419–28. https://doi.org/10.1111/j.1600-0447.2007.01066.x.
19. Arnone D, Karmegam SR, Östlundh L, Alkhyeli F, Alhammadi L, Alhammadi S, et al. Risk of suicidal behavior in patients with major depression and bipolar disorder – a systematic review and meta-analysis of registry-based studies. Neurosci Biobehav Rev. 2024;159:105594. https://doi.org/10.1016/j.neubiorev.2024.105594.
20. Holma KM, Haukka J, Suominen K, Valtonen HM, Mantere O, Melartin TK, et al. Differences in incidence of suicide attempts between bipolar I and II disorders and major depressive disorder. Bipolar Disord. 2014;16(6):652–61. https://doi.org/10.1111/bdi.12195.
21. Costa LS, Alencar ÁP, Neto PJN, Santos MSV, da Silva CGL, Pinheiro SFL, et al. Risk factors for suicide in bipolar disorder: a systematic review. J Affect Disord. 2015;170:237–54. https://doi.org/10.1016/j.jad.2014.09.003.
22. Sani G, Tondo L, Koukopoulos A, Reginaldi D, Kotzalidis GD, Koukopoulos AE, et al. Suicide in a large population of former psychiatric inpatients. Psychiatry Clin Neurosci. 2011;65(3):286–95. https://doi.org/10.1111/j.1440-1819.2011.02205.x.
23. Dennehy EB, Marangell LB, Allen MH, Chessick C, Wisniewski SR, Thase ME. Suicide and suicide attempts in the systematic treatment enhancement program for bipolar disorder (STEP-BD). J Affect Disord. 2011;133(3):423–7. https://doi.org/10.1016/j.jad.2011.04.036.
24. Seo H-J, Wang H-R, Jun T-Y, Woo YS, Bahk W-M. Factors related to suicidal behavior in patients with bipolar disorder: the effect of mixed features on suicidality. Gen Hosp Psychiatry. 2016;39:91–6. https://doi.org/10.1016/j.genhosppsych.2015.12.005.
25. Cui L, Zhu Y, Li Y, Zhou J, Xu G, Pan M, et al. A national survey of suicidality and non-suicidal self-injury in bipolar disorder: insights from network analysis. BMC Psychiatry. 2025;25(1):297. https://doi.org/10.1186/s12888-025-06750-2.
26. Dome P, Rihmer Z, Gonda X. Suicide risk in bipolar disorder: a brief review. Medicina (Kaunas). 2019;55(8) https://doi.org/10.3390/medicina55080403.
27. Baldessarini RJ, Tondo L, Pinna M, Nuñez N, Vázquez GH. Suicidal risk factors in major affective disorders. Br J Psychiatry. 2019;215(4):621–6. https://doi.org/10.1192/bjp.2019.167.
28. Hansson C, Joas E, Pålsson E, Hawton K, Runeson B, Landén M. Risk factors for suicide in bipolar disorder: a cohort study of 12 850 patients. Acta Psychiatr Scand. 2018;138(5):456–63. https://doi.org/10.1111/acps.12946.
29. Miola A, Tondo L, Pinna M, Contu M, Baldessarini RJ. Suicidal risk and protective factors in major affective disorders: a prospective cohort study of 4307 participants. J Affect Disord. 2023;338:189–98. https://doi.org/10.1016/j.jad.2023.06.018.
30. Persons JE, Coryell WH, Solomon DA, Keller MB, Endicott J, Fiedorowicz JG. Mixed state and suicide: is the effect of mixed state on suicidal behavior more than the sum of its parts? Bipolar Disord. 2018;20(1):35–41. https://doi.org/10.1111/bdi.12538.
31. Macellaro M, Cafaro R, Kelly CM, Ostacher MJ, Dell'Osso B, Lyu J, et al. The influence of depressive and manic symptoms on suicidal ideation in mixed mood states. Int J Bipolar Disord. 2025;13(1):23. https://doi.org/10.1186/s40345-025-00390-x.
32. Bezerra SF, Galvão-de-Almeida A, Studart P, Martins DF Jr, Caribé AC, Schwingel PA, et al. Suicide attempts

in bipolar I patients: impact of comorbid personality disorders. Braz J Psychiatry. 2017;39(2):133–9. https://doi.org/10.1590/1516-4446-2016-1982.
33. Hawton K, Sutton L, Haw C, Sinclair J, Harriss L. Suicide and attempted suicide in bipolar disorder: a systematic review of risk factors. J Clin Psychiatry. 2005;66(6):693–704. https://doi.org/10.4088/jcp.v66n0604.
34. Harris EC, Barraclough B. Suicide as an outcome for mental disorders. A meta-analysis. Br J Psychiatry. 1997;170:205–28. https://doi.org/10.1192/bjp.170.3.205.
35. Carls-Diamante S, Atanasova N. Psychoneural reduction revised: the case of suicidality in bipolar disorder. Eur J Neurosci. 2025;61(1):e16640. https://doi.org/10.1111/ejn.16640.
36. Pike CK, Burdick KE, Millett C, Lipschitz JM. Perceived loneliness and social support in bipolar disorder: relation to suicidal ideation and attempts. Int J Bipolar Disord. 2024;12(1):8. https://doi.org/10.1186/s40345-024-00329-8.
37. Dempsey RC, Dodd AL, Gooding PA, Jones SH. The types of psychosocial factors associated with suicidality outcomes for people living with bipolar disorder: a scoping review. Int J Environ Res Public Health. 2024;21(5):525.
38. Brent DA, Mann JJ. Familial pathways to suicidal behavior–understanding and preventing suicide among adolescents. N Engl J Med. 2006;355(26):2719–21. https://doi.org/10.1056/NEJMp068195.
39. Manchia M, Hajek T, O'Donovan C, Deiana V, Chillotti C, Ruzickova M, et al. Genetic risk of suicidal behavior in bipolar spectrum disorder: analysis of 737 pedigrees. Bipolar Disord. 2013;15(5):496–506. https://doi.org/10.1111/bdi.12088.
40. Bengoechea-Fortes SP, Ramírez-Expósito MJ, Martínez-Martos JM. Suicide, neuroinflammation and other physiological alterations. Eur Arch Psychiatry Clin Neurosci. 2024;274(5):1037–49. https://doi.org/10.1007/s00406-023-01584-z.
41. Giurgiuca A, Nemes B, Schipor S, Caragheorgheopol A, Boscaiu V, Cozman D, et al. Cortisol levels and suicide in bipolar I disorder. Acta Endocrinologica (Bucharest). 2017;13(2):188.
42. Zhong S, Chen P, Lai S, Zhang Y, Chen G, He J, et al. Hippocampal dynamic functional connectivity, HPA Axis activity, and personality trait in bipolar disorder with suicidal attempt. Neuroendocrinology. 2024;114(2):179–91. https://doi.org/10.1159/000534033.
43. Nery-Fernandes F, Quarantini LC, Guimarães JL, de Oliveira IR, Koenen KC, Kapczinski F, et al. Is there an association between suicide attempt and delay of initiation of mood stabilizers in bipolar I disorder? J Affect Disord. 2012;136(3):1082–7. https://doi.org/10.1016/j.jad.2011.10.046.
44. Undurraga J, Baldessarini RJ, Valenti M, Pacchiarotti I, Vieta E. Suicidal risk factors in bipolar I and II disorder patients. J Clin Psychiatry. 2012;73(6):778–82. https://doi.org/10.4088/JCP.11m07041.
45. Grover S, Avasthi A, Chakravarty R, Dan A, Chakraborty K, Neogi R, et al. Factors associated with lifetime suicide attempts: findings from the bipolar disorder course and outcome study from India (BiD-CoIN study). Nord J Psychiatry. 2023;77(3):227–33. https://doi.org/10.1080/08039488.2022.2083231.
46. Isometsä E, Sund R, Pirkola S. Post-discharge suicides of inpatients with bipolar disorder in Finland. Bipolar Disord. 2014;16(8):867–74. https://doi.org/10.1111/bdi.12237.
47. Clements C, Morriss R, Jones S, Peters S, Roberts C, Kapur N. Suicide in bipolar disorder in a national English sample, 1996–2009: frequency, trends and characteristics. Psychol Med. 2013;43(12):2593–602. https://doi.org/10.1017/s0033291713000329.
48. Ghaemi SN, Hsu DJ, Soldani F, Goodwin FK. Antidepressants in bipolar disorder: the case for caution. Bipolar Disord. 2003;5(6):421–33. https://doi.org/10.1046/j.1399-5618.2003.00074.x.
49. McElroy SL, Kotwal R, Kaneria R, Keck PE Jr. Antidepressants and suicidal behavior in bipolar disorder. Bipolar Disord. 2006;8(5 Pt 2):596–617. https://doi.org/10.1111/j.1399-5618.2006.00348.x.
50. Valentí M, Pacchiarotti I, Rosa AR, Bonnín CM, Popovic D, Nivoli AM, et al. Bipolar mixed episodes and antidepressants: a cohort study of bipolar I disorder patients. Bipolar Disord. 2011;13(2):145–54. https://doi.org/10.1111/j.1399-5618.2011.00908.x.
51. Viktorin A, Lichtenstein P, Thase ME, Larsson H, Lundholm C, Magnusson PK, et al. The risk of switch to mania in patients with bipolar disorder during treatment with an antidepressant alone and in combination with a mood stabilizer. Am J Psychiatry. 2014;171(10):1067–73. https://doi.org/10.1176/appi.ajp.2014.13111501.
52. Patel R, Reiss P, Shetty H, Broadbent M, Stewart R, McGuire P, et al. Do antidepressants increase the risk of mania and bipolar disorder in people with depression? A retrospective electronic case register cohort study. BMJ Open. 2015;5(12):e008341. https://doi.org/10.1136/bmjopen-2015-008341.
53. Hogg S, Ansari S, Masood Q, Agius M, Rihmer Z. Are SSRIs responsible for precipitating suicidal ideation in teenagers with 'subsyndromal' bipolar affective disorder who have been misdiagnosed with unipolar depression? Psychiatr Danub. 2016;28(Suppl-1):79–82.
54. Keramatian K, Chithra NK, Yatham LN. The CANMAT and ISBD guidelines for the treatment of bipolar disorder: summary and a 2023 update of evidence. Focus (Am Psychiatr Publ). 2023;21(4):344–53. https://doi.org/10.1176/appi.focus.20230009.
55. Jeong J-H, Bahk W-M, Woo YS, Yoon B-H, Lee JG, Kim W, et al. Korean medication algo-

rithm project for bipolar disorder 2022: comparisons with other treatment guidelines. Clin Psychopharmacol Neurosci. 2023;21(1):32–48. https://doi.org/10.9758/cpn.2023.21.1.32.
56. Fountoulakis KN, Fountoulakis NK, Antoniadis D.Challengesinthedevelopmentoftreatmentguidelines for bipolar disorder. Front Psychiatry. 2025;16–2025 https://doi.org/10.3389/fpsyt.2025.1564004.
57. Leon AC, Fiedorowicz JG, Solomon DA, Li C, Coryell WH, Endicott J, et al. Risk of suicidal behavior with antidepressants in bipolar and unipolar disorders. J Clin Psychiatry. 2014;75(7):720–7. https://doi.org/10.4088/JCP.13m08744.
58. Park JH, Nuñez NA, Gardea-Resendez M, Gerberi DJ, Breitinger S, Veldic M, et al. Short term second-generation antidepressant monotherapy in acute depressive episodes of bipolar II disorder: a systematic review and meta-analysis. Psychopharmacol Bull. 2022;52(2):45–72.
59. Nielsen RE. Switching concerns: bipolar disorder and the antidepressant dilemma. Acta Psychiatr Scand. 2024;150(3):123–5. https://doi.org/10.1111/acps.13738.
60. Orsolini L, Latini R, Pompili M, Serafini G, Volpe U, Vellante F, et al. Understanding the complex of suicide in depression: from research to clinics. Psychiatry Investig. 2020;17(3):207–21. https://doi.org/10.30773/pi.2019.0171.
61. Malone KM, Oquendo MA, Haas GL, Ellis SP, Li S, Mann JJ. Protective factors against suicidal acts in major depression: reasons for living. Am J Psychiatry. 2000;157(7):1084–8. https://doi.org/10.1176/appi.ajp.157.7.1084.
62. Darvishi N, Farhadi M, Azmi-Naei B, Poorolajal J. The role of problem-solving skills in the prevention of suicidal behaviors: a systematic review and meta-analysis. PLoS One. 2023;18:e0293620. https://doi.org/10.1371/journal.pone.0293620.
63. Fernández-Rocha ML, García-Izquierdo M, Ríos-Rísquez MI. Psychological resilience and suicide attempt in patients with bipolar disorder: an exploratory study. J Am Psychiatr Nurses Assoc. 2024;30(1):44–51. https://doi.org/10.1177/10783903211050682.
64. Goldschmied JR, Palermo E, Yocum A, McInnis M, Gehrman P. The relationship between sleep and circadian patterns with risk for suicide in bipolar disorder varies by subtype. J Psychiatr Res. 2025;181:23–8. https://doi.org/10.1016/j.jpsychires.2024.11.030.
65. Wenzel A, Jager-Hyman S. Cognitive therapy for suicidal patients: current status. Behav Ther (NY). 2012;35(7):121–30.
66. Izadi N, Mitchell RHB, Giacobbe P, Nestor S, Steinberg R, Amini J, et al. Suicide assessment and prevention in bipolar disorder: how current evidence can inform clinical practice. Focus (Am Psychiatr Publ). 2023;21(4):380–8. https://doi.org/10.1176/appi.focus.20230011.
67. Hawton K, Lascelles K, Pitman A, Gilbert S, Silverman M. Assessment of suicide risk in mental health practice: shifting from prediction to therapeutic assessment, formulation, and risk management. Lancet Psychiatry. 2022;9(11):922–8. https://doi.org/10.1016/s2215-0366(22)00232-2.
68. Berman AL, Silverman MM. Near term suicide risk assessment: a commentary on the clinical relevance of protective factors. Arch Suicide Res. 2020;24(sup2):S370–S80. https://doi.org/10.1080/13811118.2019.1612804.
69. Alda M, Manchia M. Personalized management of bipolar disorder. Neurosci Lett. 2018;669:3–9. https://doi.org/10.1016/j.neulet.2017.12.005.
70. Chen T-Y, Kamali M, Chu C-S, Yeh C-B, Huang S-Y, Mao W-C, et al. Divalproex and its effect on suicide risk in bipolar disorder: a systematic review and meta-analysis of multinational observational studies. J Affect Disord. 2019;245:812–8. https://doi.org/10.1016/j.jad.2018.11.093.
71. Yatham LN, Kennedy SH, Parikh SV, Schaffer A, Bond DJ, Frey BN, et al. Canadian network for mood and anxiety treatments (CANMAT) and International Society for Bipolar Disorders (ISBD) 2018 guidelines for the management of patients with bipolar disorder. Bipolar Disord. 2018;20(2):97–170. https://doi.org/10.1111/bdi.12609.
72. Jon D-I, Woo YS, Seo J-S, Lee JG, Jeong J-H, Kim W, et al. The Korean medication algorithm project for bipolar disorder (KMAP-BP): changes in preferred treatment strategies and medications over 16 years and five editions. Bipolar Disord. 2020;22(5):461–71. https://doi.org/10.1111/bdi.12902.
73. Zuschlag ZD. Second-generation antipsychotics and suicide: a commentary. J Clin Psychiatry. 2021;82(5):35372.
74. Pompili M, Baldessarini RJ, Forte A, Erbuto D, Serafini G, Fiorillo A, et al. Do atypical antipsychotics have Antisuicidal effects? A hypothesis-generating overview. Int J Mol Sci. 2016;17(10) https://doi.org/10.3390/ijms17101700.
75. Calabrese JR, Paul E, Keck J, Macfadden W, Minkwitz M, Ketter TA, Weisler RH, et al. A randomized, double-blind, placebo-controlled trial of quetiapine in the treatment of bipolar I or II depression. Am J Psychiatry. 2005;162(7):1351–60. https://doi.org/10.1176/appi.ajp.162.7.1351.
76. Suppes T, Vieta E, Liu S, Brecher M, Paulsson B. Maintenance treatment for patients with bipolar I disorder: results from a north American study of quetiapine in combination with lithium or divalproex (trial 127). Am J Psychiatry. 2009;166(4):476–88. https://doi.org/10.1176/appi.ajp.2008.08020189.
77. Ahearn EP, Chen P, Hertzberg M, Cornette M, Suvalsky L, Cooley-Olson D, et al. Suicide attempts in veterans with bipolar disorder during treatment with lithium, divalproex, and atypical anti-

psychotics. J Affect Disord. 2013;145(1):77–82. https://doi.org/10.1016/j.jad.2012.07.015.
78. Shen Z, Gao D, Lv X, Wang H, Yue W. A meta-analysis of the effects of ketamine on suicidal ideation in depression patients. Transl Psychiatry. 2024;14(1):248. https://doi.org/10.1038/s41398-024-02973-1.
79. Wilkowska A, Cubała WJ. Short-term ketamine use in bipolar depression: a review of the evidence for short-term treatment management. Front Psych. 2023;14:1322752. https://doi.org/10.3389/fpsyt.2023.1322752.
80. Abbar M, Demattei C, El-Hage W, Llorca P-M, Samalin L, Demaricourt P, et al. Ketamine for the acute treatment of severe suicidal ideation: double blind, randomised placebo controlled trial. BMJ. 2022;376:376.
81. Fancy F, Rodrigues NB, Di Vincenzo JD, Chau EH, Sethi R, Husain MI, et al. Real-world effectiveness of repeated ketamine infusions for treatment-resistant bipolar depression. Bipolar Disord. 2023;25(2):99–109. https://doi.org/10.1111/bdi.13284.
82. Mutz J. Brain stimulation treatment for bipolar disorder. Bipolar Disord. 2023;25(1):9–24.
83. World Health Organization. Live life: an implementation guide for suicide prevention in countries: executive summary.

Part III

Treatment

Pros and Cons: The Usefulness of Antidepressants in Bipolar Depressive Episodes

13

Jeong Seok Seo and Kwanghun Lee

Overview of Bipolar Depression

When a patient first presents to a psychiatrist with mania, the diagnosis is generally straightforward due to its distinctive clinical features, and untreated episodes rarely last longer than 3–4 months. Consequently, mania is relatively easy to recognize and, in many cases, less challenging to manage. Bipolar depression, however, presents a very different clinical challenge. Some patients fail to improve despite prolonged and intensive pharmacological interventions, while others may engage in extreme behaviors, including suicide. In such situations, a patient with bipolar I disorder may suddenly present with severe depressive symptoms and request an antidepressant saying that "I can't do anything, life is so hard, I'd rather be prescribed an antidepressant, even if it's just to make me manic switch" the doctor is left wondering, "*What should I do for the patient?*" Because bipolar depression requires a different treatment strategy than unipolar depression, which is diagnosed as major depressive disorder.

Bipolar depression requires a distinct therapeutic strategy from unipolar depression, despite both conditions currently being diagnosed using identical diagnostic criteria. This raises important clinical questions: Are unipolar and bipolar depression truly the same disorder, or are they fundamentally distinct entities? (This is discussed elsewhere in this textbook.) Can antidepressant use in bipolar depression be justified in the same way as in unipolar depression?

When treating patient with bipolar depression, clinicians may consider various strategies: discontinuing sedating medications and initiating antidepressant monotherapy; adjusting the dose of a mood stabilizer or antipsychotic before adding an antidepressant; or introducing a second mood stabilizer. In real-world clinical practice, one of the most common strategies is to add an antidepressant to existing therapy [25, 54]. However, this approach has been controversial for decades due to limited high-quality evidence supporting its efficacy and safety. While strong evidence supports long-term antidepressant maintenance therapy for relapse prevention in unipolar depression [19], whether this benefit extends to bipolar depression remains uncertain.

Bipolar disorder is a chronic and recurrent condition, with patients experiencing symptoms for approximately half of their lifetime illness duration, and depressive symptoms dominating roughly two-thirds of that time [30]. Assuming a one-year duration of symptomatic illness over the course of a lifetime, patients experience roughly 6 months without symptoms, and the remaining half of the year with mood disturbances—most

J. S. Seo (✉)
Department of Psychiatry, College of Medicine, Chung-Ang University, Gwangmyeong Hospital, Gwangmyeong, Republic of Korea
e-mail: sjs52632@daum.net

K. Lee
Lee KwangHun Mental Health Clinic, Gyeongju, Republic of Korea

W.-M. Bahk et al. (eds.), *Bipolar Disorder*, https://doi.org/10.1007/978-981-92-1323-8_13

notably, approximately 4 months with depressive symptoms during 6 months, which is why it is important to recognize and actively and appropriately treat bipolar disorder.

The clinical heterogeneity of bipolar disorder, coupled with diverse treatment options, has led to the development and regular revision of treatment guidelines worldwide since the early 2000s. These guidelines are often evidence-based but also incorporate expert consensus where empirical data are lacking. Nevertheless, the use of antidepressants in bipolar depression remains contentious. A persistent gap exists between research findings, guideline recommendations, and real clinical setting. For example, an analysis of prescription patterns in 7406 newly diagnosed bipolar patients in the United States (2000–2004) who had been medication-free for at least 6 months found that 79% were prescribed antidepressants, either as monotherapy or in combination [7]. Similarly, data from the Systematic Treatment Enhancement Program for Bipolar Disorder (STEP-BD) at Stanford University (2000–2011) showed that 39.0% of patients (46.9% of those with bipolar II and 30.8% with bipolar I) were receiving antidepressants, reflecting widespread empirical use despite the limited evidence base [28].

Although comparable data are not yet available for Korea, clinical experience suggests that prescription trends are likely similar. The enduring controversy over antidepressant use in bipolar depression can be attributed to this gap between evidence and real practice. In the following sections, we will present the principal arguments for and against their use, summarize the available evidence, and integrate recommendations from recent international clinical guidelines.

In preparing this manuscript, we endeavored to maintain a primarily neutral perspective when describing the role of antidepressants in the treatment of patients with bipolar depression. While the overall volume of the manuscript was an important consideration, we made a concerted effort to include as many relevant study findings as possible in order to allow readers to appreciate overarching research trends in this field.

As an additional comment intended to assist readers in their clinical judgment, it is noteworthy that studies expressing predominantly skeptical views were largely conducted from the 1990s to the early 2000s and typically investigated a more limited range of antidepressant agents than those available today. In contrast, studies reporting more favorable outcomes have generally been published in later periods or are based on meta-analyses incorporating a broader body of evidence.

We believe that an understanding of these temporal and methodological trends is an important factor to consider when evaluating the potential benefits and risks of antidepressants as a treatment option for bipolar depression.

Treating Bipolar Depression: Skeptics of Antidepressant Use

The controversy over the use of antidepressants in bipolar disorder began with the explosion in the use of a variety of antidepressants developed after the tetracyclic antidepressants (TCAs), which were thought to be effective and safe. Skepticism about the effects of antidepressants can be divided into two main categories: (1) lack of benefit from antidepressant use and (2) negative effects such as increased rates of manic-switching and accelerated cycling or suicidal behavior.

Lack of Benefit from Antidepressants

The argument is that there is no additional benefit from antidepressant use in bipolar depression and therefore there is a lack of evidence to justify their use.

In a 2008 double-blind, 26-week randomized controlled trial (RCT) of bipolar depression patients, the recovery rate was 23.5 versus 27.3% for those who added an antidepressant to their mood stabilizer (24/179) and 51/187 for those who combined a mood stabilizer with a placebo (23.5 vs. 27.3%). There was no significant difference in mania conversion rates between the two groups, and the authors concluded that there was no benefit to combining antidepressants, although longer-term future studies are needed [46].

An analysis of data from STEP-BD of the US National Institute of Mental Health (NIMH) came to a similar conclusion that there is no benefit to antidepressants in bipolar disorder [24]. In this study, patients with depressive episodes and two or more manic symptoms were divided into two groups: those taking mood stabilizers or atypical antipsychotics with adjunctive antidepressants (n = 136) and without antidepressants (n = 152). Time to recovery was expected to be faster in the antidepressant group, but there was no difference in time to recovery between the two groups. Short-term follow-up of 3 months showed that the antidepressant group had a higher number of manic symptoms on subsequent manic episodes. In summary, the results suggest that the use of antidepressants in bipolar disorder may not be beneficial to recovery and may actually be detrimental to subsequent mania.

However, both study designs compared the effects of adding antidepressants to existing medications, meaning that a randomized controlled trial of antidepressant monotherapy is needed to determine whether antidepressants are beneficial. While the primary outcome was to compare the antidepressant effectiveness of quetiapine versus paroxetine in bipolar depression, McElroy et al. [36] found no significant improvement in depressive symptoms in 8 weeks of paroxetine alone compared to placebo in bipolar patients with depressive episodes (n = 740) or bipolar II (n = 740).

A meta-analysis by Hu et al. [29], which examined 19 studies involving 2587 patients receiving adjunctive antidepressants with antipsychotics, demonstrated a modest improvement in depressive symptoms with a small effect size of 0.13 (95% confidence interval [CI], −0.24 to −0.02), but finally no significant difference in response rate compared to placebo (response rate of antidepressant (AD) group and placebo group = 48 vs. 43%).

In contrast, findings from Ghaemi et al. [20] raised concerns about the risk–benefit ratio of adjunctive antidepressant therapy. While they found a 27% efficacy in preventing recurrent depressive episodes, the risk of manic switching was substantially higher at 72% (number needed to harm (NNH) = 7.18, number needed to treat [NNT] = 11.2). Furthermore, when compared to mood stabilizer monotherapy, adjunctive antidepressants showed no significant preventive effect on depressive relapse (relative risk [RR] = 0.84; 95% CI, 0.56–1.27; NNT = 16), nor did they increase the risk of manic switch (RR = 1.37; 95% CI, 0.81–2.33; NNH = 16). Based on these findings, the authors concluded that antidepressants provided no net clinical benefit.

Similarly, Sidor and Macqueen [52] conducted a meta-analysis of five acute phase trials (n = 3407) conducted between 2003 and 2009, each lasting 16 weeks or less. Their results also revealed no superiority of antidepressants over placebo in bipolar depression, and no increased risk of manic switch. It is worth noting, however, that this meta-analysis did not include studies involving duloxetine. Moreover, although the antidepressant effect approached statistical significance ($p = 0.06$), it showed a strong trend.

More recently, Yatham et al. [64] conducted long-term outcomes in a double-blind trial involving 209 patients who had recovered from a bipolar depressive episode. Participants initially received escitalopram or bupropion for 8 weeks; thereafter, one group (n = 90) continued antidepressants for 52 weeks, while the other (n = 87) was switched to placebo. The study found no significant clinical benefit in preventing depressive recurrence between the prolonged treatment group and the short-term group, further questioning the utility of sustained antidepressant use in bipolar depression.

Claims of Negative Effects of Antidepressants

Increased Risk of Manic Switching

The potential for antidepressants to induce (hypo) manic switching has been a controversial issue of investigation since the 1970s. Several studies have reported this risk [1, 3, 12, 13, 32, 34, 43, 55]. In the early 2000s, short-term trials (≤10 weeks) examining lamotrigine [14], imipramine [39], and moclobemide [53] reported manic switch rates of 3–8%, 6–11%, and 4%, respectively. These rates were considerably lower than the 44% switch rate reported in the STEP-BD data [58].

Supporting these findings, Post et al. [42] observed a 13% switch rate during 10 weeks of antidepressant use in the acute depressive phase, which increased to 33% over one year in responders. Similarly, Rouillon et al. [45] reported switch rates of 51, 28, and 23% in the imipramine monotherapy, lithium plus imipramine, and lithium plus placebo groups, respectively. These results suggest that TCAs may pose a higher risk of mania conversion, particularly when used without mood stabilizers.

Among these, the STEP-BD study [58] requires cautious interpretation, as it was based on patient self-reports. Still, it reported high odds ratios for manic switching associated with various antidepressants: 7.80 for TCAs, 3.73 for selective serotonin reuptake inhibitors (SSRIs), and 4.28 for bupropion, indicating that antidepressants are a potential risk factor for manic episodes.

Further evidence comes from a meta-analysis of six studies (n = 1383) that evaluated second-generation antidepressants (paroxetine, fluoxetine, bupropion, agomelatine, and citalopram) added to mood stabilizers or antipsychotics [37]. This meta-analysis found small but statistically significant improvements in depressive symptoms (effect size, 0.165, 95% CI, 0.051–0.278, p = 0.004). However, there were no significant differences in clinical response (RR = 1.158, p = 0.371) or remission rates (RR = 1.220, p = 0.243) compared to placebo. Notably, while acute treatment did not significantly elevate manic switch risk (RR = 0.926, p = 0.753), the risk became significant during the 52-week extension phase (RR = 1.774, 95% CI, 1.018–3.091, p = 0.043).

Adding to this concern, Pacchiarotti et al. [40] directly compared 138 patients treated with antidepressant monotherapy versus combination therapy with mood stabilizers. The monotherapy group exhibited significantly higher rates of manic conversion (p = 0.005) and suicide attempts (p = 0.0041), underscoring the risks of using antidepressants without adequate mood stabilization.

This trend is further supported by a systematic review by Barnuti et al. [10], which analyzed 32 studies and reported antidepressant-induced manic switch rates ranging from 17.3% to 48.8%. Despite variations due to study design or definitions, the overall literature suggests that the rate of manic switch associated with antidepressants likely falls between 8% and 44%.

However, there are several important considerations in interpreting antidepressant-induced manic switching risk.

1. *Spontaneous manic switching in the natural course*
   It is essential to distinguish between spontaneous manic episodes and those triggered by antidepressants. Tondo et al. [56] reported similar rates of switching between natural course of bipolar disorder (13.8%) and antidepressant exposure (15.3%), suggesting that the difference may not be substantial. Likewise, Lewis and Winokur [32] reported a 41% incidence of spontaneous mania in unmedicated patients. Additionally, Sidor and MacQueen [52] found similar switching rates (~8%) in both antidepressant and placebo groups, indicating no clear causal relationship.
2. *Heterogeneity of antidepressants*
   It is misleading to generalize findings across all antidepressants. Different classes and agents have varying risk profiles. For instance, while TCAs are consistently linked to higher manic switch rates, bupropion appears relatively safer [9]. A Korean survey [47] also revealed differing expert preferences for antidepressant types in bipolar depression, reflecting this heterogeneity.
3. *Patient-level vulnerability factors*
   Beyond pharmacologic class, individual vulnerability may play a crucial role. Early onset of illness [2] and a higher number of past depressive episodes [51] have been associated with increased risk. Moreover, Cassidy et al. [15] proposed the existence of a subgroup of patients who are inherently more susceptible to antidepressant-induced mood switching.

As noted, estimates of antidepressant-induced manic switching vary widely. However, if switching rates lie between 15% and 40%, one must demonstrate a significantly higher rate—beyond what occurs naturally—to definitively attribute such episodes to antidepressant use.

Acceleration of Cycling

Another area of concern regarding antidepressant use in bipolar disorder is the potential for cycle acceleration. Wehr and Goodwin [61] hypothesized that antidepressants may hasten the cycling of mood episodes, thereby worsening long-term treatment outcomes and prognosis. Although estimates vary across studies, the risk of cycle acceleration with long-term antidepressant use has been reported to range from 26% to 51% [3, 31, 44].

Increased Risk of Suicidality

A further area of concern in the use of antidepressants for bipolar depression is the potential for increased suicidality. Several studies have reported heightened risks of suicidal ideation and behavior during antidepressant treatment. A meta-analysis of short-term pharmacotherapy trials found that antidepressants were associated with increased suicidal ideation [31] and suicide attempts [16]. Similarly, data from the STEP-BD study highlighted the elevated risk of suicidality in patients with bipolar disorder. In one analysis, suicidal ideation was reported to be four times more common in patients with mixed episodes who were receiving antidepressants [22]. Another report from 2005 STEP-BP data that 25% of patients taking antidepressants experienced suicidal ideation, compared to only 13% of those not receiving antidepressants [23].

Moreover, a retrospective study by Yerevanian et al. [65] involving 405 patients compared suicidal behavior (including suicidal ideation, suicide attempts, and successful suicides) per 100 patients per year. The results revealed that patients receiving antidepressant monotherapy had a markedly higher rate (25.92 events per 100 patient-years) compared to those on mood stabilizer monotherapy (3.48 events), indicating a seven- to eightfold increased risk. These findings suggest that antidepressants may significantly elevate the likelihood of suicidal behavior over the course of treatment.

In summary, the cumulative evidence raises significant concerns regarding the use of antidepressants in bipolar disorder. Not only is there a lack of consistent evidence supporting their efficacy, but their use has also been associated with potential risks—including manic switching, cycle acceleration, and increased suicidality—that may ultimately compromise long-term treatment outcomes and prognosis.

Treating Bipolar Depression: Arguments in Favor of Antidepressants

Despite ongoing debate and concerns about the safety of antidepressants in bipolar disorder, several counterarguments have been proposed. These suggest that the negative impact of antidepressants on treatment outcomes may be overstated, or that, under certain conditions, antidepressants may provide meaningful therapeutic benefits. The following section examines evidence supporting the use of antidepressants in the management of bipolar depression.

Positive Effects of Antidepressants on Bipolar Depression

Tondo et al. [57] conducted a large-scale analysis of antidepressant treatment outcomes in 1036 patients with bipolar I, bipolar II, and major depressive disorder who were experiencing a major depressive episode. The study aimed to test the hypothesis that antidepressant response would be more favorable in bipolar depression (types I and II) than in unipolar depression.

Among all patients, 84.8% (878/1036) received antidepressant treatment, including 58.9% of those with bipolar I, 80.1% with bipolar II, and 91.4% with unipolar depression. The remaining 15.2% (158 patients) were not prescribed antidepressants. Notably, patients who did not receive antidepressants experienced significantly poorer outcomes: they had 3.1 times more manic recurrences, spent 2.7 times more time in (hypo)mania, and spent 1.9 times more time in depressive states compared to those who received antidepressants. These findings suggest a potential clinical benefit associated with antidepressant use.

Further analysis revealed differences in the types of antidepressants used. In patients with bipolar depression, newer antidepressants—including bupropion, mirtazapine, SSRIs, and serotonin–noradrenaline reuptake inhibitors (SNRIs)—were more commonly prescribed, while TCAs were used more frequently in unipolar depression ($p = 0.002$). In terms of efficacy, the response rates were highest in bipolar II (77.0%), followed by bipolar I (71.6%) and unipolar depression (61.7%). Similarly, remission rates were 54.0% in bipolar II, 50.6% in bipolar I, and 40.8% in unipolar depression.

The risk of (hypo)manic switch within 3 months also differed by diagnostic group: 15.8% in bipolar II, 8.6% in bipolar I, and 0.56% in unipolar depression. Based on these results, the authors concluded that antidepressant treatment—particularly newer agents—may be effective in bipolar depression, especially when used selectively and for short durations, either as monotherapy or in combination with mood stabilizers.

A systematic review and meta-analysis by Gijsman et al. [21] examined 12 short-term trials of antidepressant treatment in bipolar depression, encompassing a total of 1088 patients. The analysis found that the antidepressant group demonstrated significantly higher response (mean 86%) and remission (mean 41%) rates compared to placebo or control groups. Interestingly, the rate of manic switch was slightly lower in the antidepressant group (3.8%) than in the placebo group (4.7%). However, it is important to note that this meta-analysis included a study on olanzapine monotherapy, which has been criticized for potential selection bias and lack of equivalency across treatment arms.

A subsequent meta-analysis by Vázquez et al. [60] provided further evidence. From a database of 1250 clinical trials, the authors selected 10 studies ($n = 571$) that met strict inclusion criteria: (1) at least 10 patients with an acute major depressive episode of bipolar I or II disorder, (2) randomized treatment design, (3) use of antidepressants either as monotherapy or adjunctively, (4) placebo-controlled, (5) double-blind design, and (6) exclusion of special populations such as adolescents or elderly patients. In this analysis, the response rate in the antidepressant group was 44.8% (256/571), compared to 33.4% (288/861) in the placebo group, yielding a response rate ratio (RR) of 1.43—indicating a statistically significant advantage for antidepressants over placebo.

Taken together, these findings support the efficacy of antidepressants in the treatment of bipolar depression. Moreover, newer antidepressants appear to offer a more favorable safety profile compared to older agents such as tricyclic antidepressants (TCAs).

Antidepressants and Manic Switch

One of the key counterarguments raised by proponents of antidepressant use in bipolar depression concerns the presumed causal relationship between antidepressants and manic switching. Specifically, they question whether mania can be clearly attributed to antidepressant treatment rather than to the natural course of bipolar disorder, and whether the risk has been accurately quantified using observational, retrospective, or self-reported data.

As discussed earlier, naturalistic studies have estimated rates of switch from bipolar depression to mania ranging from 8% to 44%, with a recent systematic review by Barnuti et al. (2023) reporting similar rates between 17.3% and 48.8%.

Baldessarini et al. [8] conducted a large-scale systematic review involving 51 studies and 95,786 patients. The authors reported an 8.18% rate of manic switch during antidepressant monotherapy over a median follow-up of 2.3 years. Additionally, a meta-analysis of 10 studies found that the risk of manic switch was 2.6 times higher with antidepressants. However, the study also reported that only 3.29% of patients initially diagnosed with unipolar depression were later rediagnosed as bipolar, suggesting that diagnostic misclassification may confound interpretations of causality between antidepressant use and manic conversion.

Further support for this interpretation comes from prospective studies. Bauer et al. [11] asked 182 bipolar outpatients to track daily mood fluctuations using a 100-point self-report scale over 4 months; results showed no significant association between antidepressant use and increased manic symptoms. Similarly, Young et al. [66] found no difference in manic switch rates when comparing patients treated with mood stabilizers alone to those receiving a combination of mood stabilizers and antidepressants over 6 weeks.

Taken together, these findings suggest that antidepressant use does not consistently increase the risk of manic switching beyond the rates observed in the natural course of bipolar disorder. Even if a slight increase were present, it should be weighed against the potential therapeutic benefits of antidepressant treatment.

Benefits of Antidepressants

Another argument in favor of antidepressant use is that early discontinuation may lead to an increased risk of depressive relapse. Altshuler et al. [5] found that patients who discontinued antidepressants shortly after remission had significantly higher rates of depressive episode recurrence compared to those who continued combination therapy with mood stabilizers and antidepressants (odds ratio = 3.13, $p = 0.007$). In a one-year prospective study [4] using data from the Stanley Foundation Bipolar Network, 71% of patients who discontinued antidepressants within 6 months experienced a relapse, compared to only 36% of those who continued treatment, further supporting the protective role of sustained antidepressant use.

Supporting this view, Amsterdam et al. [6] reviewed 18 studies and reported therapeutic benefits of antidepressants in bipolar disorder. In particular, they found that venlafaxine was more effective than lithium in treating bipolar II depression, with no significant difference in manic switch rates. This suggests that antidepressant monotherapy may be both effective and relatively safe in this subgroup.

A meta-analysis by Liu et al. [33], which included 14 studies ($n = 692$) selected from a pool of 1508, found that antidepressant use—either alone or in combination with mood stabilizers—significantly reduced the incidence of new depressive episodes compared with mood stabilizers or placebo (RR = 0.64, 95% CI [0.49–0.83], $p = 0.0009$). Although the difference was not statistically significant when comparing antidepressants alone to mood stabilizers alone (RR = 0.71, $p = 0.09$), the data still favored antidepressants. The number needed to treat (NNT) was 12.5 for combination therapy and 3.3 for antidepressants alone. While the risk of manic switch was slightly elevated (RR = 1.26 for combination therapy; RR = 1.11 for monotherapy), the authors concluded that antidepressants were effective in preventing depressive relapse and that the risk of manic conversion was lower than with placebo.

Evidence regarding the optimal duration of antidepressant therapy remains limited. However, a study by Fu et al. [18] found that patients who continued antidepressants, such as SSRIs, SNRIs, trazodone, bupropion, and mirtazapine for more than 6 months after remission, had a lower risk of depressive recurrence over a two-year period (hazard ratio = 0.61, $p < 0.01$) compared to those who discontinued earlier. The authors recommended continuation for 9–12 months to maintain remission.

Tundo et al. [59] compared 111 patients with unipolar depression and 86 with bipolar depression who received 12 weeks of acute pharmacotherapy with antidepressants added to mood stabilizers or atypical antipsychotics. They found no significant differences in response rates, remission rates, or symptom improvement between the two groups. Moreover, among the bipolar group, there was no increased risk of manic switch, mixed episodes, relapse, or suicidal behavior over the one-year follow-up period. These results support the effectiveness and safety of antidepressants in both acute and one-year maintenance treatment.

In summary, while concerns regarding the risk of antidepressant-induced mood instability remain valid, the accumulating evidence suggests that the benefits—such as reduced relapse rates, symptom improvement, and lower dropout—should not be underestimated. Careful and sustained use of antidepressants, especially in appropriate subgroups, may offer meaningful clinical advantages in the treatment of bipolar depression.

Recommendations of Clinical Guidelines on Antidepressant Use in the Treatment of Bipolar Depression

Canadian Network for Mood and Anxiety Treatments (CANMAT)

CANMAT 2013 [62]

According to the CANMAT 2013 guidelines, antidepressant monotherapy is not recommended for the treatment of bipolar depression. Instead, Adjunctive antidepressants are considered a first-line option. The initial (Step 1) recommendation involves the use of divalproex or an atypical antipsychotic—such as olanzapine, risperidone, aripiprazole, or ziprasidone. If there is an inadequate response, the addition of an antidepressant is suggested as Step 2.

Furthermore, if the first-line treatment consisted of lamotrigine, lithium, quetiapine, or a combination of olanzapine and an SSRI, and the response remains insufficient, then adjunctive other antidepressants may be added as Step 3. Among antidepressants, SSRIs with the exception of paroxetine due to its higher risk of mood destabilization, and bupropion were preferred,

The guideline also emphasizes the importance of carefully weighing the potential benefits of antidepressant use against the risk of adverse effects in clinical decision-making.

CANMAT 2018 [63]

Similar to the previous guideline, antidepressants were recommended only as a second-line option, to be used as adjunctive therapy when first-line treatments are insufficient.

Guideline for Treating Bipolar Disorder, British Association for Psychopharmacology 2016 (BAP 2016) [26]

The BAP 2016 guidelines recommend considering quetiapine, lurasidone, or olanzapine for the treatment of acute bipolar depression. Although the olanzapine–fluoxetine combination (OFC) is the only antidepressant officially licensed for this indication, it is not uncommon for antidepressants to be used off-label in bipolar depression, often based on extrapolated evidence from unipolar depression. In such cases, the guidelines recommend that antidepressants be used only in combination with mood-stabilizing agents such as dopamine antagonists, lithium, or valproate.

Given the limited evidence supporting the long-term efficacy of antidepressants in bipolar disorder, the guidelines further advise discontinuing antidepressants within 12 weeks following remission of the depressive episode.

World Federation of Societies of Biological Psychiatry Guideline 2010 (WFSBP 2010) [27]

According to the WFSBP 2010 guidelines, quetiapine was the only agent recommended as monotherapy with the highest level of evidence (Recommendation Grade [RG] 1). Other agents recommended for monotherapy included fluoxetine, lamotrigine, olanzapine, and valproate, all categorized as RG 3, while paroxetine was explicitly not recommended.

For combination therapy, the olanzapine–fluoxetine combination (OFC) received an RG 3 recommendation, whereas combinations such as sertraline with lithium or valproate, and venlafaxine with lithium or valproate, were classified as RG 4.

The guideline defined Recommendation Grades as follows:

- *RG 1*: Superiority over placebo in at least two randomized controlled trials (RCTs), or superiority/equivalence to a comparator in one RCT.
- *RG 3*: Limited but positive evidence from controlled studies.
- *RG 4*: Evidence derived from uncontrolled trials, case reports, or expert consensus.

At the time of publication, fluoxetine was considered the antidepressant with the strongest evidence base among available options. It was recommended as monotherapy at RG 3 and, in general, antidepressants were advised to be used only in combination with mood-stabilizing agents in the treatment of bipolar depression.

National Institute for Health and Clinical Excellence (NICE) Guideline 2006 and 2023 [37]

The 2006 NICE guideline stated that the treatment of acute depressive episodes in bipolar disorder is generally similar to that of unipolar depression. However, the long-term use of antidepressants in maintenance treatment was discouraged due to their potential to induce manic episodes or rapid cycling.

Key recommendations included:

1. *For patients not currently receiving a mood stabilizer*:
   - Initiate a combination of a mood stabilizer and an antidepressant.
   - If antidepressant monotherapy is prescribed, the patient should be counseled on the risk of mania and the benefits of adding a mood stabilizer.
   - If the patient refuses a mood stabilizer, close clinical monitoring is essential.
   - If a manic episode occurs during antidepressant treatment, the antidepressant should be discontinued immediately.
   - Antidepressants should not be routinely continued after remission, as there is no clear evidence of relapse prevention and there remains a risk of manic switching.
2. *For patients already on mood stabilizers*:
   - Evaluate the dose and adjust if necessary when a depressive episode occurs.
3. *For mild depressive episodes*:
   - Observe for up to two weeks. If symptoms worsen, treat similarly to moderate or severe depression.
4. *For moderate to severe depressive episodes:*
   - Prefer SSRIs over TCAs.
   - If the current mood stabilizer is not an antipsychotic, consider adding quetiapine.
5. *Avoid antidepressants* in patients with rapid cycling, recent hypomania, or recent functionally impairing mood fluctuations.
6. *Discontinuation of antidepressants* should be considered once remission is achieved and sustained for at least 8 weeks.

NICE Guideline 2023

The updated 2023 guideline took a more conservative stance regarding antidepressant use. Antidepressants were not recommended for patients with moderate to severe bipolar depression. Instead, the following strategies were advised:

1. *If the patient is not currently taking medication*:
   - Consider initiating treatment with olanzapine or lamotrigine.
   - If there is no response to olanzapine–fluoxetine combination (OFC) or quetiapine, consider adding lamotrigine.
2. *If the patient is already taking lithium or valproate:*
   - Check serum drug levels and adjust to optimal therapeutic ranges.
   - If symptoms persist, consider adding OFC or quetiapine as the next treatment step.

Korean Medication Algorithm for Bipolar Disorder (KMAP-BP)

The Korean Medication Algorithm for Bipolar Disorder (KMAP-BP) is a clinical guidelines developed jointly by the Korean Society for

Depressive and Bipolar Disorders and the Korean Society of Psychopharmacology. Since its initial publication in 2002, the guidelines have been revised every 4 years based on expert consensus from Korean mood disorder experts. This section focuses specifically on expert opinions and recommendations regarding the use of antidepressants in bipolar depression.

KMAP-BP 2010 [47]

In the 2010 edition, Korean experts classified bipolar depressive episodes into mild, moderate, and severe categories, with or without psychotic features. Antidepressant monotherapy was not recommended as an initial strategy. Instead, combination treatment with mood stabilizers or atypical antipsychotics was favored. Following remission of depressive symptoms, 69.2–89.2% of the experts recommended discontinuing antidepressants after a short period of continuation, ranging from 4.5 to 16 weeks.

KMAP-BP 2014 [48]

The 2014 revision continued to recommend antidepressants only in combination with other psychotropic agents as a first-line strategy. A slightly higher proportion of experts (71.9–93.7%) endorsed the use of antidepressants for a limited duration, ranging from 8 to 27 weeks. Among available antidepressants in Korea, escitalopram (25.3%), bupropion (24.7%), and sertraline (13.4%) were most preferred, based on their antidepressant efficacy and relatively lower risk of inducing manic episodes.

KMAP-BP 2018 [49]

In the 2018 update, the combination of antidepressants with other agents was recommended as a second-line treatment for mild-to-moderate and severe depressive episodes without psychotic features. However, in severe episodes with psychotic features, the combination of antidepressants and atypical antipsychotics was considered a first-line strategy. The majority of experts (76.0–95.1%) supported using antidepressants for a duration ranging from 7 to 22 weeks.

KMAP-BP 2022 [50]

In the 2022 revision, recommendations remained largely similar to the 2018 version. Notably, even in psychotic depressive episodes, the use of antidepressants in combination therapy was downgraded to a second-line strategy, indicating a slight decline in expert preference. Between 73.6% and 86.2% of experts recommended discontinuing antidepressants after 9.3–26 weeks of use.

Across several versions of the KMAP-BP series, Korean mood disorder experts consistently do not recommend antidepressants as monotherapy for bipolar depression. Instead, they support adjunctive use depending on the severity and clinical context, typically for a defined period before discontinuation. The preferred duration of antidepressant continuation generally ranged between 4.5 and 27 weeks across the different surveys.

Recommendations from the International Society for Bipolar Disorder (ISBD)

Due to the limited evidence supporting the use of antidepressants in bipolar depression, the International Society for Bipolar Disorders (ISBD) convened a task force to develop 12 consensus-based recommendations, grounded in a comprehensive literature review and expert opinion [41].

Acute Treatment

1. Adjunctive antidepressants may be used for an acute bipolar I or II depressive episode when there is a history of previous positive response to antidepressants.
2. Adjunctive antidepressants should be avoided for an acute bipolar I or II depressive episode with two or more concomitant core manic symptoms in the presence of psychomotor agitation or rapid cycling.

Maintenance Treatment

3. Maintenance treatment with adjunctive antidepressants may be considered if a patient relapses into a depressive episode after stopping antidepressant therapy.

Monotherapy

4. Antidepressant monotherapy should be avoided in bipolar I disorder.
5. Antidepressant monotherapy should be avoided in bipolar I and II depression with two or more concomitant core manic symptoms.

Switch to Mania, Hypomania, or Mixed States and Rapid Cycling

6. Bipolar patients starting antidepressants should be closely monitored for signs of hypomania or mania and increased psychomotor agitation, in which case antidepressants should be discontinued.
7. The use of antidepressants should be discouraged if there is a history of past mania, hypomania, or mixed episodes emerging during antidepressant treatment.
8. Antidepressant use should be avoided in bipolar patients with a high mood instability (i.e., a high number of episodes) or with a history of rapid cycling.

Use in Mixed States

9. Antidepressants should be avoided during manic and depressive episodes with mixed features.
10. Antidepressants should be avoided in bipolar patients with predominantly mixed states.
11. Previously prescribed antidepressants should be discontinued in patients currently experiencing mixed states.

Drug Class

12. Adjunctive treatment with norepinephrine-serotonin reuptake inhibitors or tri- and tetracyclics should be considered only after other antidepressants have been tried, and should be closely monitored because of an increased risk of mood switch or destabilization.

In summary, antidepressants should be avoided whenever possible in patients with a history of antidepressant-induced mania or hypomania, predominant mixed features, or recent rapid cycling. If their use is deemed necessary, they should be prescribed with caution. Both patients and caregivers (when appropriate) should be educated about early warning signs of mood switching or cycle acceleration, and antidepressant treatment should be promptly discontinued if such symptoms emerge. Antidepressant monotherapy should not be used to treat depressive episode in patients with bipolar I disorder.

2020 Australian and New Zealand Psychiatric Association Guidelines [35]

First-line treatment prioritizes mood modulators (lithium, lamotrigine, valproate) alone or atypical antipsychotics (quetiapine, lurasidone, cariprazine) alone.

General Considerations

1.1. The use of antidepressants in the treatment of bipolar disorder should be overseen by a psychiatrist where possible.

1.2. The clinical risks versus benefits of antidepressants in treating bipolar depression should be determined on an individual basis.

Treatment

1.3. Adjunctive antidepressant therapy should be used cautiously in the treatment of bipolar depression when there is a history of antidepressant-induced mania, current or predominant mixed features, or a history of rapid cycling.

1.4. Antidepressant monotherapy should be avoided in bipolar disorder.

Treatment Emergent Affective Switch (TEAS)

1.5. Upon commencing antidepressants, patients with bipolar disorder should be closely monitored for symptoms of mania, and if

these emerge, then antidepressant therapy should be discontinued.
Psychoeducation should be provided so that patients can identify early warning signs of mania and/or mixed symptoms.

1.6. Antidepressant therapy should be avoided in bipolar disorder patients with a history of rapid cycling and/or a high level of mood instability.
1.7. The prescription of antidepressants should consider any past history of a treatment emergent affective switch (TEAS).

The use of antidepressants in the treatment of bipolar disorder should be directed by a psychiatrist whenever possible.

The decision to use an antidepressant for bipolar depression should be based on a risk–benefit comparison tailored to the patient's individual circumstances.

The use of adjunctive antidepressants should be very cautious in patients with a history of antidepressant-induced mania, current or predominant mixed symptoms, or rapid cycling.

Antidepressant monotherapy should be avoided in bipolar disorder.

Once started, patients should be closely monitored for symptoms of (hypo)mania, and antidepressant treatment should be discontinued if symptoms of (hypo)mania occur. Patients should be educated to recognize early warning signs of mania and/or mixed symptoms.

Avoid antidepressants in patients with a history of rapid cycling and/or severe mood instability.

Past mood episodes should be checked when prescribing antidepressants.

Closing Thoughts

The evolution of antidepressant research in bipolar depression can be broadly divided into three distinct eras:

1. The 1970s and 1980s, when tricyclic antidepressants (TCAs) were the primary focus;
2. The subsequent SSRI and SNRI era; and.
3. The more recent period marked by investigations into novel agents such as mirtazapine, agomelatine, and vortioxetine.

While earlier studies involving TCAs emphasized the risks associated with antidepressant use—particularly manic switching and mood destabilization—subsequent research, especially with newer antidepressants, has increasingly focused on evaluating their therapeutic potential and safety.

Notably, the majority of randomized controlled trials (RCTs)—which form the foundation for meta-analyses—have examined SSRIs such as fluoxetine and paroxetine, and other agents like bupropion and agomelatine. This allows for comparison of clinical efficacy and safety across various antidepressant classes in bipolar depression.

Therefore, rather than making binary judgments for or against antidepressant use in bipolar depression, it is more appropriate to individualize treatment decisions. This includes evaluating the unique pharmacological profiles and effectiveness of each antidepressant, considering the patient's clinical characteristics, current medications, and any underlying medical conditions.

In other words, a one-size-fits-all approach is inadequate. As emphasized by Fico and Vieta [17], antidepressant selection should be personalized—aiming to identify which patients are most likely to benefit, and under what clinical circumstances.

In conclusion, when faced with a patient experiencing a bipolar depressive episode who pleads, *"Please help me, please make me feel up!"* the following steps are recommended:

1. *Clarify the diagnosis*: Explain the key differences between bipolar and unipolar depression, particularly in terms of antidepressant response and treatment trajectory.
2. *Evaluate potential benefits*: Carefully weigh the potential clinical benefit of adding an antidepressant in the context of the patient's current symptom profile.

3. *Educate the patient*: Provide psychoeducation regarding possible risks, such as manic or hypomanic switching and mixed states.
4. *Select appropriately*: Choose an antidepressant based on individual clinical history, co-occurring medical conditions, gender, and prior treatment response.
5. *Explore alternatives*: Consider other evidence-based treatment strategies, such as atypical antipsychotics, neuromodulation techniques, or agents like esketamine.
6. *Titrate cautiously*: Initiate antidepressants at a low dose, titrate gradually, and closely monitor for therapeutic response and adverse effects.

Declarations

Competing Interests The author(s) has no competing interests to declare that are relevant to the content of this manuscript.

Ethics Approval The author(s) declares that this manuscript does not include primary research with human participants.

The author(s) declares that this manuscript does not include primary studies involving animals.

References

1. Akiskal HS, Khani MK, Scott-Strauss A. Cyclothymic temperament disorders. Psychiatr Clin. 1979;2:527–54.
2. Akiskal HS, Hantouche EG, Allilaire JF, Sechter D, Bourgeois ML, Azorin JM, et al. Validating antidepressant-associated hypomania (bipolar III): a systematic comparison with spontaneous hypomania (bipolar II). J Affect Disord. 2003;73:65–74.
3. Altshuler LL, Post RM, Leverich GS, Mikalauskas K, Rosoff A, Ackerman L. Antidepressant-induced mania and cycle acceleration: a controversy revisited. Am J Psychiatry. 1995;152:1130–8.
4. Altshuler L, Suppes T, Black D, Nolen W, Keck PE, Frye M, et al. Impact of antidepressant discontinuation after acute remission from bipolar depression on rates of depressive relapse on 1-year follow-up. Am J Psychiatry. 2003;160:1252–62.
5. Altshuler L, Kiriakos L, Calcagno J, Goodman R, Gitlin M, Frye M, et al. The impact of antidepressant discontinuation versus antidepressant continuation on 1-year risk for relapse of bipolar depression: a retrospective chart review. J Clin Psychiatry. 2001;62:612–6.
6. Amsterdam JD, Wang C, Shwarz M, Shults J. Venlafaxine versus lithium monotherapy of rapid and non-rapid cycling patients with bipolar II major depressive episode: a randomized, parallel group, open-label trial. J Affective Disord. 2009;112:219–30.
7. Baldessarini R, Henk H, Sklar A, Chang J, Leahy L. Psychotropic medications for patients with bipolar disorder in the United States: polytherapy and adherence. Psychiatr Serv. 2008;59:1175–83.
8. Baldessarini RJ, Faedda GL, Offidani E, Vázquez GH, Marangoni C, Serra G, et al. Antidepressant-associated mood-switching and transition from unipolar major depression to bipolar disorder: a review. J Affect Disord. 2013;148:129–35.
9. Baldessarini RJ. Chemotherapy in psychiatry. 3rd ed. New York: Springer Press; 2013.
10. Barbutia M, Menculinib G, Verdolinic N, Pacchiarottic I, Kotzalidisd GD, Tortorellab A, Vietac E, Perugia G. A systematic review of manic/hypomanic and depressive switches in patients with bipolar disorder in naturalistic settings: the role of antidepressant and antipsychotic drugs. Eur Neuropsychopharmacol. 2023;73:1–15.
11. Bauer M, Rasgon N, Grof P, Glenn T, Lapp M, Marsh W, et al. Do antidepressants influence mood patterns? A naturalistic study in bipolar disorder. Eur Psychiatry. 2006;21:262–9.
12. Benazzi F. Antidepressant-associated hypomania in out-patient depression: a 203-case study in private practice. J Affect Disord. 1997;46:73–7.
13. Bunney WE, Murphy DL, Goodwin FK, Borge GF. The switch process from depression to mania: relationship to the ten- drugs which alter brain amines. Lancet. 1970;1:1022–7.
14. Calabrese JR, Bowden CL, Sachs GS, Ascher JA, Monaghan E, Rudd GD. A double-blind placebo-controlled study of lamotrigine monotherapy in outpatients with bipolar I depression. J Clin Psychiatry. 1999;60:79–88.
15. Cassidy F, Ahearn EP, Carroll BJ. Symptom profile consistency in recurrent manic episodes. Compr Psychiatry. 2002;43:179–81.
16. Fergusson D, Doucette S, Glass KC, Shapiro S, Healy D, Hebert P, et al. Association between suicide attempts and selective serotonin reuptake inhibitors: systematic review of randomized controlled trials. BMJ. 2005;330:396.
17. Fico G, Vieta E. Antidepressant use in bipolar disorder: shifting focus from 'whether' to 'whom'. Eur Neuropsychopharmacol. 2024;84:1–2.
18. Fu AZ, Christensen DB, Hansen RA, Liu GG. Second-generation antidepressant discontinuation and depressive relapse in adult patients with bipolar depression: results of a retrospective database analysis. Clin Ther. 2006;28:979–89.
19. Geddes J, Carney SM, Davies C, Furukawa TA, Kupfer DJ, Frank E, et al. Relapse prevention with antidepressant drug treatment in depressive disorders: a systematic review. Lancet. 2003;361:653–61.

20. Ghaemi SN, Wingo AP, Filkowski MA, Baldessarini RJ. Long-term antidepressant treatment in bipolar disorder: meta-analyses of benefits and risks. Acta Psychiatr Scand. 2008;118:347–56.
21. Gijsman HJ, Geddes JR, Rendell JM, Nolen WA, Goodwin GM. Antidepressants for bipolar depression: a systematic review of randomized, controlled trials. Am J Psychiatry. 2004;161:1537–47.
22. Goldberg JF, Garno JL, Kocsis JH, Leon AC, Portera L, Whiteside JE. Correlates of suicidal ideation in dysphoric mania. J Affect Disord. 1999;56:75–81.
23. Goldberg JF, Allen MH, Miklowitz DA, Bowden CL, Endick CJ, Chessick CA, et al. Suicidal ideation and pharmacotherapy among STEP-BD patients. Psychiatr Serv. 2005;56:1534–40.
24. Goldberg JF, Perlis RH, Ghaemi SN, Calabrese JR, Bowden CL, Wisniewski S, et al. Adjunctive antidepressant use and symptomatic recovery among bipolar depressed patients with concomitant manic symptoms: findings from the STEP-BD. Am J Psychiatry. 2007;164:1348–55.
25. Goldberg JF, Brooks JO III, Kurita K, Hoblyn JC, Ghaemi SN, Perlis RH, et al. Depressive illness burden associated with complex polypharmacy in patients with bipolar disorder: findings from the STEP-BD. J Clin Psychiatry. 2009;70:155–62.
26. Goodwin GM, Haddad PM, Ferrier IN, Aronson JK, Barnes T, Cipriani A, et al. Evidence-based guidelines for treating bipolar disorder: revised third edition recommendations from the British Association for Psychopharmacology. J Psychopharmacol. 2016;30:495–553.
27. Grunze H, Vieta E, Goodwin GM, Bowden C, Licht RW, Möller HJ, Kasper S, WFSBP Task Force On Treatment Guidelines For Bipolar Disorders. The world federation of societies of biological psychiatry (WFSBP) guidelines for the biological treatment of bipolar disorders: update 2010 on the treatment of acute bipolar depression. World J Biol Psychiatry. 2010;11:81–109.
28. Hooshmand F, Do D, Shah S, Gershon A, Park DY, Kim H, et al. Differential prevalence and demographic and clinical correlates of antidepressant use in American bipolar I versus bipolar II disorder patients. J Affect Disord. 2018;234:74–9.
29. Hu Y, Zhang H, Wang H, Wang C, Kung S, Li C. Adjunctive antidepressants for the acute treatment of bipolar depression: a systematic review and meta-analysis. Psychiatry Res. 2022;311(February):114468. https://doi.org/10.1016/j.psychres.2022.114468.
30. Judd LL, Akiskal HS, Schettler PJ, Endicott J, Maser J, Solomon DA, et al. The long-term natural history of the weekly symptomatic status of bipolar I disorder. Arch Gen Psychiatry. 2002;59:530–7.
31. Khan A, Khan S, Kolts R, Brown WA. Suicide rates in clinical trials of SSRIs, other antidepressants, and placebo: analysis of FDA reports. Am J Psychiatry. 2003;160:790–2.
32. Lewis J, Winokur G. The induction of mania: a natural history study with controls. Arch Gen Psychiatry. 1982;39:303–6.
33. Liu B, Zhang Y, Fang H, Liu J, Liu T, Li L. Efficacy and safety of long-term antidepressant treatment for bipolar disorders – a meta-analysis of randomized controlled trials. J Affect Disord. 2017;223:41–8.
34. Maj M, Pirozzi R, Magliano L, Bartoli L. The prognostic significance of "switching" in patients with bipolar disorder: a 10-year prospective follow-up study. Am J Psychiatry. 2002;159:1711–7.
35. Malhi GS, Bell E, Boyce P, Bassett D, Berk M, Bryant R, et al. The 2020 Royal Australian and New Zealand college of psychiatrists clinical practice guidelines for mood disorders: bipolar disorder summary. Bipolar Disord. 2020;22:805–21. https://doi.org/10.1111/bdi.13036.
36. McElroy SL, Weisler RH, Chang W, Olausson B, Paulsson B, Brecher M, Agambaram V, Merideth C, Nordenhem A, Young AH, EMBOLDEN II (Trial D1447C00134) Investigators. A double-blind, placebo-controlled study of quetiapine and paroxetine as monotherapy in adults with bipolar depression (EMBOLDEN II). J Clin Psychiatry. 2010;71:163–74.
37. McGirr A, Vöhringer PA, Ghaemi SN, Lam RW, Yatham LN. Safety and efficacy of adjunctive second-generation antidepressant therapy with a mood stabiliser or an atypical antipsychotic in acute bipolar depression: a systematic review and meta-analysis of randomised placebo-controlled trials. Lancet Psychiatry. 2016;3(12):1138–46. https://doi.org/10.1016/S2215-0366(16)30264-4.
38. National Institute for Health and Clinical Excellence (NICE). Bipolar disorder. The management of bipolar disorder in adults, children and adolescents, in primary and secondary care 2006. www.nice.org.uk/CG038.
39. Nemeroff CB, Evans DL, Gyulai L, Sachs GS, Bowden CL, Gergel IP, et al. Double-blind, placebo-controlled comparison of imipramine and paroxetine in the treatment of bipolar depression. Am J Psychiatry. 2001;158:906–12.
40. Pacchiarotti I, Valentí M, Colom F, Rosa AR, Nivoli AM, Murru A, et al. Differential outcome of bipolar patients receiving antidepressant monotherapy versus combination with an antimanic drug. J Affect Disord. 2011;129:321–6.
41. Pacchiarotti I, Bond DJ, Baldessarini RJ, Nolen WA, Grunze H, Licht RW, et al. The International Society for Bipolar Disorders (ISBD) task force report on antidepressant use in bipolar disorders. Am J Psychiatry. 2013;170:1249–62.
42. Post RM, Altshuler LL, Frye MA, Suppes T, Rush AJ, Keck PE Jr, et al. Rate of switch in bipolar patients prospectively treated with second-generation antidepressants as augmentation to mood stabilizers. Bipolar Disord. 2001;3:259–65.
43. Prien RF, Klett CJ, Caffey EM. Lithium carbonate and imipramine in prevention of affective episodes. Arch Gen Psychiatry. 1973;29:420–5.

44. Quitkin FM, Kane J, Rifkin A, Ramos-Lorenzi JR, Nayak DV. Prophylactic lithium carbonate with and without imipramine for bipolar I patients. Arch Gen Psychiatry. 1981;38:902–7.
45. Rouillon F, Lejoyeux M, Filteau MJ. Unwanted effects of long term treatment. In: Montomery SA, Rouillon FA, editors. Long term treatment of depression. New York: Wiley; 1992.
46. Sachs GS, Nierenberg AA, Calabrese JR, Marangell LB, Wisniewski SR, Gyulai L, et al. Effectiveness of adjunctive antidepressant treatment for bipolar depression. N Engl J Med. 2007;356:1711–22.
47. Seo JS, Joo YH, MD2, Bahk WM, Yoon BH, Kim W, Min KJ, Lee E, Jon DI, Ahn YM, Lee JG, Kim BS, Shin YC. Korean medication algorithm for bipolar disorder 2010: depressive episode. J Kor Soc Dep Bipol Disord 2011:9:96–102.
48. Seo JS, Bahk WM, Lee JG, Woo YS, Jeong JH, Kim MD, et al. Korean medication algorithm for bipolar disorder 2014(III): depressive episode. Korean J Psychopharmacol. 2014;25:68–78.
49. Seo JS, Bahk WM, Yoon BH, Jon DI, Kim W, Lee JG, et al. Korean medication algorithm for bipolar disorder 2018: depressive episode. Mood Emot. 2018;16:1–12.
50. Seo JS, Woo YS, Bahk WM, Jeong JH, Yoon BH, Choo IH, et al. Korean medication algorithm project for bipolar disorder 2022: depressive episode. J Korean Neuropsychiatr Assoc. 2022;61(2):123–32. https://doi.org/10.4306/jknpa.2022.61.2.123.
51. Serretti A, Artioli P, Zanardi R, Rossini D. Clinical features of antidepressant associated manic and hypomanic switches in bipolar disorder. Prog Neuro-Psychopharmacol Biol Psychiatry. 2003;27:751–7.
52. Sidor MM, Macqueen GM. Antidepressants for the acute treatment of bipolar depression: a systematic review and meta-analysis. J Clin Psychiatry. 2011;72:156–67.
53. Silverstone T. Moclobemide vs imipramine in bipolar depression: a multicentre double-blind clinical trial. Acta Psychiatr Scand. 2001;104:104–9.
54. Simon NM, Otto MW, Weiss RD, Bauer MS, Miyahara S, Wisniewski SR, et al. Pharmacotherapy for bipolar disorder and comorbid conditions: baseline data from STEP-BD. J Clin Psychopharmacol. 2004;24:512–20.
55. Strober M, Carlson G. Bipolar illness in adolescents with major depression: clinical, genetic, and psychopharmacologic predictors in a three-to-four year prospective follow-up investigation. Arch Gen Psychiatry. 1982;39:549–55.
56. Tondo L, Va'zquez G, Baldessarini RJ. Mania associated with antidepressant treatment: comprehensive meta-analytic review. Acta Psychiatr Scand. 2010;121:404–14.
57. Tondo L, Baldessarini RJ, Vázquez G, Lepri B, Visioli C. Clinical responses to antidepressants among 1036 acutely depressed patients with bipolar or unipolar major affective disorders. Acta Psychiatr Scand. 2013;127:355–64.
58. Truman CJ, Goldberg JF, Ghaemi SN, Baldassano CF, Wisniewski SR, Dennehy EB, et al. Self-reported history of manic/hypomanic switch associated with antidepressant use: data from the systematic treatment enhancement program for bipolar disorder (STEP-BD). J Clin Psychiatry. 2007;68:1472–9.
59. Tundo A, Musetti L, Grande CD, de Filippis C, Proietti L, Cambiali E, Franceschini C, Dell'Osso L. Is short-term antidepressant treatment effective and safe in bipolar depression? Results from an observational multicenter study. Hum Psychopharmacol Clin Exp. 2021;36:e2773. https://doi.org/10.1002/hup.2773.
60. Vázquez GH, Tondo L, Undurraga J, Baldessarini RJ. Overview of antidepressant treatment of bipolar depression. Int J Neuropsychopharmacol. 2013;16:1673–85.
61. Wehr TA, Goodwin FK. Can antidepressants cause mania and worsen the course of affective illness? Am J Psychiatry. 1987;144:1403–11.
62. Yatham LN, Kennedy SH, Parikh SV, Schaffer A, Beaulieu S, Alda M, O'Donovan C, Macqueen G, McIntyre RS, Sharma V, Ravindran A, Young LT, Milev R, Bond DJ, Frey BN, Goldstein BI, Lafer B, Birmaher B, Ha K, Nolen WA, Berk M. Canadian network for mood and anxiety treatments (CANMAT) and International Society for Bipolar Disorders (ISBD) collaborative update of CANMAT guidelines for the management of patients with bipolar disorder: update 2013. Bipolar Disord. 2013;15:1–44.
63. Yatham LN, Kennedy SH, Parikh SV, Schaffer A, Bond DJ, Frey BN, et al. Canadian network for mood and anxiety treatments (CANMAT) and International Society for Bipolar Disorders (ISBD) 2018 guidelines for the management of patients with bipolar disorder. Bipolar Disord. 2018;20:97–170.
64. Yatham LN, Arumugham SS, Kesavan M, BEAM-BD trial group, et al. Duration of adjunctive antidepressant maintenance in bipolar I depression. N Engl J Med. 2023;389(5):430–40. https://doi.org/10.1056/NEJMoa2300184.
65. Yerevanian BI, Koek RJ, Mintz J, Akiskal HS. Bipolar pharmacotherapy and suicidal behavior part 2. The impact of antidepressants. J Affect Disord. 2007;103:13–21.
66. Young LT, Joffe RT, Robb JC, MacQueen GM, Marriott M, Patelis-Siotis I. Double-blind comparison of addition of a second mood stabilizer vs. An antidepressant to an initial mood stabilizer for treatment of patients with bipolar depression. Am J Psychiatry. 2000;157:124–6.

Comparative Analysis of Bipolar Disorder Treatment Guidelines

14

Chan-Mo Yang and Won-Myong Bahk

Traditionally, in the treatment of psychiatric disorders, clinicians have used a variety of therapeutic techniques, including medication, based on their individual clinical experience and knowledge. However, over the past 40 years, as the etiological theories of psychiatric disorders have been partially revised and new drugs with various mechanisms have been introduced into clinical practice, it has become increasingly difficult to select and effectively use appropriate medications based solely on subjective clinical experience and knowledge [1]. Among psychiatric disorders, bipolar disorder has been particularly challenging for clinicians in selecting appropriate therapeutic agents because its clinical presentation and treatment response vary depending on the type of episode—such as manic, depressive, or mixed episodes—as well as on the specific diagnosis and subtypes. To overcome these difficulties, the field of psychiatry has been developing and utilizing treatment guidelines and algorithms based on evidence-based medicine, which has rapidly advanced since the 1990s. Notably, for bipolar disorder, treatment guidelines and algorithms for pharmacotherapy began to be developed in the United States and other countries starting in the 1990s, earlier than for other psychiatric disorders. In Korea, the Korean Medication Algorithm Project for Bipolar Disorder 2002 (KMAP-BP 2002) was first developed in 2002, and its usefulness has been confirmed through clinical studies [2–5].

International treatment guidelines or algorithms for bipolar disorder include the American Psychiatric Association Practice Guideline for Bipolar Disorder (APA-BP) [6, 7], the Expert Consensus Guideline for Bipolar Disorder (ECG-BP) [8], the Texas Implementation of Medication Algorithm (TIMA) [9, 10], the Royal Australian and New Zealand College of Psychiatrists Clinical Practice Guidelines for Mood Disorders (RANZCP) [11–13], Evidence-Based Guidelines for Treating Bipolar disorder: Recommendations from the British Association for Psychopharmacology (BAP) [14–16], the Canadian Network for Mood and Anxiety Treatments Guidelines for the Management of Patients with Bipolar Disorder (CANMAT) [17–24], The International College of Neuro-Psychopharmacology Treatment Guidelines for Bipolar Disorder in Adults (CINP-BD) [25], The World Federation Society of Biological Psychiatry Guideline for Biological Treatment of Bipolar Disorder (WFSBP) [26–32], and the

C.-M. Yang (✉)
Department of Psychiatry, Wonkwang University Hospital, School of Medicine, Wonkwang University, Iksan, Republic of Korea
e-mail: ychanmo@wku.ac.kr

W.-M. Bahk
Woo and Bahk Psychiatry Clinic, Seoul, Republic of Korea

Department of Psychiatry, College of Medicine, The Catholic University of Korea, Seoul, Republic of Korea

W.-M. Bahk et al. (eds.), *Bipolar Disorder*, https://doi.org/10.1007/978-981-92-1323-8_14

National Institute for Health and Clinical Experience Clinical Guideline (NICE) [31, 33, 34]. These treatment guidelines must be continuously revised to reflect new evidence on the efficacy and safety of each drug, in line with changes in the diagnosis of bipolar disorder and the development of new therapeutic agents. However, among these, the ECG-BP has not been revised since 2000 [8], the APA-BP since 2002 [7], and TIMA since 2005 [10]. In contrast, the KMAP-BP, published in Korea, has been revised every 4 years since its initial publication in 2002, with subsequent editions in 2006 [35], 2010 [36], 2014 [37], and 2018 [38], and the KMAP-BP 2022 was released in the first half of 2022 [39]. Therefore, this chapter aims to compare the recently revised international treatment guidelines—namely RANZCP (2020) [13], CINP-BD (2017) [25], and CANMAT (2021 and 2023) [23]—with the domestic guideline, KMAP-BP 2022.

Before comparing these guidelines, it is crucial to understand the fundamental reasons for their divergence. These differences arise not only from varying clinical interpretations but also from (1) evidence appraisal methodology (e.g., CINP-BD's multi-faceted rating vs. CANMAT's RCT-weighted evidence levels vs. KMAP-BP's expert consensus scoring); (2) national drug availability (e.g., the noted lack of asenapine and cariprazine in Korea); and (3) local clinical practice or cultural prescribing patterns (e.g., the earlier preference for combination therapy noted in KMAP-BP). This comparative analysis, therefore, operates with the understanding of these heterogeneous frameworks.

The International College of Neuro-Psychopharmacology Treatment Guidelines for Bipolar Disorder in Adults (CINP-BD 2017)

This guideline, overseen by The International College of Neuro-Psychopharmacology (CINP), was developed to provide guidelines and algorithms for the treatment of adult bipolar disorder in primary and secondary care settings. To achieve this, evidence was gathered by searching for randomized controlled trials (RCTs), post-hoc analyses of RCTs, meta-analyses, review articles, and existing treatment guideline literature. The results are presented with levels of evidence, categorized into efficacy, safety, and tolerability. Furthermore, it also provides a level of recommendation for each pharmacotherapy, integrating this evidence with clinical considerations. The levels of evidence and recommendation applied in the CINP-BD are shown in Table 14.1.

Table 14.1 Levels of evidence and recommendation based on efficacy and tolerability

Domain	Level	Adapted definition	Practical interpretation
Efficacy	1	Supported by at least two adequately sized, high-quality, placebo-controlled RCTs; if findings are mixed, the number of positive studies must outweigh the number of negative studies	Strongest efficacy signal
	2	Supported by at least one randomized, double-blind, placebo-controlled RCT. This level also includes cases supported only by a positive meta-analysis, or studies failing to meet Level 1 criteria (e.g., small sample size, lack of placebo control)	Probable benefit, but the database is smaller or less consistent
	3	Derived from controlled trials without a placebo group or from post-hoc analyses	Possible benefit that should be interpreted cautiously
	4	Supported only by uncertain evidence or by RCTs of insufficient quality	Insufficient basis for a firm efficacy claim
	5	Negative study results	Not supported for efficacy

(continued)

Table 14.1 (continued)

Domain	Level	Adapted definition	Practical interpretation
Safety/tolerability	1	Excellent: Adverse effects are uncommon, usually transient, and unlikely to threaten overall medical status or life	Favorable tolerability profile
	2	Intermediate: Adverse effects may be more frequent or persistent and can burden patients, but they are generally manageable and not typically life-threatening with usual monitoring	Acceptable with monitoring
	3	Suboptimal: Adverse effects can be persistent, clinically burdensome, medically compromising, or occasionally serious	Problematic tolerability; careful risk-benefit review is needed
Overall recommendation	1	Efficacy support at Level 1 or 2 and tolerability/safety at Level 1	Preferred option when clinically appropriate
	2	Efficacy support at Level 1 or 2 and tolerability/safety at Level 2	Reasonable option with monitoring
	3	Efficacy support at Level 3 and tolerability/safety at Level 1 or 2	Alternative when stronger options are unsuitable
	4	Efficacy support at Level 4 and tolerability/safety at Level 3	Low-priority option
	5	Negative efficacy evidence (Level 5)	Not recommended

Note. This table is an adapted and reorganized summary, not a direct reproduction. Source framework: Fountoulakis KN, Yatham L, Grunze H, et al. The International College of Neuro-Psychopharmacology (CINP) Treatment Guidelines for Bipolar Disorder in Adults (CINP-BD-2017), Part 2: Review, Grading of the Evidence, and a Precise Algorithm. Available at: https://pmc.ncbi.nlm.nih.gov/articles/PMC5409012/

Canadian Network for Mood and Anxiety Treatments Guidelines for the Management of Patients with Bipolar Disorder (CANMAT 2023) and with Mixed Presentation (CANMAT 2021)

These treatment guidelines from Canada are based on extensive literature reviews and research findings and were first developed in 1997 [20]. They were revised using the same methodology in 2005 [19], and full revisions reflecting new evidence were subsequently published in 2007 [21], 2009 [18], 2013 [17], 2018 [22], and 2023 [23]. In 2021, guidelines for mixed presentations were also released [24]. Since 2013, the CANMAT guidelines have been jointly researched and developed with the International Society for Bipolar Disorders, making them one of the most rapidly updated international treatment guidelines.

The CANMAT categorizes the level of evidence from 1 to 4. *Level 1* represents the strongest evidence and requires a meta-analysis with narrow confidence intervals, replicated double-blind studies, or at least one RCT with a placebo or active comparator group of 30 or more subjects. *Level 2* requires a meta-analysis with wide confidence intervals or at least one double-blind RCT with a placebo or active comparator group of 30 or more subjects. *Level 3* requires at least one double-blind RCT with a placebo or active comparator group of 10–29 subjects, or results from healthcare administrative data such as health insurance databases. *Level 4* refers to evidence from non-controlled studies, expert opinion, or anecdotal reports.

Meanwhile, the level of therapeutic recommendation is categorized as first-line, second-line, third-line, and "not recommended," presented according to each clinical situation. A *first-line* recommendation requires Level 1 or 2 evidence for efficacy, clinical support for safety/tolerability, and no risk of medication-induced mood switch. A *second-line* recommendation requires at least Level 3 evidence for efficacy, clinical support for safety/tolerability, and a low risk of medication-induced mood switch. A *third-*

line recommendation requires at least Level 4 evidence for efficacy and clinical support for safety/tolerability. "*Not recommended*" applies when there is Level 1 evidence of inefficacy, or Level 2 evidence of inefficacy combined with expert consensus.

For each clinical situation, the CANMAT guidelines present the first, second, and third therapeutic choices, as well as not-recommended medications, in clearly explained tables alongside algorithms.

The Royal Australian and New Zealand College of Psychiatrists Clinical Practice Guidelines for Mood Disorders (RANZCP 2020)

The RANZCP Clinical Practice Guidelines for Mood Disorders, published in 2020 [13], is a revision of the guidelines published in 2015 [11]. It primarily presents evidence-based recommendations, but if the evidence is insufficient, it also provides recommendations based on expert consensus. In the RANZCP 2020, the treatment classification was changed from the 0–4 stages of the previous edition to a new system: "*Actions*," which are essential treatments in all cases; "*Choices*," which are applicable treatments if "Actions" are insufficient; and "*Alternatives*," which are other treatments that may be considered.

The Korean Medication Algorithm Project for Bipolar Disorder (KMAP-BP 2022)

The KMAP-BP was first developed in 2002 [40], and has since been revised at four-year intervals, with updated editions published in 2006 [35], 2010 [36], 2014 [37], and 2018 [38]. The latest 2022 edition was published in March 2022 [39]. The KMAP-BP was developed through expert surveys to reflect the local clinical situation in Korea, where sufficient evidence-based data can be lacking. In each question of the survey, experts were asked to evaluate the appropriateness of treatment strategies or medication choices using a modified nine-point scale. A consensus was considered reached for an item if a chi-square test showed that the scores did not have a random distribution.

Furthermore, based on the 95% confidence interval of the scores, each option was classified into one of three categories: first-line/preferred choice, second-line/alternate choice, or third-line/usually inappropriate. Among the second-line options, those whose confidence interval overlapped with the borderline for a first-line choice (6.5 points) were classified as "high second-line." Based on this, guideline tables were created to show the preferred treatment strategies for major clinical situations. These tables then formed the basis for discussions on controversial issues by a review committee, with final decisions being made by the KMAP-BP executive committee.

The KMAP-BP addresses the various clinical situations encountered in the pharmacotherapy of patients with bipolar disorder within the Korean clinical context, and it contains expert-recommended treatments for them. Therefore, a key feature of the KMAP-BP is its role in providing clinicians with information on the appropriateness of various treatment strategies that can be chosen when treating patients.

Comparison of Treatment Guidelines in Clinical Situations

Manic Episode

Initial Treatment Strategy (Table 14.2)

The CINP-BD 2017 recommended monotherapy with aripiprazole (ARI), paliperidone (PAL), quetiapine (QUE), risperidone (RIS), or valproate (VAL). It also recommended monotherapy with asenapine (ASN) and cariprazine (CAR), which are not yet available in Korea. The RANZCP 2020 recommended monotherapy with ARI, ASN, RIS, QUE, or CAR as first-line treatment. Unlike the CINP-BD 2017 and the RANZCP 2020, which recommended monotherapy as the first-line treatment, the CANMAT 2023 also presents combination therapy as a first-

Table 14.2 Comparison of treatment guidelines for the initial treatment and maintenance treatment of manic and depressive episodes

Treatment guideline	Manic episode	Depressive episode	Maintenance treatment
CINP-BD 2017	ARI, PAL, QUE, RIS, VAL, ASN, CAR	LUR, QUE	LIT, ARI, OLZ, PAL, QUE, RIS, RIS-LAI
CANMAT 2023	Mono with LIT, QUE, VAL, ASN, ARI, PAL, RIS, CAR combination therapy with VAL/ LIT+QUE/ARI/RIS/ASN	QUE, LIT, LMT (Mono or Adj), LUR (Mono or Adj)	Mono with LIT, QUE, VAL, LMT, ASN, ARI, ARI-LAI combination therapy with QUE/ARI+LIT/VAL
RANZCP 2020	ARI, ASN, RIS, QUE, CAR, LIT, VAL, MS+AAP	LIT, LMT, VAL, QUE, LUR, CAR	Any mood episode: LIT, VAL, QUE, ASN, LIT/VAL+QUE, LIT+ARI mania: ARI depression: LMT
KMAP-BP 2022	Nonpsychotic: combination therapy with VAL/LIT+OLZ/QUE/ RIS/ ARI Mono with VAL/LIT/OLZ/ QUE psychotic: combination therapy with VAL/LIT+OLZ/QUE/ RIS/ ARI Mono with OLZ/QUE/RIS/ ARI	Mild to moderate: Momo with LIT/VAL/ ARI/QUE/ LMT combination therapy with VAL/LIT+LMT/ARI/ OLZ/QUE, LMT+ARI/ OLZ/QUE Nonpsychotic severe: combination therapy with VAL/LIT+LMT/ARI/ OLZ/QUE LMT+ARI/OLZ/QUE psychotic severe: combination therapy with VAL/LIT/AD/ LMT+QUE/OLZ/ARI	Mania: Mono with MS/ARI/QUE/ OLZ combination therapy with MS +ARI/QUE/OLZ Depression: Mono with MS/LMT/AAP, combination therapy with MS+AAP/LMT, AAP+LMT, MS+AAP+LMT

CANMAT 2023: Canadian Network for Mood and Anxiety Treatments Guidelines for the Management of Patients with Bipolar Disorder, CINP-BD 2017: The International College of Neuro-Psychopharmacology Treatment Guidelines for Bipolar Disorder in Adults, KMAP-BP 2022: Korean Medication Algorithms for Bipolar Disorder 2018, RANZCP 2020: The Royal Australian and New Zealand College of Psychiatrists Clinical Practice Guidelines for Mood Disorders
AAP atypical antipsychotics, *ARI* aripiprazole, *ASN* asenapine, *CAR* cariprazine, *HAL* haloperidol, *LAI* long-acting injection, *LIT* lithium, *LMT* lamotrigine, *LUR* lurasidone, *MS* mood stabilizer, *OLZ* olanzapine, *PAL* paliperidone, *QUE* quetiapine, *RIS* risperidone, *VAL* valproate, *Adj* adjunctive treatment, *Mono* monotherapy

line strategy. It recommended both monotherapy with lithium (LIT), QUE, VAL, ASN, ARI, PAL, RIS, or CAR, and combination therapy pairing LIT or VAL with QUE, ARI, RIS, or ASN, as first-line strategies. Furthermore, based on recent meta-analysis results, Level 1 evidence has been presented showing that combination therapy with a mood stabilizer (MS) and an antipsychotic is more effective than monotherapy in controlling manic symptoms, and it was emphasized that combination therapy should be given priority consideration in clinical practice. The KMAP-BP 2022 distinguished between mania with and without psychotic features. For both conditions, MS and atypical antipsychotics (AAP) combination therapy was recommended as the top-priority treatment, while AAP monotherapy was a first-line strategy. MS monotherapy was only a first-line strategy for mania without psychotic features. The drugs recommended for monotherapy in KMAP-BP 2022 were LIT, VAL, QUE, olanzapine (OLZ), and ARI for nonpsychotic mania, and OLZ, QUE, ARI, and RIS for psychotic mania. For combination therapy, combining LIT or VAL with OLZ, QUE, ARI, or RIS was recommended. Notably, for psychotic mania, the combination of LIT with QUE or OLZ, and VAL with QUE, were the top-priority treatments.

One key difference among the guidelines for the initial treatment of a manic episode is whether to prioritize monotherapy, as in the CINP-BD 2017 and the RANZCP 2020, or to also recommend combination therapy as an initial treatment, as in the CANMAT 2023 and the KMAP-BP 2022. Proponents of recommending combination therapy argue that the choice between monotherapy and combination therapy should be based on patient characteristics, such as symptom severity, past treatment response, tolerability to previous combination therapy, and treatment adherence [23]. Furthermore, there are differences in the recommendation level for OLZ. While OLZ was recommended for initial treatment in the KMAP-BP 2022, it is recommended for later stages of treatment in the CINP-BD 2017, the CANMAT 2023, and the RANZCP 2020. This difference appears to stem from the varying emphasis each guideline places on efficacy versus safety/tolerability, as OLZ has robust evidence for its efficacy but also has limitations regarding its safety and tolerability profile [23].

Comparison of Treatment Guidelines in Clinical Situations

For an insufficient response to initial treatment, the CINP-BD 2017 recommended trying monotherapy with another agent from the initial treatment options. If the response was still inadequate, it recommended monotherapy with OLZ, LIT, carbamazepine (CBZ), haloperidol (HAL), or ziprasidone (ZIP), or combining LIT or VAL with ASN, ARI, HAL, or OLZ. Additionally, it suggested that combining VAL with a typical antipsychotic, allopurinol, or celecoxib could be considered. If the response remained insufficient, it recommended combining LIT or VAL with QUE or RIS.

The CANMAT 2023 recommended first considering monotherapy or combination therapy with LIT, VAL, or an AAP that was not used previously. Specifically, based on recent Level 1 evidence that combination therapy with a mood stabilizer and an antipsychotic is more effective than monotherapy for improving manic symptoms, augmenting with combination therapy is more actively recommended than switching monotherapies. Second-line recommendations include monotherapy with OLZ, CBZ, ZIP, or HAL, and combination therapy with OLZ and LIT or VAL, or LIT and VAL. If the response is still insufficient, third-line recommendations include monotherapy with chlorpromazine, clozapine (CLZ), or tamoxifen, or combination therapy with CLZ, tamoxifen, or CBZ/oxcarbazepine. Additionally, combining HAL or tamoxifen with LIT or VAL can also be considered. In cases of insufficient response to initial AAP monotherapy, the RANZCP 2020 recommended adding LIT or VAL. Subsequent steps included monotherapy with CBZ, ZIP, HAL, or OLZ. If the response was still inadequate, it recommended adding LIT or VAL to OLZ.

The KMAP-BP 2022 presented treatment strategies based on the previous treatment step. For an insufficient response to initial MS or AAP monotherapy, it recommended switching to MS + AAP combination therapy or switching the existing MS or AAP to a different AAP. If AAP monotherapy was insufficient for a patient with psychotic features, adding another AAP was also recommended. If an insufficient response was seen after initial MS + AAP combination therapy in a patient without psychotic features, the recommendation was to switch the existing AAP or MS, or to add another MS or AAP. For psychotic mania, it recommended adding another AAP or switching the existing one; however, if there was a partial response to the existing combination, adding another MS was also an option to consider. Furthermore, for later stages, the KMAP-BP 2022 recommended considering a combination of LIT or VAL with two AAPs, as well as a combination of LIT, VAL, and two AAPs.

Unlike the international guidelines, the KMAP-BP 2022 sometimes recommends combining three or more drugs for an insufficient response to initial treatment. This may be because the limited availability of newer drugs like ASN and CAR in Korea necessitates using various combinations of existing medications. It may also reflect a preference among Korean clinicians for the potential therapeutic benefits of combination therapy [41], despite the limitations regarding safety and tolerability. Another distinctive feature is that the CANMAT 2023 and the CINP-BD 2017 recommend the use of agents not traditionally used in psychiatry but which have recently shown evidence of antimanic effects—such as allopurinol [42], celecoxib [43], and tamoxifen [44]—at a relatively earlier stage of treatment.

Depressive Episode

Initial Treatment Strategy (Table 14.2)

The CINP-BD 2017 recommended only lurasidone (LUR) or QUE monotherapy as first-line treatment. The RANZCP 2020 recommended monotherapy with MS(LIT, lamotrigine (LMT), or VAL) or AAP(QUE, LUR, or CAR), but prioritized MS over AAPs. In the CANMAT 2023 guidelines, CAR was newly included as a first-line treatment in addition to monotherapy with QUE, LIT, LMT, and LUR; combination therapy with LUR and LMT was also maintained as a first-line recommendation. Notably, CAR, which had been a second-line treatment in 2018 due to limited clinical experience, has been upgraded to a first-line treatment based on the results of three recent RCTs. Combination therapy with QUE and LIT still has limited evidence but can be considered based on clinical judgment. Additionally, for second-line treatment, the new drug lumateperone (LUM) was added alongside divalproex, antidepressant (AD, selective serotonin reuptake inhibitor [SSRI] or bupropion) combination therapy, electroconvulsive therapy (ECT), and olanzapine-fluoxetine combination therapy. LUM has recently demonstrated superior antidepressant effects compared to placebo in an RCT, with favorable safety results also being reported. The KMAP-BP 2022 subdivided clinical situations and presented treatment strategies accordingly. For mild-to-moderate depressive episodes, it recommended monotherapy with an MS (LIT or VAL), LMT, or an AAP, or combination therapy with MS + AAP or AAP + LMT. For severe depressive episodes without psychotic features, it recommended combination therapy using two agents from among MS, AAP, and LMT. For depressive episodes with psychotic features, it recommended combination therapy with MS + AAP or AAP + LMT, with MS + AAP being the top-priority treatment. For monotherapy, LIT, LMT, VAL, ARI, QUE, and OLZ were recommended for episodes both with and without psychotic features. For combination therapy in depressive episodes with psychotic features, the recommended AAPs were ARI, QUE, OLZ, and RIS.

A commonality across several guidelines was the preference for QUE, and international guidelines also recommended LUR at a high level. Additionally, many guidelines recommended LMT as either monotherapy or combination therapy; the KMAP-BP 2022 and the CANMAT 2023 recommended it for both, while the RANZCP 2020 recommended it for monotherapy. The efficacy of LMT monotherapy for bipolar depression can be controversial, as four double-blind RCTs failed to show a significant difference from placebo on the primary outcome variables [45]. However, subsequent studies pointed out methodological issues in these earlier trials, such as dosing, and suggested that the short study durations may not have accounted for the long titration period required for LMT to reach an effective dose, thus potentially masking its efficacy [46]. Furthermore, LMT's recommendation for bipolar depression can be interpreted as a result of comprehensively considering its superior efficacy reported in some monotherapy and combination therapy studies [47–49], along with its excellent safety and tolerability profile.

Another difference is that VAL (among MSs) and ARI (among AAPs) are recommended at a relatively high level in KMAP-BP 2022 but are less favored in the international guidelines. Based on studies reporting that ARI monotherapy was not superior to placebo, the CANMAT 2023 and the CINP-BD 2017 list ARI as a third-line agent for combination therapy and do not recommend it for monotherapy [50, 51]. However, a meta-analysis synthesizing multiple studies showed its potential efficacy in bipolar depression [52, 53]. Furthermore, the increasing use of low-dose ARI for bipolar depression in Korea also suggests its potential effectiveness. As for VAL, it was a first-line choice in the KMAP-BP 2022 and the RANZCP 2020, but a second-line choice in the

CANMAT 2023 and a third-line choice in the CINP-BD 2017. These latter guidelines point out that although some small-scale RCTs and a meta-analysis have reported its effectiveness over placebo, the strength of the evidence is weak due to the small number of subjects.

Insufficient Response to Initial Treatment

For an insufficient response, the CINP-BD 2017 primarily recommended OLZ monotherapy, OLZ + fluoxetine combination therapy, combination of an MS with LUR, modafinil, or pramipexole, combination of LIT with LMT or pioglitazone, or combination therapy with escitalopram or fluoxetine. If the response was still insufficient, it recommended monotherapy with VAL, LIT, ARI, LMT, imipramine, or phenelzine, or combination therapy of LIT with L-sulpiride. Subsequent options included tranylcypromine or LIT monotherapy, venlafaxine combination therapy, combination of an MS with armodafinil or ketamine, or LIT+fluoxetine/LMT.

In the CANMAT 2023 guidelines, VAL monotherapy, or combination therapy of an SSRI or bupropion with LIT, VAL, or an AAP is recommended. If the response remains insufficient, OLZ or CBZ monotherapy, or combination therapies involving ARI, armodafinil, ASN, eicosapentaenoic acid (EPA), ketamine, levothyroxine, modafinil, N-acetylcysteine (NAC), pramipexole, an SNRI, or an MAOI were suggested. Notably, the 2023 edition newly mentioned the use of lurasidone (LUR), CAR, and LUM, and also emphasized the potential use of esketamine. When initial treatment was not sufficiently effective, the RANZCP 2020 primarily recommended combination therapy with an MS, AAP, and/or antidepressants (ADs). It recommended combinations such as MS and AAP, two MSs, MS and AD, or AAP and AD, but did not recommend combining two AAPs. A triple-combination therapy of MS, AAP, and AD was recommended as a next step. Subsequent options included CBZ or OLZ monotherapy, or adjunctive treatments such as ASN, modafinil/armodafinil, pramipexole, or levothyroxine.

The KMAP-BP 2022 provided stratified recommendations. For no response to initial MS monotherapy, it recommended switching the MS to LMT or another MS, or adding LMT or an AAP; for a partial response, it recommended adding an AAP, LMT, or another MS. For no response to AAP monotherapy, it recommended adding LMT or an MS, or switching to an MS or LMT; for a partial response, it recommended adding an MS, LMT, or another AAP. For no response after initial LMT monotherapy, it recommended switching to or adding an MS or AAP; for a partial response, adding an AAP or MS was recommended. For no response to MS and AAP combination therapy, it recommended switching the MS or AAP, switching the MS to LMT, or adding LMT, an AAP, or an MS; for a partial response, it recommended switching the AAP or adding LMT, an AAP, or an MS. For no or partial response to AAP and LMT combination therapy, it recommended switching the AAP or adding an MS or another AAP. For no or partial response to MS and AD combination therapy, adding an AAP or LMT was recommended; for no response, switching the MS to LMT or another MS was also an option, while for a partial response, adding another MS was recommended. For no response to MS and LMT combination therapy, the recommended methods were to add an AAP, switch LMT to an AAP, or switch the MS; for a partial response, adding an AAP was recommended. For patients with psychotic features showing no or partial response to AAP + AD, it recommended adding an MS, LMT, or an AAP, and for no response, switching the AAP to a different one. If the response to these treatments remains insufficient, it suggested considering the use of CLZ or adding buspirone, thyroid hormone, or psychostimulants.

In summary, the evidence for treatment-resistant bipolar depression is still insufficient, leading to some differences among the various guidelines. The international guidelines suggest various combination therapies involving ADs, MSs, and AAPs, as well as dopamine-acting agents like armodafinil, modafinil, psychostimulants, and pramipexole. Furthermore, the CINP-BD 2017 and the CANMAT 2023 suggest considering agents not typically used for bipolar disorder but for which evidence has recently emerged, such as pioglitazone, L-sulpiride, EPA, and N-acetylcysteine (NAC).

Pioglitazone is an insulin sensitizer used for type 2 diabetes that acts on the peroxisome proliferator-activated nuclear receptor gamma. Insulin resistance and its associated inflammatory responses are known to be related to mood [54], and one double-blind study reported its effectiveness in bipolar depression [55]. L-sulpiride is a D2 receptor antagonist, also supported by one double-blind study [56]. The antidepressant effect of EPA has been reported in meta-analyses [57, 58]. NAC is used as a health supplement with antioxidant functions and is being studied for various psychiatric disorders through mechanisms such as modulating oxidative stress, neurogenesis, and apoptosis; one double-blind study has reported its efficacy in bipolar depression [59]. The antidepressant effects of ketamine and esketamine in depression, including bipolar depression, have also been demonstrated in several recent studies [60, 61]. However, due to the short duration of their antidepressant effect and insufficient long-term safety data, their use should be considered for cases with severe symptoms, high suicide risk, and non-response to other treatments.

Mixed Episode

The CINP-BD 2017 provided the same recommendations as for a manic episode, but specified that for a mixed episode meeting Diagnostic and Statistical Manual of Mental Disorders, fourth Edition (DSM-IV) diagnostic criteria, OLZ and fluoxetine combination therapy or ZIP monotherapy was recommended. The RANZCP 2020 recommended LIT, VAL, or QUE. The CANMAT 2021 had no first-line choice for manic episodes with mixed features, but recommended ASN, CAR, ARI, or VAL as second-line choices. For depressive episodes with mixed features, there was also no first-line choice, with CAR or LUR recommended as second-line choices.

The KMAP-BP 2022 recommended MS and AAP combination therapy as the top-priority treatment for mixed mania, with AAP or MS monotherapy as other first-line choices. For mixed depression, it recommended MS or AAP monotherapy, or combining any two agents from among MS, AAP, and LMT. If manic and depressive symptoms were of similar severity, MS and AAP combination therapy or AAP and MS monotherapy was prioritized.

For an insufficient response to treatment, the KMAP-BP 2022 provided further stratified recommendations. In mixed mania, if initial MS monotherapy was insufficient, adding an AAP was the top-priority treatment, with adding another MS also being a first-line strategy. If initial AAP monotherapy was insufficient, it recommended adding an MS or another AAP. If initial MS and AAP combination therapy was insufficient, it recommended adding an MS or AAP, switching the MS to another MS or an AAP, or switching the AAP to another AAP.

In mixed depression with an insufficient response to ongoing MS monotherapy, the second-step strategies included adding an AAP, LMT, or another MS as first-line options. For an insufficient response to ongoing AAP monotherapy, it recommended adding an MS, LMT, or another AAP. For an insufficient response to MS and AAP combination therapy, it recommended adding an MS, AAP, or LMT, or switching the AAP or MS. After MS and LMT combination therapy, it recommended adding an AAP or switching the MS to an AAP. For an insufficient response to MS and AD combination therapy, it recommended adding an AAP or LMT, or switching the AD to an AAP. For an insufficient response to AAP and LMT combination therapy, it recommended adding an MS or AAP, or switching the AAP. If AAP and AD combination therapy was used, it recommended adding an MS or LMT, and if LMT monotherapy was used, it recommended adding an AAP or MS.

The international guidelines provide only limited recommendations for mixed features. This is because most of the evidence comes from analyses of subgroups within studies targeting manic populations or from secondary analyses, and sufficient primary evidence has not yet been accumulated.

Rapid Cycling

The CINP-BD 2017 does not recommend any specific therapeutic agents for rapid cycling. The CANMAT 2023 states that for manic symptoms in rapid cycling, there is no evidence that any particular drug is more effective than others among the first-line treatments. However, it notes that combination therapy may be more appropriate than monotherapy, while also mentioning that one double-blind study showed that a three-drug combination was not superior to a two-drug combination. For depressive symptoms in rapid cycling, it states that there is still no clear evidence, and that medication should be chosen based on its efficacy in the acute and maintenance treatment of depressive symptoms. It also notes that while LIT, VAL, OLZ, and QUE all show similar maintenance efficacy, LMT has been reported to show no difference from placebo in the maintenance treatment of rapid-cycling bipolar disorder.

Compared to other guidelines, which only make general statements due to insufficient evidence, the KMAP-BP 2022 offers more detailed recommendations based on its advantage of using expert consensus. For treatment-naïve patients with rapid-cycling mania, it recommended MS and AAP combination therapy, MS monotherapy, or AAP monotherapy. For the depressive state, it recommended MS and AAP combination therapy, AAP monotherapy, MS monotherapy, AAP and LMT combination therapy, or MS and LMT combination therapy. For patients with rapid-cycling mania who had an insufficient response to MS monotherapy, adding an AAP was the top-priority treatment, and adding another MS was a first-line strategy. For patients with rapid-cycling depression who had been treated with MS and AD combination therapy, it recommended adding an AAP or LMT.

Maintenance Treatment and Long-Term Prophylaxis (Table 14.2)

The CINP-BD 2017 recommended initiating monotherapy by selecting from LIT, ARI, OLZ, PAL, QUE, RIS, or RIS-long acting injection (LAI), taking into account the predominant polarity. For an insufficient response, the next step recommended was to add fluoxetine, LMT, or LIT to the previous medication, again considering the predominant polarity. It also recommended combination therapies of LIT+CBZ, QUE + LIT or VAL, or OLZ or ARI with an MS. If the effect was still insufficient, it recommended trying a previously unused agent from among RIS-LAI, VAL, CBZ, or NAC. In subsequent steps, it suggested adding previously unused drugs—even those effective in acute episodes but with insufficient evidence for maintenance—or considering the use of LIT+LMT, or venlafaxine or HAL.

The CANMAT 2023 guidelines stated that monotherapy with LIT, QUE, VAL, and LMT has the clearest evidence, and noted that ASN has also been reported to be effective in preventing manic and depressive episodes. It also stated that ARI or ARI-LAI could be considered a first-line option due to its efficacy in preventing mood episodes and, specifically, manic episodes. In addition, QUE+LIT/VAL and ARI+LIT/VAL were also presented as first-line choices. For subsequent steps, it was recommended to switch to or combine agents that were recommended for initial treatment but not yet used. Later-stage agents were recommended for consideration only in cases where the response remained insufficient even after multiple trials of the initially recommended drugs. Agents that could be used at this stage included OLZ, RIS-LAI, CBZ, PAL, ZIP, and LUR. If the response to these was also insufficient, it was stated that ARI+LMT, OLZ+fluoxetine, CLZ, or gabapentin could also be used. The RANZCP 2020 recommended LIT, VAL, QUE, and ASN monotherapy, as well as combination therapy of LIT/VAL with QUE, and LIT with ARI. In addition, it recommended the use of ARI to prevent manic relapse and LMT to prevent depressive relapse.

The KMAP-BP 2022 presented separate recommendations based on the polarity of the previous episode. For maintenance treatment strategy after a manic episode, it recommended MS monotherapy, AAP monotherapy, or MS and AAP combination therapy. When initiating maintenance treatment after remission from an acute depressive episode, it recommended MS and AAP or LMT combination therapy, LMT, AAP, or MS monotherapy, AAP and LMT combination therapy, or a combination of two MSs.

A notable difference among the various maintenance treatment guidelines is the recommendation level for OLZ. While other guidelines present OLZ as a first-line choice for maintenance, the CANMAT 2023 recommends it only when other treatments are ineffective. This appears to be due to an emphasis on the safety issues of OLZ, such as metabolic side effects, which is particularly important given the long-term nature of maintenance treatment for bipolar disorder, even though OLZ has proven efficacy in preventing both manic and depressive episodes [62].

Recommendations for LAI agents also differ somewhat. While the CINP-BD 2017 stated that only the efficacy of RIS-LAI for maintenance treatment was established by RCTs, the CANMAT 2023, based on more recent study results, recommended ARI-LAI as a first-line choice. This was based on its efficacy in preventing manic episodes and all mood episodes (though not depressive episodes) [63] and its relatively stable tolerability and safety profile.

Bipolar II Disorder

The CINP-BD 2017 and the RANZCP 2020 did not provide separate recommendations for bipolar II disorder. The CANMAT 2023 guidelines recommended QUE or LUR as first-line choices, and listed LIT, LMT, sertraline, venlafaxine, and bupropion as second-line choices. For maintenance treatment of bipolar II disorder, the guidelines presented QUE, LIT, LMT, and LUR as first-line choices, venlafaxine as a second-line choice, and recommended CBZ, VAL, other ADs, and RIS as third-line choices. The KMAP-BP 2022 recommended MS or AAP monotherapy and MS and AAP combination therapy for hypomanic episodes, with a particular priority on LIT, VAL, QUE, OLZ, and ARI. The KMAP-BP 2022 stated that treatment strategies for depressive episodes should differ between bipolar I and bipolar II disorder. For the treatment of bipolar II depression, it recommended MS, AAP, or LMT monotherapy, or MS and AAP combination therapy. If an AD is used, it recommended choosing bupropion, sertraline, or escitalopram. For the maintenance treatment of bipolar II disorder, the first-line choices after a hypomanic episode were VAL, LIT, ARI, QUE, OLZ, or RIS monotherapy, or MS and AAP combination therapy. After a depressive episode, the first-line choices were MS, AAP, or LMT monotherapy, or a combination of any two of these three agents. Among the AAPs, ARI was especially recommended as a top-priority treatment, with OLZ and QUE also recommended as first-line choices.

The most significant divergence regarding bipolar II disorder (BD-II) is the existence of specific recommendations. The CINP-BD and the RANZCP do not provide separate guidelines, whereas the CANMAT and the KMAP-BP offer detailed recommendations. This reflects a growing clinical focus on BD-II, particularly its depressive predominance. Notably, the CANMAT includes antidepressants (e.g., sertraline) as second-line options for depression, while the KMAP-BP, if using an antidepressant, favors agents like bupropion and generally emphasizes MS and AAP monotherapy or combination.

Specific Populations

International treatment guidelines also provide recommendations for specific situations, such as for children and adolescents, the elderly, pregnant women, and comorbid conditions, although the level of detail varies. However, the RANZCP 2020 only provides a general description of the diagnosis and treatment of pediatric bipolar disorder and borderline personality disorder and does not recommend specific treatment strategies. The CINP-BD 2017 recommended the use of injectable HAL or OLZ for severe agitation and stated that injectable clonazepam or lorazepam could be used concurrently with antipsychotics. During pregnancy, it recommended reducing the medication dosage several weeks before delivery. It stated that LIT, VAL, CBZ, and LMT at doses exceeding 200 mg/day have a risk of teratogenicity and recommended against the use of VAL and CBZ in all cases. For patients who had been using LIT, it noted that the past risk of cardiac malformations was overestimated [64]; therefore, LIT could be used if the patient is informed and consents. During pregnancy, an AAP or LMT at a dose of 200 mg/day or less was considered appropriate, but it was also pointed out that the evidence for their safety is still insufficient.

In the CANMAT 2023 guidelines, the recommendation to consider discontinuing typical antipsychotics or RIS for women wishing to conceive—due to the risk of prolactin increase interfering with ovulation and pregnancy—was maintained; however, the principle of "monotherapy at the lowest possible dose" for treatment during pregnancy was more clearly emphasized. Furthermore, the use of VAL was strongly advised against for women during pregnancy, of childbearing age, and in adolescence, with CBZ also being presented as a contraindicated drug. For breastfeeding, the existing recommendation that QUE and OLZ are relatively safe was maintained. For the treatment of mania in children/adolescents, LIT, RIS, ARI, ASN, and QUE were recommended, which is the same as in 2018. However, for the treatment of depression, the 2023 edition, while maintaining LUR monotherapy as the top priority, specified that LIT and LMT could be used adjunctively. For maintenance treatment, ARI, LIT, and VAL were recommended, and the 2023 edition reinforced the potential use of LMT and QUE for maintenance treatment in the adolescent population. For the treatment of elderly patients, LIT and VAL monotherapy were recommended for mania, with the 2023 edition adding a caution regarding the risk of metabolic syndrome with the use of OLZ and QUE. For depression, the recommendation for QUE and LUR monotherapy was maintained, with an increased emphasis on the use of LMT. The recommendation for LIT, LMT, and VAL for maintenance treatment remains the same. Furthermore, the CANMAT 2023 expanded upon the 2018 edition with more specific recommendations for psychiatric and physical comorbidities such as substance use disorders, anxiety disorders, and personality disorders. For example, it specified that for comorbid anxiety disorders, benzodiazepine monotherapy should be avoided, and AAP or MS-based treatment should be prioritized. In contrast, a distinctive feature of the KMAP-BP 2022 is that it provides therapeutic guidance based on expert consensus for various clinical situations that may be encountered in actual practice, even if the evidence is insufficient. For example, in the case of significant weight gain associated with medication, education on exercise and diet was the top-priority treatment, with metformin, topiramate, orlistat, bupropion, liraglutide, naltrexone, or naltrexone/bupropion (Contrave) presented as second-line choices. If weight gain occurred while using an MS or AAP, switching to an AAP with less risk of weight gain was recommended, and the use of LMT, ARI, or ZIP was suggested if weight gain is a concern. In case of increased prolactin during antipsychotic use, reducing the current medication's dosage was recommended. If a benign skin rash occurred during LMT use, discontinuing the medication was recommended.

For mania in elderly patients, the KMAP-BP 2022 recommended ARI, QUE, OLZ, RIS, LIT, or VAL monotherapy. For depression, it recommended ARI, QUE, OLZ, LMT, LIT, or VAL monotherapy, or a combination of two agents from among MS, AAP, and LMT. If an AD had to be used, escitalopram or bupropion was presented as the first-line choice. For mania in children, AAP monotherapy or MS and AAP combination therapy were recommended as first-line choices; among AAPs, ARI and RIS were first-line, and among MSs, VAL was first-line. For depressive episodes in children, AAP monotherapy or MS and AAP combination therapy were recommended; among AAPs, ARI was the top-priority treatment and RIS was a first-line drug, but there was no first-line MS, with VAL, LIT, and LMT being preferred as second-line drugs. For the treatment of mania in adolescents, MS and AAP combination therapy was the top-priority treatment, with MS or AAP monotherapy as a first-line strategy; recommended MSs were LIT and VAL, and recommended AAPs were ARI, QUE, and RIS. For depression in adolescents, AAP monotherapy and MS and AAP combination therapy were recommended as first-line strategies; among AAPs, ARI was the top-priority treatment, with

RIS and QUE as first-line drugs, and among MSs, LIT and VAL were recommended. In addition to these, the KMAP-BP 2022 also presents expert consensus-based recommendations for various other comorbid conditions.

Recommendations for special populations highlight the scope and methodological focus of each guideline. The CANMAT provides detailed, evidence-based recommendations for key life-cycle groups, including pregnancy, youth, and the elderly. In contrast, the KMAP-BP demonstrates a unique strength by addressing not only these groups but also providing specific, expert consensus-based strategies for practical clinical challenges that often lack robust evidence, such as managing medication-induced weight gain or hyperprolactinemia.

Conclusion

While most treatment guidelines present similar recommendations, some differences appear to stem from varying perspectives on whether to place greater emphasis on the efficacy or the safety of each drug. This difference in perspective is particularly prominent in the case of VAL and OLZ. Furthermore, it is also highly suggestive that various treatment guidelines are gradually moving away from traditional drug classifications like mood stabilizers or antipsychotics and are instead making recommendations based on the characteristics of individual drugs. In the future, it may be more appropriate to make therapeutic choices based on the mechanism of action and research results of each drug, rather than on traditional drug classifications. Additionally, while there may be some differences between BD I and conditions like BD II, rapid cycling, and the mixed features introduced in DSM-V in terms of drug response and selection, the evidence is still insufficient and there is no clear consensus among the guidelines. Therefore, future clinical drug research from this perspective is deemed necessary.

An additional point to mention is that the domestic guideline, KMAP-BP, has long favored both monotherapy and combination therapy for initial treatment, whereas most foreign guidelines prioritized monotherapy. Recently, however, these foreign guidelines have also begun to recommend combination therapy from the initial stages. This serves as evidence that expert consensus-based guidelines like the KMAP-BP reflect actual clinical practice and real-world aspects more rapidly than evidence-based guidelines. It can be interpreted that evidence-based studies are now being conducted that meet these real-world situations and needs, thereby supporting the opinions of experts. Therefore, more research based on clinical experience is needed in the future, and it is hoped that through this, treatment guidelines that include more practical recommendations will continue to be presented to help clinicians and patients.

Furthermore, it is highly suggestive that guidelines are gradually moving away from traditional drug classifications like MS or AAP instead making recommendations based on the characteristics of individual drugs. This aligns with the emerging paradigm of the neuroscience-based nomenclature (NbN), which classifies psychotropic medications based on their pharmacological mechanism and targets rather than their approved indication or traditional class. For example, agents classified as "antipsychotics" but acting as dopamine D2/D3 partial agonists, like aripiprazole and cariprazine, show efficacy in not only mania but also depression, highlighting the importance of this mechanism-based approach. In the future, therapeutic choices based on the mechanism of action and research results of each drug will likely become more appropriate than those based on traditional drug classifications.

Declarations

Competing Interests The author(s) has no competing interests to declare that are relevant to the content of this manuscript.

Ethics Approval The author(s) declares that this manuscript does not include primary research with human participants.

The author(s) declares that this manuscript does not include primary studies involving animals.

References

1. Frances AJ, Kahn DA, Carpenter D, Docherty JP, Donovan SL. The expert consensus guidelines for treating depression in bipolar disorder. J Clin Psychiatry. 1998;59(Suppl 4):73–9.
2. Kim CH, Min KJ, Shin YC, Yoon BH, Cho HS, Jon DI, et al. Feasibility of Korean medication algorithm for bipolar disorder (I): global assessment. Korean J Psychopharmacol. 2005;16:225–33.
3. Shin YC, Bahk WM, Kim CH, Min KJ, Yoon BH, Cho HS, et al. Feasibility of Korean medication algorithm for bipolar disorder (II): choice of medications. Korean J Psychopharmacol. 2005;16:285–91.
4. Jon DI, Bahk WM, Shin YC, Kim CH, Min KJ, Yoon BH, et al. Feasibility of Korean medication algorithm for bipolar disorder (III): treatment response and tolerability. Korean J Psychopharmacol. 2005;16:292–300.
5. Bahk WM, Shin YC, Jon DI, Yoon BH, Kim DJ, Ahn YM, et al. Korean medication algorithm for bipolar disorder (I). Korean J Psychopharmacol. 2002;13:205–21.
6. American Psychiatric Association. Practice guideline for the treatment of patients with bipolar disorder. Am J Psychiatry. 1994;151(12 Suppl):1–36.
7. American Psychiatric Association. Practice guideline for the treatment of patients with bipolar disorder (revision). Am J Psychiatry. 2002;159(4 Suppl):1–50.
8. Sachs GS, Printz DJ, Kahn DA, Carpenter D, Docherty JP. The expert consensus guideline series: medication treatment of bipolar disorder 2000. Postgrad Med. 2000;Spec No 1:1–104.
9. Suppes T, Swann AC, Dennehy EB, Habermacher ED, Mason M, Crismon ML, et al. Texas medication algorithm project: development and feasibility testing of a treatment algorithm for patients with bipolar disorder. J Clin Psychiatry. 2001;62(6):439–47.
10. Suppes T, Dennehy EB, Hirschfeld RM, Altshuler LL, Bowden CL, Calabrese JR, et al. The Texas implementation of medication algorithms: update to the algorithms for treatment of bipolar I disorder. J Clin Psychiatry. 2005;66:870–86.
11. Malhi GS, Bassett D, Boyce P, Bryant R, Fitzgerald PB, Fritz K, et al. Royal Australian and New Zealand College of Psychiatrists clinical practice guidelines for mood disorders. Aust N Z J Psychiatry. 2015;49(12):1087–206.
12. Malhi GS, Outhred T, Morris G, Boyce PM, Bryant R, Fitzgerald PB, et al. Royal Australian and New Zealand College of Psychiatrists clinical practice guidelines for mood disorders: bipolar disorder summary. Med J Aust. 2018;208(5):219–25.
13. Malhi GS, Bell E, Bassett D, Boyce P, Bryant R, Hazell P, et al. The 2020 Royal Australian and New Zealand College of Psychiatrists clinical practice guidelines for mood disorders. Aust N Z J Psychiatry. 2021;55(1):7–117.
14. Goodwin GM, British Association for Psychopharmacology. Evidence-based guidelines for treating bipolar disorder: revised second edition--recommendations from the British Association for Psychopharmacology. J Psychopharmacol. 2009;23(4):346–88.
15. Goodwin GM, Consensus Group of the British Association for Psychopharmacology. Evidence-based guidelines for treating bipolar disorder: recommendations from the British Association for Psychopharmacology. J Psychopharmacol. 2003;17(2):149–73. discussion 147
16. Goodwin GM, Haddad PM, Ferrier IN, Aronson JK, Barnes T, Cipriani A, et al. Evidence-based guidelines for treating bipolar disorder: revised third edition recommendations from the British Association for Psychopharmacology. J Psychopharmacol. 2016;30(6):495–553.
17. Yatham LN, Kennedy SH, Parikh SV, Schaffer A, Beaulieu S, Alda M, et al. Canadian Network for Mood and Anxiety Treatments (CANMAT) and International Society for Bipolar Disorders (ISBD) collaborative update of CANMAT guidelines for the management of patients with bipolar disorder: update 2013. Bipolar Disord. 2013;15(1):1–44.
18. Yatham LN, Kennedy SH, Schaffer A, Parikh SV, Beaulieu S, O'Donovan C, et al. Canadian Network for Mood and Anxiety Treatments (CANMAT) and International Society for Bipolar Disorders (ISBD) collaborative update of CANMAT guidelines for the management of patients with bipolar disorder: update 2009. Bipolar Disord. 2009;11(3):225–55.
19. Yatham LN, Kennedy SH, O'Donovan C, Parikh S, MacQueen G, McIntyre R, et al. Canadian Network for Mood and Anxiety Treatments (CANMAT) guidelines for the management of patients with bipolar disorder: consensus and controversies. Bipolar Disord. 2005;7(Suppl 3):5–69.
20. Sharma V, Yatham LN, Haslam DR, Silverstone PH, Parikh SV, Matte R, et al. Continuation and prophylactic treatment of bipolar disorder. Can J Psychiatr. 1997;42(Suppl 2):92S–100S.
21. Yatham LN, Kennedy SH, O'Donovan C, Parikh SV, MacQueen G, McIntyre RS, et al. Canadian Network for Mood and Anxiety Treatments (CANMAT) guidelines for the management of patients with bipolar disorder: update 2007. Bipolar Disord. 2006;8(6):721–39.
22. Yatham LN, Kennedy SH, Parikh SV, Schaffer A, Bond DJ, Frey BN, et al. Canadian Network for Mood and Anxiety Treatments (CANMAT) and International Society for Bipolar Disorders (ISBD) 2018 guidelines for the management of patients with bipolar disorder. Bipolar Disord. 2018;20(2):97–170.
23. Keramatian K, Chithra NK, Yatham L. The CANMAT and ISBD guidelines for the treatment of bipolar disorder: summary and a 2023 update of evidence. Focus (Am Psychiatr Publ). 2023;21(4):344–53.
24. Yatham LN, Chakrabarty T, Bond DJ, Schaffer A, Beaulieu S, Parikh SV, et al. Canadian Network for Mood and Anxiety Treatments (CANMAT) and International Society for Bipolar Disorders (ISBD)

recommendations for the management of patients with bipolar disorder with mixed presentations. Bipolar Disord. 2021;23(8):767–88.
25. Fountoulakis KN, Grunze H, Vieta E, Young A, Yatham L, Blier P, et al. The International College of Neuro-Psychopharmacology (CINP) Treatment Guidelines for Bipolar Disorder in Adults (CINP-BD-2017), part 3: the clinical guidelines. Int J Neuropsychopharmacol. 2017;20(2):180–95.
26. Grunze H, Vieta E, Goodwin GM, Bowden C, Licht RW, Moller HJ, et al. The World Federation of Societies of Biological Psychiatry (WFSBP) guidelines for the biological treatment of bipolar disorders: update 2012 on the long-term treatment of bipolar disorder. World J Biol Psychiatry. 2013;14(3):154–219.
27. Grunze H, Vieta E, Goodwin GM, Bowden C, Licht RW, Moller HJ, et al. The World Federation of Societies of Biological Psychiatry (WFSBP) guidelines for the biological treatment of bipolar disorders: update 2010 on the treatment of acute bipolar depression. World J Biol Psychiatry. 2010;11(2):81–109.
28. Grunze H, Vieta E, Goodwin GM, Bowden C, Licht RW, Moller HJ, et al. The World Federation of Societies of Biological Psychiatry (WFSBP) guidelines for the biological treatment of bipolar disorders: update 2009 on the treatment of acute mania. World J Biol Psychiatry. 2009;10(2):85–116.
29. Grunze H, Kasper S, Goodwin G, Bowden C, Moller HJ. WFSBP Task Force on Treatment Guidelines for Bipolar Disorders. The World Federation of Societies of Biological Psychiatry (WFSBP) guidelines for the biological treatment of bipolar disorders, part III: maintenance treatment. World J Biol Psychiatry. 2004;5(3):120–35.
30. Grunze H, Kasper S, Goodwin G, Bowden C, Baldwin D, Licht RW, et al. The World Federation of Societies of Biological Psychiatry (WFSBP) guidelines for the biological treatment of bipolar disorders, part II: treatment of mania. World J Biol Psychiatry. 2003;4(1):5–13.
31. Grunze H, Kasper S, Goodwin G, Bowden C, Baldwin D, Licht R, et al. World Federation of Societies of Biological Psychiatry (WFSBP) guidelines for biological treatment of bipolar disorders. Part I: treatment of bipolar depression. World J Biol Psychiatry. 2002;3(3):115–24.
32. Grunze H, Vieta E, Goodwin GM, Bowden C, Licht RW, Azorin JM, et al. The World Federation of Societies of Biological Psychiatry (WFSBP) guidelines for the biological treatment of bipolar disorders: acute and long-term treatment of mixed states in bipolar disorder. World J Biol Psychiatry. 2018;19(1):2–58.
33. National Institute for Health and Clinical Excellence. Bipolar disorder: the management of bipolar disorder in adults, children and adolescents, in primary and secondary care. Leicester: British Psychological Society; 2006. 592 p
34. National Institute for Health and Care Excellence (NICE). Bipolar disorder: assessment and management, NICE guideline; no. 185. London: NICE; 2018.
35. Jon DI, Bahk WM, Yoon BH, Shin YC, Cho HS, Lee E, et al. Revised Korean medication algorithm for bipolar disorder. World J Biol Psychiatry. 2009;10(4 Pt 2):846–55.
36. Shin YC, Min KJ, Yoon BH, Kim W, Jon DI, Seo JS, et al. Korean medication algorithm for bipolar disorder: second revision. Asia Pac Psychiatry. 2013;5(4):e1–11.
37. Woo YS, Lee JG, Jeong JH, Kim MD, Sohn I, Shim SH, et al. Korean medication algorithm project for bipolar disorder: third revision. Neuropsychiatr Dis Treat. 2015;11:493–506.
38. Woo YS, Bahk WM, Lee JG, Jeong JH, Kim MD, Sohn I, et al. Korean medication algorithm project for bipolar disorder 2018 (KMAP-BP 2018): fourth revision. Clin Psychopharmacol Neurosci. 2018;16(4):434–48.
39. Woo YS, Bahk WM, Jeong JH, Lee JG, Kim W, Sohn I, et al. Korean medication algorithm project for bipolar disorder 2022, fifth revision: an executive summary. Clin Psychopharmacol Neurosci. 2022;20(4):747–61.
40. The Executive Committee of Korean Medication Algorithm Project for Bipolar Disorder. The Korean medication guideline for bipolar disorder. Seoul: Choong-Ang-Moonwhasa; 2002.
41. Glue P, Herbison P. Comparative efficacy and acceptability of combined antipsychotics and mood stabilizers versus individual drug classes for acute mania: network meta-analysis. Aust N Z J Psychiatry. 2015;49(12):1215–20.
42. Chen AT, Malmstrom T, Nasrallah HA. Allopurinol augmentation in acute mania: a meta-analysis of placebo-controlled trials. J Affect Disord. 2018;226:245–50.
43. Arabzadeh S, Ameli N, Zeinoddini A, Rezaei F, Farokhnia M, Mohammadinejad P, et al. Celecoxib adjunctive therapy for acute bipolar mania: a randomized, double-blind, placebo-controlled trial. Bipolar Disord. 2015;17(6):606–14.
44. Talaei A, Pourgholami M, Khatibi-Moghadam H, Faridhosseini F, Farhoudi F, Askari-Noghani A, et al. Tamoxifen: a protein kinase C inhibitor to treat mania: a systematic review and meta-analysis of randomized, placebo-controlled trials. J Clin Psychopharmacol. 2016;36(3):272–5.
45. Calabrese JR, Huffman RF, White RL, Edwards S, Thompson TR, Ascher JA, et al. Lamotrigine in the acute treatment of bipolar depression: results of five double-blind, placebo-controlled clinical trials. Bipolar Disord. 2008;10(2):323–33.
46. Unholzer S, Haen E. Retrospective analysis of therapeutic drug monitoring data for treatment of bipolar disorder with lamotrigine. Pharmacopsychiatry. 2015;48(6):296.
47. Calabrese JR, Bowden CL, Sachs GS, Ascher JA, Monaghan E, Rudd GD. A double-blind placebo-

controlled study of lamotrigine monotherapy in outpatients with bipolar I depression. Lamictal 602 Study Group. J Clin Psychiatry. 1999;60(2):79–88.
48. van der Loos ML, Mulder PG, Hartong EG, Blom MB, Vergouwen AC, de Keyzer HJ, et al. Efficacy and safety of lamotrigine as add-on treatment to lithium in bipolar depression: a multicenter, double-blind, placebo-controlled trial. J Clin Psychiatry. 2009;70(2):223–31.
49. Young AH, McElroy SL, Bauer M, Philips N, Chang W, Olausson B, et al. A double-blind, placebo-controlled study of quetiapine and lithium monotherapy in adults in the acute phase of bipolar depression (EMBOLDEN I). J Clin Psychiatry. 2010;71(2):150–62.
50. Cruz N, Sanchez-Moreno J, Torres F, Goikolea JM, Valenti M, Vieta E. Efficacy of modern antipsychotics in placebo-controlled trials in bipolar depression: a meta-analysis. Int J Neuropsychopharmacol. 2010;13(1):5–14.
51. Selle V, Schalkwijk S, Vazquez GH, Baldessarini RJ. Treatments for acute bipolar depression: meta-analyses of placebo-controlled, monotherapy trials of anticonvulsants, lithium and antipsychotics. Pharmacopsychiatry. 2014;47(2):43–52.
52. Fountoulakis KN, Kontis D, Gonda X, Yatham LN. A systematic review of the evidence on the treatment of rapid cycling bipolar disorder. Bipolar Disord. 2013;15(2):115–37.
53. Vieta E, Valenti M. Pharmacological management of bipolar depression: acute treatment, maintenance, and prophylaxis. CNS Drugs. 2013;27(7):515–29.
54. Kemp DE, Schinagle M, Gao K, Conroy C, Ganocy SJ, Ismail-Beigi F, et al. PPAR-gamma agonism as a modulator of mood: proof-of-concept for pioglitazone in bipolar depression. CNS Drugs. 2014;28(6):571–81.
55. Zeinoddini A, Sorayani M, Hassanzadeh E, Arbabi M, Farokhnia M, Salimi S, et al. Pioglitazone adjunctive therapy for depressive episode of bipolar disorder: a randomized, double-blind, placebo-controlled trial. Depress Anxiety. 2015;32(3):167–73.
56. Bocchetta A, Bernardi F, Burrai C, Pedditzi M, Del Zompo M. A double-blind study of L-sulpiride versus amitriptyline in lithium-maintained bipolar depressives. Acta Psychiatr Scand. 1993;88(6):434–9.
57. Sarris J, Mischoulon D, Schweitzer I. Omega-3 for bipolar disorder: meta-analyses of use in mania and bipolar depression. J Clin Psychiatry. 2012;73(1):81–6.
58. Grosso G, Pajak A, Marventano S, Castellano S, Galvano F, Bucolo C, et al. Role of omega-3 fatty acids in the treatment of depressive disorders: a comprehensive meta-analysis of randomized clinical trials. PLoS One. 2014;9(5):e96905.
59. Berk M, Copolov DL, Dean O, Lu K, Jeavons S, Schapkaitz I, et al. N-acetyl cysteine for depressive symptoms in bipolar disorder–a double-blind randomized placebo-controlled trial. Biol Psychiatry. 2008;64(6):468–75.
60. Romeo B, Choucha W, Fossati P, Rotge JY. Meta-analysis of short- and mid-term efficacy of ketamine in unipolar and bipolar depression. Psychiatry Res. 2015;230(3):682–8.
61. Rodolico A, Cutrufelli P, Di Francesco A, Aguglia A, Catania G, Concerto C, et al. Efficacy and safety of ketamine and Esketamine for unipolar and bipolar depression: an overview of systematic reviews with meta-analysis. Front Psych. 2024;15:1325399.
62. Tohen M, Calabrese JR, Sachs GS, Banov MD, Detke HC, Risser R, et al. Randomized, placebo-controlled trial of olanzapine as maintenance therapy in patients with bipolar I disorder responding to acute treatment with olanzapine. Am J Psychiatry. 2006;163(2):247–56.
63. Calabrese JR, Sanchez R, Jin N, Amatniek J, Cox K, Johnson B, et al. Efficacy and safety of aripiprazole once-monthly in the maintenance treatment of bipolar I disorder: a double-blind, placebo-controlled, 52-week randomized withdrawal study. J Clin Psychiatry. 2017;78(3):324–31.
64. Yacobi S, Ornoy A. Is lithium a real teratogen? What can we conclude from the prospective versus retrospective studies? A review. Isr J Psychiatry Relat Sci. 2008;45(2):95–106.

Biological Non-pharmacological Treatments for Bipolar Disorder

15

Min-Kyu Song and Jonghun Lee

Introduction

Bipolar disorder (BD) is a leading cause of disability worldwide, characterized by recurrent manic/hypomanic and depressive episodes and high medical comorbidity [1, 2]. Despite guideline-concordant pharmacotherapy and psychotherapy, many patients fail to remit, relapse frequently, or cannot tolerate medications, underscoring the role of biological non-pharmacological treatments (BNPTs). The diverse clinical roles and indications for major BNPTs in BD are summarized in Table 15.1 [4, 7, 9–31, 34–41]. BNPTs modulate dysfunctional frontolimbic circuits, neuroplasticity, neuroinflammation, and circadian systems implicated in BD pathophysiology [3–6]. Contemporary guidelines (APA 2023; CANMAT/ISBD 2023; NICE 2022; WFSBP 2020) increasingly incorporate BNPTs for treatment-resistant bipolar depression (TRBD), mixed states, rapid cycling, catatonia, suicidality, and for special groups such as pregnancy or older age [4, 6–8]. For clinical clarity, biological non-pharmacological treatments can be broadly categorized according to their evidence base and guideline endorsement into established, emerging, and investigational modalities. This framework is intended to help clinicians rapidly assess clinical relevance and appropriate placement within longitudinal bipolar care.

Table 15.1 Roles of major non-pharmacological modalities in bipolar disorder

Modality	Typical clinical role (summary)	Evidence status/ Recommendation
ECT	Severe depression, mania, catatonia	Established; first-line in severe or urgent cases (APA, CANMAT, ISBD) [7, 9–12, 34, 35]
rTMS	Bipolar depression	Established; adjunctive/second-line [4, 13–17]
tDCS	Bipolar depression	Emerging; adjunctive [18, 19]
BLT	Bipolar depression	Established; adjunctive (with mood stabilizer) [20–22, 30, 31]
VNS	Chronic TRBD	Investigational/ limited guideline endorsement [25, 29, 37]
DBS	Refractory BD	Investigational; research setting only [26–28]
Sleep deprivation	Rapid antidepressant effect	Emerging; adjunctive, high switch risk [23, 24, 38–40]

ECT electroconvulsive therapy, *rTMS* repetitive transcranial magnetic stimulation, *tDCS* transcranial direct current stimulation, *DBS* deep brain stimulation, *VNS* vagus nerve stimulation, *BLT* bright light therapy

M.-K. Song (✉)
Department of Psychiatry, St. Mary's Gong-Gam Mental Health Clinic, Siheung, Republic of Korea
e-mail: somtt0714@gmail.com

J. Lee
Department of Psychiatry, School of Medicine, Daegu Catholic University, Daegu, Republic of Korea

W.-M. Bahk et al. (eds.), *Bipolar Disorder*, https://doi.org/10.1007/978-981-92-1323-8_15

Electroconvulsive Therapy (ECT)

Mechanisms and Neurobiological Rationale

ECT induces a brief, controlled generalized seizure under anesthesia. Downstream effects include normalization of subcallosal cingulate (SCC) activity, modulation of frontolimbic connectivity, monoaminergic release, GABAergic enhancement, and neurotrophic signaling (e.g., BDNF), supporting synaptic remodeling and network reset pertinent to BD [9–12, 34].

Efficacy and Indications in BD

Systematic reviews and guideline syntheses affirm robust efficacy for bipolar depression, mania, mixed states, rapid cycling, and catatonia [9, 10, 12, 34, 35]. ECT yields response rates ≥60–80% and remission ~50–60% in acute depressive episodes; it is effective and comparatively safe during pregnancy when medications are contraindicated [7, 12, 34]. It can rapidly reduce suicidal intent and severe agitation in mania.

Protocols and Parameter Choices

- *Course:* 2–3 sessions/week for 6–12 sessions; continue until maximal clinical benefit, then taper.
- *Electrode placement:* bitemporal/bifrontal (greater efficacy) versus right unilateral (better cognitive profile).
- *Pulse width/dosing:* ultrabrief (≤0.3 ms) reduces cognitive effects with possible slower onset; individualized threshold titration advised [12, 17–19].
- *Continuation/Maintenance (C-/M-ECT):* biweekly → monthly schedules reduce relapse in recurrent BD; integrate with mood stabilizers [11].

  Practical parameters for implementing ECT in patients with BD, including electrode placement and frequency, are detailed in Table 15.2 [11, 12, 17–19, 41].

Table 15.2 Practical parameter guide for ECT in BD

Choice	Typical option	Clinical note
Placement	Bitemporal/bifrontal/right unilateral	Balance efficacy vs. cognitive profile [12]
Pulse width	0.25–1.0 ms (ultrabrief ≤0.3 ms)	Shorter width → fewer cognitive effects, may need more sessions [17–19]
Frequency	2–3×/week (acute); q2–4 weeks (maintenance)	Taper based on stability [11, 12]

Safety and Cognitive Effects

Transient disorientation, headache, myalgia are common; autobiographical memory gaps persist in a minority [20]. Medical complications are rare with proper anesthesia and monitoring; ECT is feasible with pacemakers and in late pregnancy with obstetric collaboration [7, 12, 34] (Box 15.1).

Box 15.1: ECT Pre-treatment Checklist
- Medical/anesthetic evaluation; electrocardiography (ECG) and labs as indicated [12, 17]
- Informed consent covering memory risks and alternatives [20]
- Electrode placement and dosing plan (threshold titration; cognitive-sparing strategy) [12, 18, 19]
- Relapse prevention: C-/M-ECT ± pharmacotherapy; follow-up schedule [11]

Repetitive Transcranial Magnetic Stimulation (rTMS)

Mechanisms and Targets

rTMS modulates cortical excitability and network connectivity through magnetic induction. High-frequency left dorsolateral prefrontal cortex (DLPFC) (excitatory) is antidepressant; low-frequency right DLPFC may be antimanic;

imaging shows normalization of DLPFC–subgenual connectivity with response [13–17].

Protocols and Innovations

- *Standard:* 10 Hz left DLPFC, ~3000 pulses/session, 20–30 sessions over 4–6 weeks.
- *iTBS:* intermittent theta-burst (~3–5 min/session) is non-inferior to 10 Hz in major depressive disorder (MDD); increasingly used in BD depression [16].
- *Bilateral/sequential:* low frequency (LF) right + high frequency (HF) left paradigms explored for mood stabilization.
- *Accelerated schedules:* multiple daily iTBS sessions over 1–5 days are under study for rapid relief [17].
- *Maintenance:* tapered booster sessions to prevent relapse in responders.

  Commonly utilized rTMS protocols for bipolar depression are compared in Table 15.3 [13–16, 41].

Efficacy and Guideline Placement

Meta-analyses show superiority to sham with response ~40–55% and remission ~25–35% in TRBD—below ECT but with superior tolerability [14, 15]. The CANMAT/ISBD 2023 endorses rTMS as an adjunct after inadequate pharmacotherapy, particularly for depressive episodes [4]. Data for acute mania remain limited.

Table 15.3 Common rTMS protocols for bipolar depression

Protocol	Target	Pulses	Session time	Notes
10 Hz (HF-L)	Left DLPFC	3000	~37 min	Most evidence; guideline-endorsed [13–15]
1 Hz (LF-R)	Right DLPFC	1800	~20 min	Alternative/adjunct; lower seizure risk [13]
iTBS	Left DLPFC	600	~3–5 min	Time-efficient; non-inferior in MDD; promising in BD [16]

Safety and Tolerability

Scalp discomfort and transient headache are common; protocolized screening keeps seizure risk <0.1%. No consistent cognitive impairment; some studies suggest modest executive gains [13–17] (Box 15.2).

Box 15.2: rTMS Candidacy and Safety Screen

- ≥1 inadequate pharmacotherapy trial; preference for noninvasive option [4, 13]
- Exclude incompatible cranial ferromagnetics/cochlear implants.
- Review seizure risk factors (sleep deprivation, medications).

Note on Magnetic Seizure Therapy (MST): seizure induction using magnetic fields is under investigation as a potentially cognition-sparing alternative to ECT; early data are promising but limited.

Transcranial Direct Current Stimulation (tDCS)

Mechanisms and Montages

tDCS delivers 1–2 mA direct current via scalp electrodes to shift resting membrane potentials and facilitate *N-methyl-D-aspartate* (NMDA)-dependent plasticity. Anode left DLPFC/cathode right supraorbital is the common antidepressant montage [18, 19].

Efficacy and Combinations

Randomized and meta-analytic data indicate small-to-moderate benefits in bipolar depression, particularly as augmentation to pharmacotherapy (e.g., SSRIs, lithium) [18, 19]. Improvements in cognition and sleep may contribute to relapse prevention [29].

Protocols and Practicalities

- *Dose:* 1–2 mA for 20–30 min.
- *Schedule:* 5×/week for 2–6 weeks, then boosters as needed.
- *Setting:* clinic-based or remote-supervised home tDCS to improve access and adherence [29].

Safety and Limitations

Generally well tolerated (tingling, itching, mild erythema, headache). Serious adverse event (AEs) are rare with standard protocols. Effects are modest and heterogeneous; careful patient selection and adherence monitoring are important [18, 19] (Box 15.3).

> **Box 15.3: Selecting Patients for tDCS**
> - Mild–moderate bipolar depression; barriers to rTMS/ECT
> - Preference for low-cost, portable modality
> - No implanted electronic devices; healthy scalp skin

Deep Brain Stimulation (DBS)

Targets and Mechanisms

DBS delivers chronic stimulation to subcortical mood circuits: subcallosal cingulate (SCC/Area 25), ventral capsule/ventral striatum (VC/VS), nucleus accumbens (NAcc), and medial forebrain bundle (MFB). Modulation may normalize pathologic network dynamics in refractory depression, including bipolar depression [26–28].

Efficacy and Patient Selection

Open-label and controlled series show sustained response (~40–50% at 1–2 years) in carefully selected treatment-resistant cohorts; evidence in mania is sparse [27, 28, 32]. DBS is considered only after failure/intolerance of comprehensive pharmacotherapy and noninvasive neuromodulation. Despite promising long-term outcomes in highly selected cohorts, deep brain stimulation for bipolar disorder remains investigational and is currently confined to specialized research settings rather than routine clinical practice.

Safety and Programming

Surgical risks (infection, hemorrhage) and hardware complications occur infrequently. Programming is iterative over weeks–months; closed-loop approaches are emerging [26–28] (Box 15.4).

> **Box 15.4: DBS Candidate Profile (Bipolar Depression)**
> - ≥2–3 adequate mood stabilizer/antidepressant augmentation strategies plus ECT and/or rTMS failure
> - Predominantly depressive polarity; chronicity with functional impairment
> - Multidisciplinary evaluation; informed consent for investigational therapy

Vagus Nerve Stimulation (VNS)

Mechanisms

Intermittent stimulation of the left cervical vagus projects to nucleus tractus solitarius, then locus coeruleus and dorsal raphe, modulating monoaminergic tone and limbic-prefrontal circuits [29].

Efficacy and Expectations

Acute RCTs show limited short-term separation from sham, but registry data demonstrate delayed yet durable improvements over months–years in subsets with chronic TRBD or rapid cycling, particularly with concomitant pharmacotherapy [25, 29, 37]. Vagus nerve stimulation occupies an intermediate position between established and investigational therapies, with limited short-term efficacy but potential long-term benefit in chronic, treatment-resistant bipolar depression.

Safety

Common stimulation-related adverse effects: hoarseness, throat discomfort, cough, dyspnea; possible sleep-related breathing issues. Surgical complications (infection, lead issues) are uncommon. Access varies by region/indication.

Chronotherapeutics: Bright Light Therapy (BLT) and Dark/Sleep Manipulations

Rationale and Mechanisms

Circadian and sleep/wake dysregulation is central to BD. Light signals via intrinsically photosensitive retinal ganglion cells synchronize the suprachiasmatic nucleus, influencing melatonin and monoaminergic systems [20, 30, 31]. Stabilizing circadian timing can improve depressive symptoms and reduce mood instability. Chronotherapeutic interventions may provide rapid symptomatic relief; however, they require careful monitoring due to the risk of mood destabilization and should generally be used as adjunctive strategies in conjunction with mood stabilizers.

Bright Light Therapy in BD Depression

Randomized trials support *BLT* as an effective adjunct for *bipolar depression*; a notable strategy is *midday dosing* (e.g., 12:00–14:00) to mitigate manic switch risk while achieving antidepressant effects [21]. Morning 10,000 lux for ~30 min is standard in unipolar depression, but in BD, protocol individualization (midday/moderate intensity) is common [21, 22, 31]. Combine with mood stabilizers and monitor weekly for activation.

Dark Therapy/Blue-Blocking Strategies (Mania-Prone States)

Evening dark therapy and blue-blocking (amber) glasses reduce nocturnal photic input, stabilizing circadian signals and may help manic activation; integrate with sleep hygiene and consistent lights-off schedules [30, 31].

Safety and Practical Guidance

Adverse effects are usually mild (eye strain, headache, agitation if too late in day). Screen retinal disease and photosensitizing medications; educate on device distance (~50 cm), viewing angle, and eyes-open exposure without staring at LEDs [21, 31]. Key parameters and cautions for chronotherapeutic modalities in BD are presented in Table 15.4 [21, 22, 30, 31, 41].

Table 15.4 Chronotherapy parameters in BD

Modality	Typical dose	Timing	Key cautions
BLT	7000–10,000 lux × 30 min	*Midday* preferred in BD	Monitor for activation; combine with mood stabilizers [21, 22]
Sleep phase advance	1–2 h earlier bedtime/wake	Over 3–5 days	Maintain routine; avoid late light exposure [31]
Dark therapy/ blue-blocking	Amber lenses after dusk; lights-off window	Evening–night	Use consistently during mania-prone periods [30, 31]

Sleep Deprivation (Wake Therapy)

Forms and Mechanisms

Total (36–40 h), partial (first or second half of the night), or selective rapid eye movement (REM) deprivation can produce rapid antidepressant effects, likely via REM suppression and circadian phase shifts [23, 24].

Efficacy, Maintenance, and Combinations

About 40–60% of bipolar depression patients improve within 24–48 h, but ~70% relapse after recovery sleep. Combining with lithium, BLT, and phase advance ("triple chronotherapy") prolongs benefit and reduces relapse [23, 24, 38, 39].

Risks and Safeguards

Significant mania switch risk necessitates careful selection, close monitoring, and concurrent mood stabilizers. Use structured inpatient/day-hospital protocols when feasible [39, 40] (Box 15.5).

Box 15.5: Practical Wake-Therapy Bundle

- Single-night total sleep deprivation → morning phase advance → midday BLT
- Lithium continuation; daily mood/activation checks for 1–2 weeks
- Abort protocol on hypomanic signs; revert to stabilizing routine

Special Populations and Clinical Scenarios

- *Pregnancy and postpartum:* ECT is a first-line non-pharmacological option for severe depression/mania with obstetric monitoring; rTMS is considered when available; BLT can be adjunctive for postpartum depression with prudent monitoring [7, 12, 21].
- *Older adults:* ECT is effective and safe with cognitive-sparing strategies; rTMS/tDCS are well tolerated and may aid cognition [12–15, 18].
- *Rapid cycling /mixed features:* Prefer ECT; consider chronotherapy carefully due to switch risk; avoid evening BLT [9, 12, 23].

Implementation: A Practical Algorithm

1. Define episode polarity and urgency. Severe suicidality, catatonia, malignant agitation → ECT.
2. For bipolar depression (nonemergent): optimize mood stabilizers → consider rTMS (± iTBS) or tDCS; add BLT (midday) with monitoring.
3. For refractory depression: evaluate for C-/M-ECT, VNS (where available), or DBS (clinical trial/tertiary center).
4. Chronotherapy bundle for rapid relief in selected patients: sleep deprivation + phase advance + BLT under stabilizer cover.
5. Maintenance: tapered rTMS boosters or M-ECT; circadian hygiene (regular sleep/wake, light–dark schedule) to reduce relapse (Box 15.6).

Box 15.6: Contraindications and Cautions (Selected)

- *ECT:* raised intracranial pressure, unstable cardiac status (relative), recent MI—optimize first [12]
- *rTMS/tDCS:* ferromagnetic cranial implants/cochlear devices; active skin disease at electrode sites
- *BLT/chronotherapy:* retinal disease, photosensitizing drugs, high switch risk without stabilizer

Adjunctive Biological Approaches (Brief)

Evidence for exercise and nutritional interventions in BD is emerging but less robust than in unipolar depression. Meta-analyses suggest exercise improves depressive symptoms and functioning; nutritional strategies (e.g., omega-3, micronutrients) may confer modest adjunctive benefits in selected phenotypes [32, 33]. These should complement—rather than replace—core BD treatments.

Conclusion

From a longitudinal and stage-based perspective, biological non-pharmacological treatments should be integrated with pharmacotherapy rather than viewed as isolated interventions. Electroconvulsive therapy remains the treatment of choice for acute, severe, or life-threatening episodes, while rTMS and tDCS are best positioned as adjunctive options during depressive phases with partial pharmacological response. Chronotherapeutic strategies may offer rapid symptom relief but require structured stabilization and relapse-prevention planning. Maintenance approaches—including continuation ECT, booster neuromodulation sessions, and sustained circadian regulation—are essential for optimizing long-term outcomes in this chronic, recurrent disorder. Future bipolar care will increasingly emphasize personalized sequencing, multimodal integration, and stage-specific treatment strategies across the course of illness.

Declarations

Competing Interests The author(s) has no competing interests to declare that are relevant to the content of this manuscript.

Ethics Approval The author(s) declares that this manuscript does not include primary research with human participants.

The author(s) declares that this manuscript does not include primary studies involving animals.

References

1. Grande I, Berk M, Birmaher B, Vieta E. Bipolar disorder. Lancet. 2016;387(10027):1561–72.
2. Ferrari AJ, Stockings E, Khoo JP, et al. The prevalence and burden of bipolar disorder: findings from the Global Burden of Disease Study 2019. Psychol Med. 2023;53(5):2334–43.
3. Goodwin GM, Haddad PM, Ferrier IN, et al. Evidence-based guidelines for treating bipolar disorder: revised third edition recommendations from the British Association for Psychopharmacology. J Psychopharmacol. 2016;30(6):495–553.
4. Yatham LN, Kauer-Sant'Anna M, Bond DJ, et al. CANMAT and ISBD 2023 guidelines for the management of patients with bipolar disorder. Bipolar Disord. 2023;25(3):301–52.
5. Malhi GS, Bell E, Boyce P, et al. The 2020 RANZCP clinical practice guidelines for mood disorders. Aust N Z J Psychiatry. 2021;55(1):7–117.
6. Pfennig A, Bauer M, Severus E. WFSBP guidelines update 2020 on the treatment of bipolar disorders. World J Biol Psychiatry. 2020;21(3):190–250.
7. American Psychiatric Association. Practice guideline for the treatment of patients with bipolar disorder. 3rd ed. Washington, DC: APA Publishing; 2023.
8. National Institute for Health and Care Excellence. Bipolar disorder: assessment and management. NICE guideline NG222. London: NICE; 2022.
9. Kishi T, Ikuta T, Matsuda Y, et al. Efficacy and tolerability of electroconvulsive therapy for bipolar disorder: systematic review and meta-analysis. Psychol Med. 2022;52(6):1105–15.
10. Medda P, Perugi G, Zanello S, et al. Response to ECT in bipolar I, bipolar II and unipolar depression. J Affect Disord. 2015;177:114–9.
11. Sienaert P, Lambrichts L, Popleu L, et al. Maintenance electroconvulsive therapy in patients with bipolar dis-

order: a retrospective chart review. Bipolar Disord. 2021;23(2):165–73.
12. Milev RV, Giacobbe P, Kennedy SH, et al. CANMAT 2016 recommendations: ECT and neurostimulation treatments. Can J Psychiatr. 2016;61(9):561–75.
13. Mutz J, Vipulananthan V, Carter B, et al. Comparative efficacy and acceptability of non-surgical brain stimulation for mood disorders: network meta-analysis. BMJ. 2019;364:l1079.
14. Berlim MT, McGirr A, Dos Santos NR, et al. Efficacy of bilateral rTMS in bipolar depression: meta-analysis. Psychol Med. 2014;44(12):2255–62.
15. McGirr A, Voineskos D, Blumberger DM, et al. rTMS for treatment-resistant bipolar depression: systematic review and meta-analysis. Bipolar Disord. 2016;18(2):137–44.
16. Blumberger DM, Vila-Rodriguez F, Thorpe KE, et al. THREE-D trial: iTBS vs 10 Hz rTMS in depression. JAMA Psychiatry. 2018;75(11):1192–200.
17. Dell'Osso B, Camuri G, Castellano F, et al. rTMS for bipolar depression: state of the art. Expert Rev Neurother. 2020;20(9):967–75.
18. Brunoni AR, Moffa AH, Sampaio-Junior B, et al. tDCS in bipolar depression: randomized clinical trial. JAMA Psychiatry. 2017;74(9):903–10.
19. Mutz J, Edgcumbe DR, Brunoni AR, Fu CHY. Non-invasive brain stimulation for depression and bipolar disorder: updated meta-analysis. JAMA Psychiatry. 2022;79(5):424–34.
20. Alda M, McCarthy MJ. Circadian genes, circadian rhythms, and bipolar disorders. Bipolar Disord. 2023;25(2):97–109.
21. Sit DK, McGowan J, Wiltrout C, et al. Midday bright light therapy for bipolar depression: randomized double-blind trial. Am J Psychiatry. 2018;175(2):131–9.
22. Zhou X, Teng T, Zhang Y, et al. Comparative efficacy of psychotherapies, BLT, and exercise for bipolar depression: network meta-analysis. Psychol Med. 2019;49(6):773–83.
23. Benedetti F, Colombo C, Barbini B, et al. Chronotherapeutics in bipolar depression: sleep deprivation and light therapy. Psychiatr Clin North Am. 2007;30(1):85–102.
24. Dallaspezia S, Benedetti F. Sleep deprivation therapy for bipolar depression: meta-analysis. J Affect Disord. 2015;183:103–9.
25. Aaronson ST, Sears P, Ruvuna F, et al. Five-year observational outcomes with VNS vs treatment as usual in TRD. Am J Psychiatry. 2017;174(7):640–8.
26. Conway CR, Xiong W, Greenberg BD, et al. Deep brain stimulation for TRD including bipolar depression: outcomes and mechanisms. Transl Psychiatry. 2021;11:164.
27. Holtzheimer PE, Husain MM, Lisanby SH, et al. Subcallosal cingulate DBS in TRD (unipolar and bipolar): 2-year outcomes. Am J Psychiatry. 2017;174(7):640–8.
28. Lozano AM, Mayberg HS, Giacobbe P, et al. DBS for psychiatric disorders: expert consensus. Mol Psychiatry. 2019;24(1):28–39.
29. Krahl SE, Senanayake SS, Handforth A. Vagus nerve stimulation for bipolar disorder: mechanisms and evidence. CNS Drugs. 2020;34(10):1031–42.
30. Geoffroy PA, Schroder CM, Bourgin P. Chronotherapy for mood disorders: from theory to practice. Dialogues Clin Neurosci. 2019;21(1):63–72.
31. Wirz-Justice A, Benedetti F, Terman M. Chronotherapeutics for affective disorders: a clinician's manual for light and wake therapy. 2nd ed. Basel: Karger; 2013.
32. Carvalho AF, Firth J, Vieta E. Physical activity and exercise in bipolar disorder: systematic review and meta-analysis. J Affect Disord. 2020;295:105–19.
33. Sarris J, Logan AC, Akbaraly TN, et al. Nutritional medicine as adjunctive treatment in bipolar disorder: consensus and review. Lancet Psychiatry. 2015;2(7):672–85.
34. Malhi GS, Gessler D, Outhred T. The use of ECT in bipolar disorder. Curr Psychiatry Rep. 2021;23(6):34.
35. Bahji A, Hawken ER, Sepehry AA, et al. ECT beyond unipolar major depression: systematic review and meta-analysis. J ECT. 2019;35(1):4–15.
36. McIntyre RS, Cha DS, Jerrell JM, et al. Emerging neuromodulatory treatments for bipolar depression: review. Bipolar Disord. 2014;16(6):558–78.
37. Nierenberg AA, Ostacher MJ, Huffman JC, et al. VNS for treatment-resistant bipolar disorder: pilot. Bipolar Disord. 2008;10(6):826–34.
38. Benedetti F, Barbini B, Colombo C, et al. Triple chronotherapy (sleep deprivation, phase advance, BLT) in bipolar depression: controlled trial. J Clin Psychiatry. 2005;66(7):853–9.
39. Dallaspezia S, Suzuki M, Colombo C, et al. Chronotherapeutics to prevent recurrence in BD: review and meta-analysis. CNS Spectr. 2020;25(1):2–11.
40. McCarthy MJ, Wei H, Nievergelt CM, et al. Circadian predictors of response to chronotherapy in BD. Mol Psychiatry. 2019;24(3):544–53.
41. Korean Society for Depressive and Bipolar Disorders. Bipolar disorder. 4th ed. Seoul: Sigma Press; 2024.

Part IV

Miscellaneous

The Impact of Parental Bipolar Disorder on Children

16

Chan-Mo Yang and Hyung-Mo Sung

Given the high heritability of bipolar disorder, a family history is the most significant risk factor for its development. The offspring of parents with bipolar disorder are typically classified as a high-risk group. In fact, it is reported that while approximately 40% of the offspring of parents with depressive disorder are at risk for developing the disorder in adulthood, about 10% of those with a bipolar parent are at risk of developing bipolar disorder in adulthood [1]. Through large-scale cohort studies on the offspring of parents with bipolar disorder, conducted for over 20 years, it has been revealed that due to the strong family history and genetic predisposition of the disorder, there is a high incidence and a strong tendency for clustering of bipolar disorder within families [2]. These characteristics are also confirmed by various epidemiological studies on pediatric and adolescent bipolar disorder. A meta-analysis of epidemiological studies found the prevalence of pediatric bipolar disorder to be approximately 1.8%; in contrast, the prevalence among child and adolescent offspring of parents with bipolar disorder is reported to range from 8.5% to 16%, with an odds ratio of 16 [3, 4].

The offspring of parents with bipolar disorder also show a higher incidence of other psychiatric disorders compared to the general population. A recent meta-analysis on the psychopathology of these high-risk offspring revealed that, compared to a control group, the incidence of bipolar spectrum disorder was nine times higher, mood disorders other than bipolar disorder were 2.5 times higher, and anxiety disorders were more than twice as high [5]. Furthermore, the offspring of parents with bipolar disorder exhibit a higher incidence not only of bipolar disorder but also of major depressive disorder (MDD), sleep disorders, anxiety disorders, and substance use disorders [6]. Even in the absence of a formal diagnosis for a specific psychiatric disorder, the offspring of parents with bipolar disorder are known to exhibit greater psychopathology, more substance use problems, impaired neurocognitive function, structural abnormalities in cortical-subcortical connections, and neuroendocrine abnormalities compared to the offspring of parents without the disorder [4, 7].

In psychiatry, research on the offspring of parents with bipolar disorder is crucial for understanding the disorder's genetic characteristics. More recently, this research has led to attempts to improve prognosis by identifying the features of high-risk groups and implementing early interventions during the prodromal state to either prevent the disorder's onset or treat it in its initial stages. For bipolar disorder, which has a relatively well-studied genetic

C.-M. Yang (✉)
Department of Psychiatry, Wonkwang University Hospital, School of Medicine, Wonkwang University, Iksan, Republic of Korea
e-mail: ychanmo@wku.ac.kr

H.-M. Sung
Department of Psychiatry, Soonchunhyang University Gumi Hospital, College of Medicine, Soonchunhyang University, Gumi, Republic of Korea

W.-M. Bahk et al. (eds.), *Bipolar Disorder*, https://doi.org/10.1007/978-981-92-1323-8_16

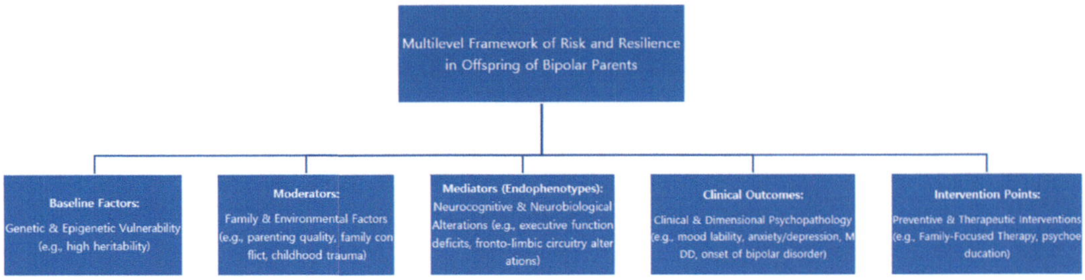

Fig. 16.1 A multilevel framework of risk and resilience in offspring of bipolar parents

basis, such studies on offspring help elucidate the gene–environment interactions related to the development of the illness and aid in developing early intervention methods for prevention and treatment. Moreover, these preventive interventions could have significant socioeconomic implications by reducing societal costs [8] (Fig. 16.1).

Why Are the Offspring of Parents with Bipolar Disorder Considered a High-Risk Group?

It is scientifically accepted that bipolar disorder has a strong genetic predisposition. Results from twin studies have shown that the concordance rate for bipolar disorder is approximately seven times higher in identical twins than in fraternal twins [9]. The heritability of bipolar disorder, as confirmed by numerous genetic studies including pedigree, twin, and adoption studies, is known to be as high as 85%. Moreover, when both parents have bipolar disorder, the risk of their offspring developing the disorder is 5.7 times higher than when only one parent is affected and 51.9 times higher than in children of unaffected parents [10, 11]. A pooled analysis of large-scale family studies also revealed a high sibling odds ratio of 6.96, with the sibling risk for bipolar disorder being higher than that for attention-deficit/hyperactivity disorder (ADHD) [12]. This strong heritability indicates that family history is the greatest risk factor for bipolar disorder, providing a solid basis for classifying the offspring of parents with the disorder as a high-risk group.

Although the heritability of bipolar disorder is higher than that of many other psychiatric disorders, the specific processes and mechanisms involved have not yet been clearly elucidated. Although efforts to identify the genes associated with the heritability of bipolar disorder are ongoing through numerous genomic studies, a specific genome or a fundamental genetic model has yet to be established. Models such as monogenic inheritance, the common variant hypothesis, multivariate threshold models, and oligogenic quasi-Mendelian modes have been proposed and are under discussion, but further research is required. Consequently, their application in clinical interventions for prevention and early treatment in the high-risk offspring of parents with bipolar disorder remains a distant prospect [13]. Findings from clinical studies on patients with bipolar disorder have been similar. For instance, a recent study analyzing multigenerational transmission trends in the offspring of parents with bipolar disorder found that while there was high concordance for psychiatric illness between parents and children, the level of risk was observed to change across generations [14]. This suggests that in the transmission of bipolar disorder across generations, various mechanisms, including epigenetic ones, may be involved in addition to purely genetic factors. This possibility warrants careful consideration in clinical and public health strategies aimed at preventing or delaying the disorder's onset in genetically predisposed individuals.

Risk Factors in the Family Environment

While it is true that genetic factors play a significant role in the development of psychopathology and psychiatric disorders in the offspring of parents with bipolar disorder, a variety of environmental factors are also known to influence their onset. Among these, factors related to the parenting practices of the affected parent seem to be particularly important. In fact, longitudinal studies on the offspring of parents with bipolar disorder have confirmed that parenting-related factors have a significant impact on their children's psychopathology [15]. In this context, the psychopathology of a mother with bipolar disorder and her quality of parenting are considered especially crucial. Maternal neglect has been proposed as a predictor for the development of mood disorders in children with a family history of the disorder. Furthermore, the mother's psychopathology can become a significant risk factor for the onset of bipolar disorder in her child by rendering her unable to provide adequate care [16, 17]. These findings suggest that providing parents with bipolar disorder with appropriate education and information on parenting, along with early interventions for both the parents and the family, could be highly beneficial for preventing or effectively treating psychopathology in their children.

Furthermore, various studies have recently been published seeking to identify other potential risk factors within the family environment. Dysfunctional family interactions are more common in families with a parent with bipolar disorder than in control families. Given this, and the higher prevalence of psychiatric disorders (including bipolar disorder) among the offspring of these parents, it is evident that the family environment—encompassing parental personality, parenting styles, and the parent-child relationship—can be a significant factor in the development of psychopathology in children [18–20]. High levels of family conflict and low cohesion are associated with higher levels of internalizing and externalizing symptoms in children, and low family cohesion has also been reported to be strongly correlated with mood disorders in offspring. The relationship between these environmental factors and a child's psychopathology has been found to be stronger in younger children [21].

Other Non-genetic Risk Factors

Although the offspring of parents with bipolar disorder are classified as a high-risk group due to strong heritability, various studies have sought to identify the specific risk and mediating factors that contribute to the actual onset of bipolar disorder or other psychiatric illnesses in these children. Unlike in schizophrenia, where parental age at the time of birth is a significant risk factor, parental age appears to be less relevant in bipolar disorder [22]; rather, the duration of the parent's illness during the child's upbringing seems to be a more critical factor. The longer the duration of the parent's bipolar disorder and the longer the child's exposure to it during their developmental years, the higher the risk for developing psychopathology. This finding also underscores the importance of actively treating the parent's bipolar disorder [23].

Long-term follow-up studies of specific regions or populations have reported anxiety disorders, depressive disorders, and behavioral disorders such as ADHD as potential prodromal symptoms or risk factors [24]. Furthermore, a longitudinal study in Canada emphasized that childhood anxiety disorders (e.g., generalized anxiety disorder, social anxiety disorder) are a predictive risk factor for the onset of mood disorders in high-risk offspring, making anxiety disorders an important target for early intervention in this group [25]. A systematic review of 21 individual cohort studies has shown that childhood anxiety disorders in these high-risk groups are associated with the subsequent onset of bipolar disorder, and recurrent substance use disorder has also been proposed as a risk factor for the development of bipolar disorder in late adolescence and early adulthood [26]. The Pittsburgh Bipolar Offspring Study (BIOS), a long-term study initiated in 2001 and running for over a decade, identified mania, depression, anxiety, mood lability, psychosocial functioning, and parental age as key factors for predicting the onset of bipolar spectrum disorder in offspring. The study also proposed a method using these factors to predict the five-year risk of developing a bipolar spectrum disorder in children with a familial risk [27].

Finally, stressful life events act as a risk factor for the onset of mood disorders, particularly in the offspring of parents with bipolar disorder, and there is evidence that passive coping styles and a harm-avoidant temperament influence the recurrence of mood episodes [2]. Furthermore, while the experience of childhood trauma is well-known to increase the risk of developing bipolar disorder in itself, it also acts as a significant risk factor for the offspring of parents with bipolar disorder and for pediatric bipolar patients with a family history of the disorder. In other words, the interaction between childhood trauma and genetic factors is presumed to further elevate the risk of developing bipolar disorder in high-risk offspring [28]. Additionally, low self-esteem and an avoidant coping style for stress in children have also been reported to be related to the onset and recurrence of mood episodes in this high-risk group [29].

In summary, the offspring of parents with bipolar disorder are classified as a high-risk group due to multiple risk factors, among which family history and genetic factors are the most potent. However, in addition to these genetic factors, various environmental factors are also influential. Key factors related to the family environment include parenting problems, dysfunctional family interactions, family conflict, and the duration of the child's exposure to the parent's bipolar disorder. Childhood anxiety disorder stands out as the most representative predictive risk factor for the onset of bipolar disorder or other psychopathology in offspring and could be a target for early intervention in this high-risk group.

Psychopathology (Categorical and Dimensional)

From the perspective of "categorical psychopathology," excluding bipolar disorder itself, the most representative psychiatric disorders that are significantly more prevalent in high-risk offspring include major depressive disorder (MDD), anxiety disorders, ADHD, and behavioral disorders. The prevalence of MDD is more than four times higher in the offspring of parents with bipolar disorder compared to those of parents without the disorder, and high-risk offspring with MDD are known to have a more than twofold increased risk of developing a substance use disorder. Prospective studies have confirmed that many high-risk offspring who are eventually diagnosed with bipolar disorder were previously diagnosed with MDD. Furthermore, when the offspring of parents with bipolar disorder exhibit depressive symptoms, they tend to have more severe depression—including atypical symptoms—and mixed manic symptoms, an earlier age of onset for MDD, and a higher rate of recurrence compared to the offspring of parents with depressive disorder [4, 30, 31]. This highlights the significance of depressive symptoms in the offspring of parents with bipolar disorder and indicates that these symptoms should be a target for active clinical treatment.

Anxiety disorders also have a high prevalence in the offspring of parents with bipolar disorder. Cross-sectional studies show an odds ratio greater than 2 compared to control groups, and the presence of an anxiety disorder in high-risk offspring acts as a risk factor for the subsequent development of bipolar disorder [4, 25]. ADHD and disruptive behavior disorder are also highly prevalent in the offspring of parents with bipolar disorder, with ADHD showing an even higher prevalence than in the offspring of parents with major depressive disorder. However, studies have reported conflicting results as to whether ADHD is a risk factor for the subsequent onset of bipolar disorder [4]. In the case of disruptive mood dysregulation disorder (DMDD), first recognized in the Diagnostic and Statistical Manual of Mental Disorders, fifth Edition (DSM-V), The Pittsburgh Bipolar Offspring Study found that a family history of bipolar disorder increased the risk for DMDD, whereas other large-scale studies found no such association [32, 33].

Numerous studies have confirmed that, irrespective of a formal psychiatric diagnosis, the offspring of parents with bipolar disorder exhibit various forms of psychopathology during childhood and adolescence. Results from The Pittsburgh Bipolar Offspring Study (BIOS) show an increased risk for ADHD and subsyndromal depressive and manic symptoms in high-risk preschool-aged children. Regardless of a psychiatric diagnosis, they also exhibited significantly more aggression, mood dysregulation, sleep problems, and somatic symptoms [34, 35]. Studies examining different developmental stages report that externalizing psychopathology is more common before puberty, whereas depressive and prodromal symptoms are more frequently observed after puberty [36]. Synthesizing these issues from a "dimensional psychopathology" perspective, the most common psychopathologies observed in the offspring of these parents include mood instability, high levels of anxiety and depression, and excessive excitability, including aggression. Such psychopathologies may represent a prodromal phenotype of bipolar disorder and are expected to be strong predictors for the future onset of bipolar disorder and other psychiatric conditions. This makes them clinically very important as targets for prevention and early treatment [4, 37].

Finally, regarding suicidality among the offspring of parents with bipolar disorder, The Pittsburgh Bipolar Offspring Study confirmed a higher risk of suicide in this group compared to the general population. This risk is further elevated by the interaction between genetic factors for bipolar disorder and childhood trauma, which underscores the critical importance of addressing psychological trauma in high risk children [38, 39].

Abnormalities in Neurocognitive Function

Studies comparing the neurocognitive function of offspring of parents with and without bipolar disorder have confirmed that the offspring of affected parents exhibit deficits across various neurocognitive domains. These neurocognitive deficits are present when compared to control groups, regardless of whether the offspring have any psychopathology, and have been confirmed to appear even before the onset of bipolar disorder or other psychiatric illnesses. Based on these differences, researchers are attempting to identify objectively measurable predictive factors or vulnerability markers for the disorder's onset by comparing offspring of parents with bipolar disorder who do and do not go on to develop the illness. This has significant clinical implications, as it could enable the identification of an ultra-high-risk subgroup within the broader high-risk group, allowing for early preventive interventions or the initiation of treatment in the earliest stages of the illness.

Early studies of neurocognitive function often sought to identify differences in intelligence, and while intelligence has been included in most neurocognitive studies, the results have not been consistent. Although some studies reported lower intelligence in the offspring of parents with bipolar disorder compared to controls, a comprehensive review of the research indicates no difference in overall intelligence between the two groups [40]. Studies using neurocognitive tests such as the Continuous Performance Test and the Wisconsin Card Sorting Test to compare the two groups have found differences in specific domains. The offspring of parents with bipolar disorder show poorer performance in sustained attention, response inhibition, verbal/visual-spatial memory, working memory, cognitive flexibility, and social cognition compared to the offspring of parents without the disorder [4]. This suggests the presence of impairments in higher-order cognitive functions, including executive function, in the offspring of parents with bipolar disorder, regardless of any current psychopathology. However, some of these neurocognitive deficits are also observed in the offspring of parents with schizophrenia and are, therefore, not specific to bipolar disorder.

More recent and interesting findings indicate that, regardless of psychopathology, the offspring of parents with bipolar disorder show deficits in neurocognitive functions related to cognitive processing speed and the immediate recall of visual memory. These deficits are particularly pronounced in offspring who later develop bipolar disorder, suggesting their potential as a vulnerability marker for its onset [41]. Similarly, abnormalities in the processing of affective information, a cognitive impairment commonly observed in both pediatric bipolar patients and the offspring of parents with bipolar disorder, are also being studied as a potential vulnerability marker [42].

Abnormalities in Neuroanatomy

Numerous studies have sought to identify neuroanatomical abnormalities in the offspring of parents with bipolar disorder. However, these neuroimaging studies are still relatively few in number, and the majority are cross-sectional, limiting them to the identification of group differences. Therefore, future longitudinal studies are needed to determine whether these observed group differences are actually related to the development of psychopathology or psychiatric disorders in the offspring.

Studies investigating structural abnormalities in various cerebral regions have yielded inconsistent results; some have reported reduced cortical thickness and smaller amygdala volumes in the offspring of parents with bipolar disorder, while others have found no differences in the hippocampus, thalamus, basal ganglia, prefrontal cortex, or pituitary gland [4, 43, 44]. One study found that adolescents with ADHD and a family history of bipolar disorder had more severe symptoms and significant reductions in the volume of the hippocampus, thalamus, and basal ganglia compared to adolescents with ADHD but no such family history [45]. More recently, a study reported that changes in cerebellar volume in adolescents with pediatric bipolar spectrum disorder and in the offspring of parents with bipolar disorder are closely related to emotional processing, suggesting that cerebellar abnormalities could be an important neurodevelopmental marker in these high-risk groups [46].

Various abnormalities have been reported in the connectivity and functional circuits of different brain regions. Studies using functional magnetic resonance imaging (fMRI) have identified several abnormalities in healthy offspring of parents with bipolar disorder, including functional changes in the frontolimbic circuit responsible for voluntary emotional regulation, reduced prefrontal–subcortical connectivity, abnormalities in the amygdala–prefrontal circuit involved in processing facial emotions, abnormalities in reward circuitry, abnormal prefrontal activation and connectivity during reward processing, and network abnormalities in key regions responsible for emotion and cognition [47–52]. Recently, the offspring of patients with bipolar disorder showed reduced fractional anisotropy (FA) in various brain regions, including the frontal and temporal lobes [53]. Changes in the frontal and temporal lobes, in particular, are closely related to emotional regulation and cognitive function, suggesting they could be considered a potential endophenotype for bipolar disorder. The uncinate fasciculus (UF), a white matter tract connecting the amygdala and the ventral prefrontal cortex, is involved in emotional regulation, and a meta-analysis based on 32 recent studies was conducted on this structure. While abnormalities in UF microstructure, particularly changes in myelination, were associated with the mechanisms of bipolar disorder, there was insufficient evidence to support its role as an endophenotype in high-risk groups [54]. Meanwhile, a meta-analysis of 57 studies on individuals with bipolar disorder and 10 studies on high-risk groups found lower FA in the corpus callosum in both groups. This suggests that abnormalities in the corpus callosum may be an endophenotype for bipolar disorder and that the disorder is associated with abnormalities in white matter tracts related to working memory performance, attention, and reward processing [55]. A recently published six-year long-term follow-up study analyzed the UF's FA in asymptomatic and symptomatic offspring of parents with bipolar disorder, as well as in a healthy control group, focusing on those who went on to develop bipolar disorder. FA in the right UF was found to predict the onset of bipolar disorder with a sensitivity of 88.9% and a specificity of 77.3% [56]. Further longitudinal research will be necessary to determine whether the various abnormalities identified through neuroimaging studies can serve as neurodevelopmental or predictive markers for the onset of bipolar disorder in high-risk individuals.

Clinical Implications and Preventive Interventions

Translating Risk to Clinical Practice: Screening and Early Intervention

The multilevel risk factors identified in offspring of parents with bipolar disorder—ranging from genetic predisposition to environmental stressors—necessitate a proactive clinical approach. Effective clinical translation requires systematic screening, targeted monitoring of prodromal symptoms, and the timely application of evidence-based psychosocial interventions.

1. *Risk Assessment and Screening Protocols*

Given the high heritability and the significant role of family history, clinicians must prioritize obtaining a thorough family history of psychiatric disorders. Screening should ideally begin in early childhood and continue longitudinally, as the manifestation of psychopathology varies by developmental stage.

- *Key Risk Markers*: Clinicians should be vigilant for prodromal signs such as mood lability, high levels of anxiety, and subsyndromal depressive symptoms, which are strong predictors of future bipolar disorder. Additionally, exposure to childhood trauma and high family conflict should be assessed as critical environmental moderators.
- *Screening Tools*: To operationalize these findings, the use of validated standardized instruments is recommended. The Kiddie Schedule for Affective Disorders and Schizophrenia can be utilized for comprehensive diagnostic assessment. For dimensional screening of internalizing and externalizing behaviors, the Child Behavior Checklist is valuable, particularly given the high prevalence of ADHD and behavioral disorders in this population. Furthermore, the Mood and Feelings Questionnaire may be employed to monitor depressive symptoms, which are often the initial presentation of mood disorders in these high-risk offspring.

2. *Hierarchy of Interventions*
   - *Psychosocial First-Line Strategy*: Before the onset of a full manic episode, psychosocial interventions are the primary recommendation. Psychoeducation for both parents and children is essential to improve illness understanding and symptom management. Family-focused therapy has demonstrated efficacy in reducing symptoms by addressing family conflict and communication, which are known environmental risk factors. Additionally, Interpersonal and Social Rhythm Therapy (IPSRT) shows promise in stabilizing sleep–wake cycles, addressing the sleep disturbances frequently observed in this group.
   - *Pharmacologic Considerations*: While pharmacotherapy is common for treating comorbid conditions like ADHD or anxiety, the use of mood stabilizers for the primary prevention of bipolar disorder in asymptomatic or prodromal youth remains a subject of ethical debate and limited evidence. Therefore, pharmacologic intervention should be carefully weighed against potential risks, prioritizing symptom-targeted treatment over prophylactic use until further longitudinal evidence is established.

Therapeutic Interventions

Although research aimed at identifying high-risk offspring of parents with bipolar disorder—those who show symptoms of mood disorders or are at high risk of onset—has shown some progress, studies on preventive treatment and early intervention for these high-risk groups have yet to yield satisfactory results. Early studies in this area primarily attempted non-pharmacological treatments such as psychotherapy, interventions involving sleep and diet, and omega-3 fatty acids. However, most of these were open-label studies with small sample sizes and have not yet provided results with sufficient evidence to support their efficacy [57].

Recently, more proactive attempts to reduce psychopathology or prevent the onset of psychiatric disorders in high-risk offspring have garnered significant attention, and various noteworthy, albeit fragmented, research findings are being reported [58]. Interventions using psychosocial treatments can include psychoeducation, cognitive-behavioral therapy (CBT), and family-focused interventions [59]. Psychoeducation helps to increase the understanding of bipolar disorder for both children and parents and teaches them methods to recognize and manage symptoms [60]. Cognitive-behavioral therapy can help children recognize and modify negative thought patterns and improve their stress management skills. There has also been research showing that family-focused therapy is effective in reducing depressive symptoms in children [61], and web-based interventions are being attempted to support the parenting of parents with bipolar disorder [62]. More specialized interventions for the offspring of parents with bipolar disorder have also been attempted recently. A study was recently published showing that applying Interpersonal and Social Rhythm Therapy (IPSRT), a form of CBT, and improving sleep quality may delay or prevent the onset of manic or hypomanic episodes [63]. More proactive therapeutic interventions for high-risk groups are also being explored, such as a study using aripiprazole, an atypical antipsychotic commonly used in the treatment of pediatric bipolar disorder. This study reported that aripiprazole had significant effects, including the reduction of manic symptoms, in high-risk children and adolescents (ages 5–17) [64].

Many children in the high-risk group receive various forms of pharmacotherapy before the onset of bipolar disorder, particularly before a manic episode. It is known that they are often prescribed medications for anxiety symptoms, depressive symptoms, or ADHD that appear prior to a manic episode, and some are also prescribed mood stabilizers. There are no consistent research findings on how the use of these medications affects the onset of bipolar disorder. Although some cross-sectional studies suggest that the use of mood stabilizers is associated with a delay in the onset of mania, more longitudinal research is needed in this area [65]. Furthermore, significant ethical debates persist among experts regarding whether the potential benefits of early psychotropic agent use outweigh the risks, particularly when interventions are based on provisional factors such as putative risk states or endophenotypes. Therefore, in addition to identifying decisive or predictive risk factors for onset, further studies and attempts are needed to elucidate the developmental trajectory of bipolar disorder and to find and apply appropriate intervention methods for each stage of the illness.

Summary and Conclusion

A synthesis of numerous studies on the offspring of parents with bipolar disorder reveals that these children not only belong to a high-risk group for developing the disorder but also exhibit various other psychopathologies and abnormalities in interpersonal functioning, personality traits, and neurocognitive and neurobiological domains. In terms of psychopathology, various issues such as somatic symptoms, sleep problems, anxiety and depressive symptoms, attention deficits, and impulsivity are more common during childhood and adolescence compared to control groups. Regarding psychiatric disorders, major mood disorders, anxiety disorders, ADHD, and behavioral disorders are more frequent. In particular, it is reported that children who experience major depressive episodes during childhood are more likely to develop bipolar disorder after adolescence. The likelihood of developing a major mood disorder is further increased by the influence of environmental factors such as dysfunctional family environments, high emotionality, and behavioral disinhibition. The offspring of parents with bipolar disorder also commonly exhibit neurocognitive deficits, particularly in areas such as audiovisual memory, cognitive flexibility, and attention. Furthermore, various neuroimaging studies have confirmed abnormalities in cortical–subcortical connections and white matter, and these subcortical abnormalities are similar to findings in patients with pediatric bipolar disorder.

Based on these previous findings, while future research elucidating the mechanisms of intergenerational transmission of bipolar disorder is important, it is also clinically imperative to conduct studies that identify an ultra-high-risk subgroup among these offspring—those at greatest risk for developing bipolar disorder and other psychopathologies—and to establish appropriate preventive measures. It is hoped that through such research, we can optimize screening methods and timing by utilizing the symptomatic, psychopathological, and neurobiological characteristics of the high-risk group, and through the establishment of individualized intervention strategies, prevent the onset of bipolar disorder and improve treatment outcomes with early intervention.

Declarations

Competing Interests The author(s) has no competing interests to declare that are relevant to the content of this manuscript.

Ethics Approval The author(s) declares that this manuscript does not include primary research with human participants.

The author(s) declares that this manuscript does not include primary studies involving animals.

References

1. Maciejewski D, Hillegers M, Penninx B. Offspring of parents with mood disorders: time for more transgenerational research, screening and preventive intervention for this high-risk population. Curr Opin Psychiatry. 2018;31(4):349–57.
2. Kemner SM, Mesman E, Nolen WA, Eijckemans MJ, Hillegers MH. The role of life events and psychological factors in the onset of first and recurrent mood episodes in bipolar offspring: results from the Dutch Bipolar Offspring Study. Psychol Med. 2015;45(12):2571–82.
3. Van Meter AR, Moreira AL, Youngstrom EA. Meta-analysis of epidemiologic studies of pediatric bipolar disorder. J Clin Psychiatry. 2011;72(9):1250–6.
4. Frías A, Palma C, Farriols N, Salvador A. Characterizing offspring of bipolar parents: a review of the literature. Actas Esp Psiquiatr. 2015;44(5):221–34.
5. Lau P, Hawes DJ, Hunt C, Frankland A, Roberts G, Mitchell PB. Prevalence of psychopathology in bipolar high-risk offspring and siblings: a meta-analysis. Eur Child Adolesc Psychiatry. 2018;27(7):823–37.
6. Duffy A, Horrocks J, Doucette S, Keown-Stoneman C, McCloskey S, Grof P. The developmental trajectory of bipolar disorder. Br J Psychiatry. 2014;204(2):122–8.
7. DelBello MP, Geller B. Review of studies of child and adolescent offspring of bipolar parents. Bipolar Disord. 2001;3(6):325–34.
8. Chang K, Steiner H, Dienes K, Adleman N, Ketter T. Bipolar offspring: a window into bipolar disorder evolution. Biol Psychiatry. 2003;53(11):945–51.
9. Kieseppä T, Partonen T, Haukka J, Kaprio J, Lönnqvist J. High concordance of bipolar I disorder in a nationwide sample of twins. Am J Psychiatry. 2004;161(10):1814–21.
10. McGuffin P, Rijsdijk F, Andrew M, Sham P, Katz R, Cardno A. The heritability of bipolar affective disorder and the genetic relationship to unipolar depression. Arch Gen Psychiatry. 2003;60(5):497–502.
11. Gottesman II, Laursen TM, Bertelsen A, Mortensen PB. Severe mental disorders in offspring with 2 psychiatrically ill parents. Arch Gen Psychiatry. 2010;67(3):252–7.
12. Wozniak J, Faraone SV, Martelon M, McKillop HN, Biederman J. Further evidence for robust familiality of pediatric bipolar I disorder: results from a very large controlled family study of pediatric bipolar I disorder and a meta-analysis. J Clin Psychiatry. 2012;73(10):1328–34.
13. Kerner B. Genetics of bipolar disorder. Appl Clin Genet. 2014;7:33–42.
14. Post RM, Altshuler LL, Kupka R, McElroy SL, Frye MA, Rowe M, et al. Multigenerational transmission of liability to psychiatric illness in offspring of parents with bipolar disorder. Bipolar Disord. 2018; https://doi.org/10.1111/bdi.12668.
15. Iacono V, Beaulieu L, Hodgins S, Ellenbogen MA. Parenting practices in middle childhood mediate the relation between growing up with a parent having bipolar disorder and offspring psychopathology from childhood into early adulthood. Dev Psychopathol. 2018;30(2):635–49.
16. Doucette S, Levy A, Flowerdew G, Horrocks J, Grof P, Ellenbogen M, et al. Early parent-child relationships and risk of mood disorder in a Canadian sample of offspring of a parent with bipolar disorder: findings from a 16-year prospective cohort study. Early Interv Psychiatry. 2016;10(5):381–9.
17. Moreno DH, Bio DS, Petresco S, Petresco D, Gutt EK, Soeiro-de-Souza MG, et al. Burden of maternal bipolar disorder on at-risk offspring: a controlled study on family planning and maternal care. J Affect Disord. 2012;143(1–3):172–8.

18. Ferreira GS, Moreira CR, Kleinman A, Nader EC, Gomes BC, Teixeira AM, et al. Dysfunctional family environment in affected versus unaffected offspring of parents with bipolar disorder. Aust N Z J Psychiatry. 2013;47(11):1051–7.
19. Nijjar R, Ellenbogen MA, Hodgins S. Sexual risk behaviors in the adolescent offspring of parents with bipolar disorder: prospective associations with parents' personality and externalizing behavior in childhood. J Abnorm Child Psychol. 2016;44(7):1347–59.
20. Lau P, Hawes DJ, Hunt C, Frankland A, Roberts G, Wright A, et al. Family environment and psychopathology in offspring of parents with bipolar disorder. J Affect Disord. 2018;226:12–20.
21. Freed RD, Tompson MC, Wang CH, Otto MW, Hirshfeld-Becker DR, Nierenberg AA, et al. Family functioning in the context of parental bipolar disorder: associations with offspring age, sex, and psychopathology. J Fam Psychol. 2015;29(1):108–18.
22. Brown A, Bao Y, McKeague I, Shen L, Schaefer C. Parental age and risk of bipolar disorder in offspring. Psychiatry Res. 2013;208(3):225–31.
23. Goodday SM, Levy A, Flowerdew G, Horrocks J, Grof P, Ellenbogen M, et al. Early exposure to parental bipolar disorder and risk of mood disorder: the flourish Canadian prospective offspring cohort study. Early Interv Psychiatry. 2018;12(1):160–8.
24. Egeland JA, Endicott J, Hostetter AM, Allen CR, Pauls DL, Shaw JA. A 16-year prospective study of prodromal features prior to BPI onset in well Amish children. J Affect Disord. 2012;142(1–3):186–92.
25. Duffy A, Horrocks J, Doucette S, Keown-Stoneman C, McCloskey S, Grof P. Childhood anxiety: an early predictor of mood disorders in offspring of bipolar parents. J Affect Disord. 2013;150(2):363–9.
26. Raouna A, Osam CS, MacBeth A. Clinical staging model in offspring of parents with bipolar disorder: a systematic review. Bipolar Disord. 2018;20(4):313–33.
27. Hafeman DM, Merranko J, Goldstein TR, Axelson D, Goldstein BI, Monk K, et al. Assessment of a person-level risk calculator to predict new-onset bipolar spectrum disorder in youth at familial risk. JAMA Psychiatry. 2017;74(8):841–7.
28. Etain B, Henry C, Bellivier F, Mathieu F, Leboyer M. Beyond genetics: childhood affective trauma in bipolar disorder. Bipolar Disord. 2008;10(8):867–76.
29. Goodday SM, Bentall R, Jones S, Weir A, Duffy A. Coping strategies and self-esteem in the high-risk offspring of bipolar parents. Aust N Z J Psychiatry. 2018; https://doi.org/10.1177/0004867418761577.
30. Vandeleur C, Rothen S, Gholam-Rezaee M, Castelao E, Vidal S, Favre S, et al. Mental disorders in offspring of parents with bipolar and major depressive disorders. Bipolar Disord. 2012;14(6):641–53.
31. Diler RS, Goldstein TR, Hafeman D, Rooks BT, Sakolsky D, Goldstein BI. Characteristics of depression among offspring at high and low familial risk of bipolar disorder. Bipolar Disord. 2017;19(5):344–52.
32. Perich T, Frankland A, Roberts G, Levy F, Lenroot R, Mitchell PB. Disruptive mood dysregulation disorder, severe mood dysregulation and chronic irritability in youth at high familial risk of bipolar disorder. Aust N Z J Psychiatry. 2017;51(12):1220–6.
33. Propper L, Cumby J, Patterson VC, Drobinin V, Glover JM, MacKenzie LE, et al. Disruptive mood dysregulation disorder in offspring of parents with depression and bipolar disorder. Br J Psychiatry. 2017;210(6):408–12.
34. Birmaher B, Axelson D, Goldstein B, Monk K, Kalas C, Obreja M, et al. Psychiatric disorders in preschool offspring of parents with bipolar disorder: the Pittsburgh Bipolar Offspring Study (BIOS). Am J Psychiatry. 2010;167(3):321–30.
35. Maoz H, Goldstein T, Axelson DA, Goldstein BI, Fan J, Hickey MB, et al. Dimensional psychopathology in preschool offspring of parents with bipolar disorder. J Child Psychol Psychiatry. 2014;55(2):144–53.
36. Morón-Nozaleda MG, Díaz-Caneja CM, Rodríguez-Toscano E, Arango C, Castro-Fornieles J, de la Serna E, et al. A developmental approach to dimensional expression of psychopathology in child and adolescent offspring of parents with bipolar disorder. Eur Child Adolesc Psychiatry. 2017;26(10):1165–75.
37. Birmaher B, Goldstein BI, Axelson DA, Monk K, Hickey MB, Fan J, et al. Mood lability among offspring of parents with bipolar disorder and community controls. Bipolar Disord. 2013;15(3):253–63.
38. Goldstein TR, Obreja M, Shamseddeen W, Axelson DA, Goldstein BI, Liao F, et al. Risk for suicidal ideation among the offspring of bipolar parents: results from the Bipolar Offspring Study (BIOS). Arch Suicide Res. 2011;15(3):207–22.
39. Wilcox HC, Fullerton JM, Glowinski AL, Benke K, Kamali M, Hulvershorn LA, et al. Traumatic stress interacts with bipolar disorder genetic risk to increase risk for suicide attempts. J Am Acad Child Adolesc Psychiatry. 2017;56(12):1073–9.
40. Klimes-Dougan B, Jeong J, Kennedy KP, Allen TA. Intellectual functioning in offspring of parents with bipolar disorder: a review of the literature. Brain Sci. 2017;7(11):143.
41. de la Serna E, Vila M, Sanchez-Gistau V, Moreno D, Romero S, Sugranyes G, et al. Neuropsychological characteristics of child and adolescent offspring of patients with bipolar disorder. Prog Neuro-Psychopharmacol Biol Psychiatry. 2016;65:54–9.
42. Bauer IE, Frazier TW, Meyer TD, Youngstrom E, Zunta-Soares GB, Soares JC. Affective processing in pediatric bipolar disorder and offspring of bipolar parents. J Child Adolesc Psychopharmacol. 2015;25(8):684–90.
43. Hanford LC, Sassi RB, Minuzzi L, Hall GB. Cortical thickness in symptomatic and asymptomatic bipolar offspring. Psychiatry Res Neuroimaging. 2016;251:26–33.
44. Akbas S, Nahir M, Pirzirenli ME, Dündar C, Ceyhan M, Sarısoy G, et al. Quantitative analysis of the amygdala, thalamus and hippocampus on magnetic

resonance images in paediatric bipolar disorders and compared with the children of bipolar parents and healthy control. Psychiatry Res Neuroimaging. 2017;270:61–7.
45. Zhu Z, Lei D, Qin K, Zhang X, Cao J, Chen C, et al. Cortical and subcortical structural differences in psychostimulant-free ADHD youth with and without a family history of bipolar I disorder: a cross-sectional morphometric comparison. Transl Psychiatry. 2023;13(1):368.
46. Saxena K, Simonetti A, Verrico CD, Zhou C, Ouyang X, Chen X, et al. Neurocognitive correlates of cerebellar volumetric alterations in youth with pediatric bipolar spectrum disorders and bipolar offspring. Curr Neuropharmacol. 2023;21(6):1367–78.
47. Ladouceur CD, Diwadkar VA, White R, Bass J, Birmaher B, Axelson DA, et al. Fronto-limbic function in unaffected offspring at familial risk for bipolar disorder during an emotional working memory paradigm. Dev Cogn Neurosci. 2013;5:185–96.
48. Singh MK, Chang KD, Kelley RG, Saggar M, Reiss AL, Gotlib IH. Early signs of anomalous neural functional connectivity in healthy offspring of parents with bipolar disorder. Bipolar Disord. 2014;16(6):678–89.
49. Singh MK, Kelley RG, Howe ME, Reiss AL, Gotlib IH, Chang KD. Reward processing in healthy offspring of parents with bipolar disorder. JAMA Psychiatry. 2014;71(10):1148–56.
50. Manelis A, Ladouceur CD, Graur S, Monk K, Bonar LK, Hickey MB, et al. Altered amygdala-prefrontal response to facial emotion in offspring of parents with bipolar disorder. Brain. 2015;138(Pt 9):2777–90.
51. Manelis A, Ladouceur CD, Graur S, Monk K, Bonar LK, Hickey MB, et al. Altered functioning of reward circuitry in youth offspring of parents with bipolar disorder. Psychol Med. 2016;46(1):197–208.
52. Roberts G, Perry A, Lord A, Frankland A, Leung V, Holmes-Preston E, et al. Structural dysconnectivity of key cognitive and emotional hubs in young people at high genetic risk for bipolar disorder. Mol Psychiatry. 2018;23(2):413–21.
53. Camkurt MA, Melicher T, Mwangi B, Atasoy HT, Ulasoglu C, Aydin M, et al. Investigation of endophenotype potential of decreased fractional anisotropy in pediatric bipolar disorder patients and unrelated offspring of bipolar disorder patients. CNS Spectr. 2022;27(6):709–15.
54. Xu E, Nguyen L, Hu R, Stavish CM, Leibenluft E, Linke JO. The uncinate fasciculus in individuals with and at risk for bipolar disorder: a meta-analysis. J Affect Disord. 2022;297:208–16.
55. Hu R, Stavish C, Leibenluft E, Linke JO. White matter microstructure in individuals with and at risk for bipolar disorder: evidence for an endophenotype from a voxel-based meta-analysis. Biol Psychiatry Cognit Neurosci Neuroimaging. 2020;5(12):1104–13.
56. Li X, Lu W, Zhang R, Liu Y, Wang Y, Chen X, et al. Integrity of the uncinate fasciculus is associated with the onset of bipolar disorder: a 6-year follow-up study. Transl Psychiatry. 2021;11(1):111.
57. Zalpuri I, Singh MK. Treatment of psychiatric symptoms among offspring of parents with bipolar disorder. Curr Treat Options Psychiatry. 2017;4(3):341–56.
58. Peay HL, Rosenstein DL, Biesecker BB. Parenting with bipolar disorder: coping with risk of mood disorders to children. Soc Sci Med. 2014;104:194–200.
59. Miklowitz DJ, Schneck CD, Singh MK, Taylor DO, George EL, Cosgrove VE, et al. Early intervention for symptomatic youth at risk for bipolar disorder: a randomized trial of family-focused therapy. J Am Acad Child Adolesc Psychiatry. 2013;52(2):121–31.
60. Youngstrom EA, Birmaher B, Findling RL. Pediatric bipolar disorder: validity, phenomenology, and recommendations for diagnosis. Bipolar Disord. 2008;10(1 Pt 2):194–214.
61. Hooley JM, Miklowitz DJ. Perceived criticism in the treatment of a high-risk adolescent. J Clin Psychol. 2017;73(5):570–8.
62. Jones SH, Jovanoska J, Calam R, Wainwright LD, Vincent H, Asar O, et al. Web-based integrated bipolar parenting intervention for parents with bipolar disorder: a randomised controlled pilot trial. J Child Psychol Psychiatry. 2017;58(9):1033–41.
63. Goldstein TR, Merranko J, Krantz M, Garcia M, Franzen P, Levenson J, et al. Early intervention for adolescents at-risk for bipolar disorder: a pilot randomized trial of interpersonal and social rhythm therapy (IPSRT). J Affect Disord. 2018;235:348–56.
64. Findling RL, Youngstrom EA, Rowles BM, Deyling E, Lingler J, Stansbrey RJ, et al. A double-blind and placebo-controlled trial of aripiprazole in symptomatic youths at genetic high risk for bipolar disorder. J Child Adolesc Psychopharmacol. 2017;27(10):864–74.
65. Chang KD, Saxena K, Howe M, Simeonova D. Psychotropic medication exposure and age at onset of bipolar disorder in offspring of parents with bipolar disorder. J Child Adolesc Psychopharmacol. 2010;20(1):25–32.

17 Historical Figures and Bipolar Disorder

Jee Hyun Ha and Sang-Yeol Lee

The definition of a historical figure is somewhat ambiguous. This is because it is necessary to distinguish between celebrities, whose names are widely known to the public, and individuals who have been historically recorded and hold sufficient significance in a particular field to be recognized by future generations. In this regard, distinguishing between historical figures requires careful consideration. The authors have defined and selected as historical figures those individuals who have been repeatedly mentioned in the fields of politics, culture, and art history, and whose names and historical value in their respective fields have been sufficiently verified by the public even after enough time has passed since their deaths. In this chapter, we will introduce figures who are presumed or confirmed to have had bipolar disorder in the political, cultural, and social spheres. We hope that this will help readers understand that bipolar disorder is not only understood from a psychopathological perspective but also as a characteristic of personality and behavior, and that it can be an advantage in achieving historical value from a contextual perspective. The diagnosis and application of bipolar disorder have not been around for very long. Therefore, the presence of bipolar disorder in historical figures can only be inferred based on retrospective interpretation.

Even if a person is an important figure in modern history, it is very rare for them to disclose their mental illness due to its nature and the stigma of revealing mental illness.

The following are what is known so far.

1. Scholars' estimations based on historical figures' behavior, direct documents such as diaries and letters, and observations from those around them.
2. Cases where experiences of psychiatric treatment or hospitalization in modern European asylums were recorded in biographies or autobiographies and published in papers or books.
3. Cases where the individual directly disclosed their condition through interviews or writings can also be included.

The authors will introduce historical figures who are estimated or confirmed to have had bipolar disorder, focusing on what is currently known.

Social and Political Sphere

King George III of England (1738–1820) was controversial during his reign due to his strange behavior. He was easily excitable and hyperactive, like bipolar disorder. Some have interpreted

J. H. Ha
Department of Psychiatry, Konkuk University Medical Center, Seoul, Republic of Korea

S.-Y. Lee (✉)
Department of Psychiatry, Wonkwang University Hospital, School of Medicine, Wonkwang University, Iksan, Republic of Korea
e-mail: psysangyeol@hanmail.net

W.-M. Bahk et al. (eds.), *Bipolar Disorder*, https://doi.org/10.1007/978-981-92-1323-8_17

his behavior as symptoms of acute porphyria, a condition he suffered from, or because of arsenic poisoning from the treatment he received. A recent study analyzed all the letters written by King George during his 60-year reign using a computer program to examine sentence structure, style, and linguistic characteristics, revealing significant differences between stable periods and acute manic episodes [1].

William Tecumseh Sherman (1820–1891), a Union general during the American Civil war, graduated near the top of his class at the United States Military Academy, but immediately left the army to start a business, which failed, leaving him heavily in debt and in a state of depression for a long time. He returned to the military and became the commander of a newly established military academy, participating in the Civil War. Leading the Union Army, he adopted an unconventional strategy of penetrating deep into Confederate-occupied territory, looting and destroying civilian property, which proved highly successful. During the war, he remained extremely sensitive, energetic, and in a heightened state of excitement. He is often referred to as the founder of modern warfare, having introduced the concept of total war. When the Civil War was at a stalemate, General Sherman used his manic creativity to create new problems and solve old ones, and a study of Sherman's life found numerous signs of bipolar disorder [2, 3].

Winston Churchill (1874–1965) was a British politician who served as Prime Minister toward the end of World War II. He experienced distinct and severe depressive episodes in his early 20s, mid-30s when he was Home Secretary, and twice in his 40s and 50s. He referred to those periods as "black dogs." Depressive episode, he experienced around the age of 35, lasted for 2–3 years. However, after recovering from depression, he became a lively, temperamental, and aggressive person. He was extremely sociable and extroverted, with quick thoughts and actions, and completed many books, leaving behind 72 works in his lifetime. US President Roosevelt is reported to have quipped that Churchill generated "a hundred ideas a day, of which at least four were good." By today's diagnostic standards, this would be close to a diagnosis of bipolar disorder type II.

Franklin Delano Roosevelt (1882–1945) was the 32nd president of the United States. He was always energetic, sociable, outgoing, and a talkative person. During his 13 years in office, he traveled by train 399 times and held press conferences twice a week in front of about 100 reporters, for a total of 1000 press conferences. He was always open-minded, curious, and humorous. Rather than being diagnosed with bipolar disorder, he is presumed to have had a manic temperament.

After contracting polio at the age of 39 and becoming disabled in his lower body, his empathy strengthened, and he became more mature.

Adolf Hitler (1889–1945) was a German politician who established the Nazi regime and initiated World War II. Emotional instability was observed in his family, including his father, indicating a familial predisposition. His friend August Kubizek noted that during his late teens to early twenties, there was a marked difference between periods of intense enthusiasm and activity and periods of inactivity. He would walk for hours, and once an idea came to mind, he would become engrossed in it, forgetting about time, sleep, and hunger. When his mood was elevated, he would talk about politics nonstop for hours and preach grandiose social reforms. On the other hand, when he was depressed, he slept a lot, ate alone, and had difficulty concentrating. Overall, grandiose thinking and excessive thoughts were frequently observed, and his impulsive nature was evident in his words, writings, and recorded films. Until he seized power in 1937, these tendencies were expressed and perceived as charisma and political creativity. Many scholars have diagnosed his mental pathology, with bipolar disorder and psychosis caused by amphetamine use frequently mentioned. His grandiose thinking and manic tendencies are additionally interpreted as having been exacerbated by amphetamine use, leading to impaired reality testing [3].

In Korea, there has been research on Prince Sado (1735–1762) of the Chosun Dynasty. After he was imprisoned in a rice chest by his father, King Yeongjo, and starved to death, his wife,

Lady Hyeongyeong, wrote a book titled "Hanjungnok" (Records of Leisure), which was analyzed to examine Prince Sado's mental pathology. In addition, the family tree of the Lee Dynasty of the Choseon Dynasty was analyzed to examine the family history of mental symptoms. As a result, behavioral and emotional changes were observed that are estimated to be depressive episodes accompanied by depressed mood and suicidal thoughts at the ages of 20 and 21, and manic episodes accompanied by irritability, elevated mood, and violent behavior in the summers of 21 and 22. Manic episodes recurred at ages 25–26, and it is estimated that psychotic symptoms such as auditory hallucinations were present at this time. Manic episodes accompanied by psychosis persisted until his death at age 27, and it appears that this was related to his death [4].

Arts and Culture

Music

Ludwig von Beethoven (1770–1827) experienced rapid mood swings, instability, and alcohol problems. He lived in isolation, including hearing loss, and suffered from persistent depression and a negative attitude toward the world. On the contrary, his confidence in his ability has been described by biographers as nearly delusional.

Despite his rapid mood swings accompanied by depression and suicidal thoughts, as well as his overall depressive mood, there is a view that he had bipolar disorder, considering factors such as the seven-year-long paranoid legal battle over custody of his nephew [5].

Italian composer Gioacchino Rossini (1792–1868) composed 39 operas by the age of 37. However, he suddenly stopped composing operas and did not release any more works for 40 years. An analysis of his biography suggests that severe symptoms of depression may have influenced this change. On the other hand, there is ample evidence to suggest that his behavior during his teenage years was indicative of manic episodes or a manic personality, and that such tendencies influenced his ability to compose many pieces in a short period during his youth. Considering these points, it can be inferred that he may have had bipolar disorder.

Robert Schumann (1810–1856) was a German composer who suffered from depression in his twenties, during which time he exhibited behavioral and emotional changes consistent with mania. During a depressive episode, he exhibited severe symptoms, including auditory hallucinations. His bipolar disorder was also evaluated based on his creative output. While he completed no more than five works per year during depressive episodes or when in a normal mood, he published 24 works in 1840 and 27 works in 1849, several times more than usual. After attempting suicide twice due to severe depression, he died in a mental hospital at the age of 46 in 1856. One of his sons also received treatment in a mental hospital for 30 years [6].

Among modern composers, there is Malcolm Arnold (1921–2006). He was known to have severe mood swings. He is famous for composing the music for the film "The Bridge on the River Kwai," which he completed in just 10 days. He is known to have been hospitalized in 1978 for bipolar disorder and alcohol problems and to have received treatment thereafter.

Literature

British poets William Blake (1757–1827) and George Gordon Byron (1788 1824) are believed to have had bipolar disorder. Alfred Tennyson (1809–1892) had a family history of mental illness, including bipolar disorder, among his father, grandfather, and siblings, and he was hospitalized in a mental institution until his death from mania.

British novelist Charles Dickens (1812–1870) suffered from periodic bouts of severe depression, during which he was unable to finish the works he was writing. In contrast, when he was active, he completed many works in a short period of time, showing a marked difference. This contrast between his work and daily activities suggests that he had bipolar disorder.

German philosopher Friedrich Nietzsche (1844–1900) is reported to have experienced grandiose delusions, including statements such as referring to himself as "a god in human form." He exhibited repeated episodes of possible mania, which reportedly led to several periods of institutional psychiatric care. Many studies suggest that he may have had bipolar disorder, while others believe that he suffered from neurosyphilis and the resulting symptoms of dementia.

Virginal Wolf (1882–1941) is known to have suffered from severe depression, though some view it as bipolar disorder. When she experienced severe depressive symptoms, she exhibited psychotic symptoms accompanied by auditory hallucinations, and she had mood instability. The fact that she exhibited depressive symptoms at an early age, around 13, after her mother's death, and attempted suicide in 1904 after her father's death, suggests bipolar disorder. She disappeared during a walk in 1941 and was later determined to have died by suicide.

American poet Ezra Pound (1885–1972) was arrested by the US military in Italy during World War II due to his anti-American and anti-Semitic broadcasts. He was later declared mentally unfit to stand trial and was confined to St. Elizabeth's Hospital in Washington, D.C., for 12 years. At the time, he reportedly exhibited delusions of grandeur and espoused ideas about constructing an ideal society. While his political activities were the primary cause of his detention, some scholars have speculated that his impulsivity, expansive thinking, hyperactivity, and tumultuous personal life may be indicative of bipolar disorder.

American novelist Ernest Hemingway (1899–1961) had a father who committed suicide, several brothers who also committed suicide, and a niece and model, Margaux Hemingway, who suffered from depression and bulimia before committing suicide. This significant family history is further highlighted by the fact that his youngest son, Gregory, was diagnosed with bipolar disorder and underwent treatment. His biographies repeatedly report that he had bipolar disorder, alcohol dependence, and head injuries, and that he exhibited borderline or narcissistic personality traits.

Hemingway's first wife, Hadley Richardson, reportedly described his mood swings as "soaring to the heavens" and appearing "ready to explode," reflecting the emotional intensity he often exhibited.

In 1924, he demonstrated prolific creativity by writing seven short stories in a single year. Biographical accounts describe him as experiencing intense mental activity and restlessness during such times, once noting that his "brain [got] to racing like a flywheel" when deeply engaged in writing.

This suggests he was in a state close to a manic episode. In the 1960s, he developed severe depressive symptoms accompanied by delusions of persecution and uncontrollable alcohol problems, eventually leading him to seek treatment. He underwent electroconvulsive therapy at the Mayo Clinic in the United States and later committed suicide after being discharged [7–9].

Sylvia Plath (1932–1963) began experiencing depression at the age of 20 and underwent multiple electroconvulsive therapy sessions, insulin coma therapy, and psychotherapy. She ultimately ended her life by suicide. Some believe she may have had bipolar II disorder, but recent research has shown that, based on detailed case analysis and modern diagnostic criteria, it is more reasonable to conclude that she had major depressive disorder with psychotic symptoms and borderline personality disorder.

Art

Spanish painter Francis Goya (1746–1828) experienced sudden hearing loss, headaches, and paralysis at the age of 46, followed by symptoms such as depression, auditory hallucinations, and confusion. Following this, he became reclusive and depressed, cohabited with a maid, fathered an illegitimate child, and painted extremely grotesque pictures, leading to the assumption that he had bipolar disorder.

Dutch painter Vincent Van Gogh (1853–1890) showed a marked difference in his artistic output between periods when he was suspected of having depression and periods when he appeared to be manic. During depressive episodes, his productivity declined significantly. He ultimately died by suicide at the age of 37. Various hypotheses have been proposed regarding his mental condition, including lead poisoning, neurosyphilis, Ménière's disease, absinthe intoxication, and temporal lobe epilepsy. However, the likelihood of an underlying bipolar disorder remains high [10].

Norwegian painter Edvard Munch (1863–1944) experienced the deaths of his mother and sister at a young age, and later suffered from severe depression, which led to his hospitalization in a psychiatric facility in Copenhagen. At the time, he complained of agoraphobia, paranoia, and depression. Some researchers have interpreted his childhood experiences of loss and fear, along with his inner depression, as unconscious motivations for his creativity. Based on his repetitive mood fluctuations and severe depressive episodes, it has been suggested that he may have had bipolar disorder [11].

American modern artist Jackson Pollock (1912–1956) is known to have led a highly impulsive and spontaneous life, as reflected in his paintings. He was described as having a capricious personality and struggling with alcoholism for much of his life. Although he reportedly underwent psychoanalysis for 3 years in his mid-twenties, many researchers believe that he may have had bipolar disorder.

Summary

We have examined historical figures who are believed to have suffered from bipolar disorder. While many were creative artists, the literature also highlights political and social figures. Since it is often impossible to verify medical diagnoses for historical figures, our understanding is necessarily limited to careful inferences based on various documents and accounts. This suggests that although bipolar disorder is a mental illness, some individuals with the condition have made remarkable contributions in various fields. Understanding this dual aspect is important in appreciating both the challenges and the potential associated with the disorder.

Declarations

Competing Interests The author(s) has no competing interests to declare that are relevant to the content of this manuscript.

Ethics Approval The author(s) declares that this manuscript does not include primary research with human participants.

The author(s) declares that this manuscript does not include primary studies involving animals.

References

1. Rentoumi V, Peters T, Conlin J, Garrard P. The acute mania of King George III: a computational linguistic analysis. PLoS ONE. 2017;12(3):e0171626.
2. Fellman M. The making of Rober E Lee. Baltimore: Johns Hopkins University Press; 2003.
3. Gaemi N. A first-rate madness. London: Penguin Press; 2011.
4. Jeong HE, Kim CY. A psychiatric approach to Prince Sado: a bipolar disorder sufferer or a victim of party strife. J Korean Neuropsychiatr Assoc. 2014;53(5):299–309.
5. Mai FM. Diagnosing genius: the life and death of beethoven. Montreal: Mcguill-Queens University Press; 2007.
6. Jamison KR. Manic-depressive illness and creativity. Sci Am. 1995;272(2):62–7.
7. Janka Z. Artistic creativity and bipolar mood disorder. Orv Hetil. 2004;145(33):1709–18.
8. Cooper C. Sylvia Plath and the depression continuum. J R Soc Med. 2003;96(6):296–301.
9. Martin C. Ernest hemingway: a psychological autopsy of a suicide. Psychiatry. 2006;69(4):351–61.
10. Perry IH. Vincent van Gogh's illness: a case record. Bull Hist Med. 1967;21:146–72.
11. Rothenberg A. Bipolar illness, creativity, and treatment. Psych Q. 2001;72(2):131–47.

Bipolar Disorder and Creativity

18

Won Kim and Young Joon Kwon

Mental Illness and Creativity

Since ancient times, humans have developed culture as a means to adapt to nature. Cultural archetypes first emerged in early religious systems responding to natural or divine forces, and the evolution of culture has paralleled the development of the human mind and way of life. Within early religious and cultural systems, human madness occupied a significant position. Madness was viewed as an extraordinary condition manifesting in certain individuals at particular times, serving as a medium between the divine/nature and the human community. Those considered to be mad—close to the divine or nature—were perceived as possessing unique, mysterious, imaginative, and sometimes fear-inducing characteristics. The long-standing notion of madness was strongly linked to the concept of genius during the Romantic period in the late eighteenth century, thereby reinforcing the association between madness and creativity. The concept of creativity is not as ancient as that of madness. It originates from the fundamental notion of divine creation—bringing something out of nothing—but has recently been reinterpreted in the context of modern ideas such as the realization of novel ideas and imagination. Creativity is also attracting growing attention as a potential for human flourishing and a guide for life's purposes. Creativity and madness have long been meaningful in human life, and vague narratives about their connection have always existed. However, scientific investigations into the relationship between creativity and madness remain limited, making it difficult to form an accurate and comprehensive understanding.

Since the modern era, madness has been redefined as mental illness, and there remains considerable interest in the relationship between creativity and psychopathology. It is quite common to speculate on the possibility of mental illness in historical figures and artists. Among the various psychiatric disorders presumed to be associated with creativity, bipolar disorder is the most frequently mentioned. This prominence is due to the mood fluctuations and dramatic behaviors characteristic of bipolar disorder, which are often linked to conventional notions of creativity. Moreover, numerous historical figures have exhibited behavioral patterns suggestive of bipolar disorder, lending further support to this association. As a result, despite numerous methodological challenges, the body of research on the relationship between bipolar disorder and creativity is relatively substantial compared to other psychiatric disorders, and includes a

W. Kim (✉)
Department of Psychiatry, Inje University Sanggye Paik Hospital, College of Medicine, Inje University, Seoul, Republic of Korea
e-mail: phrenie@naver.com

Y. J. Kwon
Department of Psychiatry, Soonchunhyang University Cheonan Hospital, College of Medicine, Soonchunhyang University, Cheonan, Republic of Korea

W.-M. Bahk et al. (eds.), *Bipolar Disorder*, https://doi.org/10.1007/978-981-92-1323-8_18

number of distinguished scholarly contributions [1]. This chapter aims to provide an overview of the existing research and discussions concerning the association between creativity and mental illness, with a particular focus on bipolar disorder.

What Is Creativity?

Although the Merriam-Webster Learner's Dictionary defines creativity simply as "the ability to make new things or think of new ideas," recent discussions in psychology and business studies have approached it more extensively in the context of human capacity development. Nevertheless, the essence of creativity remains elusive, and no standardized definition of creativity as a psychological trait has yet been established. Instead, numerous scholars have engaged in exploring the various components and dimensions that constitute creativity. Ludwig [2] identified three dimensions of creativity: the creative person, the creative process, and the creative product. Drevdahl and Cattell [3] described creative individuals as possessing intelligence, adventurousness, revolutionary thinking, and strong ego strength, while also being emotionally sensitive. Andreasen and Glick [4] later added introspectiveness and independence as further traits contributing to creativity, noting that a tangible product is ultimately required as the basis for establishing creativity. Post [5] characterized highly creative and renowned individuals as those endowed with exceptional talent, meticulousness, and persistence.

In truth, creativity is not easily distinguished from other capacities. It overlaps significantly with intelligence, innate ability, and genius. McKinnon [6] made a distinction between intelligence and creativity, arguing that while intelligence is generally a prerequisite for creativity, not all intelligent individuals are necessarily creative. Recent research on creativity has employed a variety of tools for its assessment. Some studies have used creativity scales or intelligence tests, while others have relied on academic achievement or social recognition as proxies for creativity. Clearly, however, such measures alone cannot fully capture the essence of creativity. The Lifetime Creativity Scale, which offers one of the more comprehensive operational definitions, gives higher scores to individuals who demonstrate original and extraordinary capabilities, particularly among those who have gained public recognition [7]. Yet even this scale faces limitations, as social and political influences often determine societal recognition, making it an imprecise criterion.

Mental illness, too, is a concept that resists precise definition. Nevertheless, practical definitions have been established in major diagnostic systems such as the Diagnostic and Statistical Manual of Mental Disorders (DSM) of the American Psychiatric Association, and the International Classification of Diseases (ICD) of the World Health Organization. The DSM defines mental disorder as a clinically significant behavioral or psychological syndrome that is associated with distress, disability in social or occupational functioning, or a loss of freedom. Similarly, the ICD characterizes it as a combination of symptoms or behaviors that are associated with personal distress or impairment in functioning. Both systems, therefore, adopt operational definitions that conceptualize mental illness as a constellation of symptoms linked to some form of functional impairment.

Historical Evolution of the Concept

Eccentric behaviors among artists have long been recognized, and the association between human madness and creativity has a long-standing conceptual history. In mythology, references can be found to the divine madness of the Muses, the goddesses of art. In ancient Greece, Socrates and Plato regarded madness as a state in which thought and emotion were profoundly altered, while Aristotle wrote about the relationship between melancholy, madness, and inspiration. During the Middle Ages, narrow and predominantly negative views of madness prevailed. However, the Renaissance revived interest in the connections among genius, madness, and melancholia.

The concepts of creativity and mental illness underwent dramatic shifts across different historical periods. In the eighteenth century, the Age of Reason emphasized the idea that rational thought was essential to genius. By contrast, in the nineteenth century, Romanticism came to dominate, positing that extreme emotional experiences and mental states were central to artistic inspiration and expression. Toward the late nineteenth century, the radical romantic view began to wane, and the emerging disciplines of psychology and psychiatry initiated more scholarly inquiries into the relationship between genius and madness. William James, a prominent philosopher and psychologist known to have suffered from severe depression, and Emil Kraepelin, often regarded as the father of modern psychiatry, both noted that while severe forms of manic-depressive illness could cause significant suffering and impairment, milder mood fluctuations might have beneficial aspects.

Thus, the loosely defined connection between madness and creativity, oscillating between Enlightenment rationalism and Romantic emotionalism throughout the modern period, has now reached a stage where scholarly research and a more balanced perspective are needed. While earlier discussions on psychopathology associated with creativity focused primarily on schizophrenia and depression, since the 1970s—driven by more structured research and advances in understanding bipolar disorder—bipolar disorder has increasingly been recognized as the psychiatric condition most prominently linked to creativity [1].

Renowned Artists Who Are Presumed to Have Suffered from Bipolar Disorder

There is a wealth of anecdotal evidence suggesting that many renowned artists experienced psychiatric illnesses or spent significant portions of their lives in mental institutions. Among writers alone, numerous figures—such as William Faulkner, F. Scott Fitzgerald, Ernest Hemingway, Eugene O'Neill, Virginia Woolf, and Tennessee Williams—are known to have had histories of psychiatric hospitalization. Although it is difficult to retrospectively diagnose deceased artists due to the lack of objective documentation and changes in diagnostic criteria over time, several individuals—such as Virginia Woolf, Robert Schumann, Lord Byron, and Vincent van Gogh—are widely regarded as having almost certainly suffered from bipolar disorder. Their lives and works have sparked continued interest in the potential association between bipolar disorder and creativity.

Virginia Woolf, a central figure of twentieth-century British modernism and the originator of the stream-of-consciousness novel, is known to have experienced severe mood fluctuations and episodes of psychosis throughout her life. Her vivid depictions of sleepless nights and her descriptions of navigating emotional extremes are now understood by many scholars as clear indicators of bipolar disorder. Woolf ultimately died by suicide at the age of 59, drowning herself in a river. Robert Schumann, one of the leading composers of the Romantic era, reportedly experienced unstable emotional states beginning in his twenties. By his thirties, he alternated between periods of intense creative productivity and episodes of profound depression. In his forties, he attempted suicide by throwing himself into the Rhine River. Though he survived, he was subsequently institutionalized and died in the mental hospital. Lord Byron, a quintessential Romantic poet, was similarly known for intense emotional volatility, marked by profound melancholy and passionate outbursts. The case of Vincent van Gogh, who famously mutilated his own ear during a state of extreme emotional distress, is often cited as a paradigmatic example of the dramatic behavior associated with artistic temperament.

These cases have served to reinforce the longstanding, romanticized notion of a mysterious link between madness and creativity. For many years, this theme has captivated public imagination. However, with the advancement of psychiatry and psychology, such ambiguous ideas have gradually begun to take on more precise form. As emotion and creative potential are essential to understanding human nature, interest in this topic continues to persist despite the inherent difficulties of empirical investigation.

Studies on the Association Between Bipolar Disorder and Creativity

The empirical study of creativity and psychopathology represents an attempt to recast the ancient question of "madness and genius" in scientific terms. From Plato's notion of divine inspiration to Romantic conceptions of suffering as the source of art, this association has long attracted philosophical reflection. Modern psychiatry and psychology have sought to translate these intuitions into testable hypotheses, examining whether creative achievement and bipolar vulnerability share common temperamental, cognitive, or neurobiological features.

Despite these efforts, the number of methodologically rigorous studies remains relatively small, and their findings are often inconsistent. Investigating this relationship poses inherent challenges: creativity itself is difficult to define and measure, psychiatric diagnoses change over time, and historical materials are often incomplete. Nonetheless, the available literature—though limited—offers valuable insights, as outlined in the following sections according to their principal methodological approaches.

Biographical Studies of Eminent Figures

Analyses of the lives of historically significant individuals have long been a source of speculation regarding the role of extreme affective states—such as mania and depression—in shaping their achievements. These biographical studies can highlight patterns of behavior and emotional fluctuation, but they also carry unavoidable limitations. Accounts are filtered through the perspectives of authors, constrained by the materials available—letters, diaries, memoirs—and influenced by the cultural attitudes prevailing at the time of writing. For example, during eras dominated by Romantic ideals, public and scholarly narratives often embraced the notion that artists were naturally prone to melancholy or psychological turmoil, making detached assessment especially difficult. Diagnostic interpretation adds another layer of complexity. In the early and mid-twentieth century, psychiatric attention to bipolar disorder focused primarily on manic episodes, with depressive phases receiving comparatively less emphasis. Psychotic features, such as hallucinations, often led to an initial misdiagnosis of schizophrenia. Only more recently have clinical definitions broadened to encompass the full range of bipolar presentations, allowing for more systematic retrospective analysis of historical figures.

The tradition of examining mental illness among celebrated creators dates back to the late nineteenth and early twentieth centuries. Early commentators often asserted that artistic genius was frequently accompanied by mood instability, and that psychiatric symptoms were common among family members as well. One widely cited observation suggested that, among eminent individuals, painters and poets showed higher rates of psychiatric disturbance than scientists or politicians [8]. By the latter half of the twentieth century, more structured inquiries appeared. A German study of 113 artists and their relatives revealed that about one-third met criteria for psychiatric disorder, a rate notably higher than that of the general population. Poets showed the highest prevalence (50%), followed by musicians (38%), painters (18%), and architects (17%). Family histories often included cyclothymia, suicide, and bipolar disorder [9]. Although methodological constraints—such as reliance on retrospective accounts—limit the certainty of these findings, the general pattern across studies suggests that eminent artists, compared with other occupational groups, have elevated rates of psychiatric hospitalization, psychotic symptoms, and suicide.

Several biographical investigations have specifically targeted mood disorders. In a systematic review of 36 distinguished English-speaking poets, Jamison [10] reported that 17% had been hospitalized for psychiatric illness, 22% experienced psychotic symptoms, and 6% had died by suicide—figures well above population norms.

Structured Interview Research in Artists

From the 1970s onward, researchers began supplementing biographical evidence with direct interviews of living artists and matched control participants. These studies, using standardized diagnostic tools, have been able to capture more objective data on lifetime mood patterns, co-occurring disorders, and creative output. In one early study, Andreasen and Canter [11] assessed 30 writers and found that 80% met lifetime criteria for a mood disorder—major depressive disorder in 37%, bipolar I disorder in 13%, and bipolar II disorder in 30%. In contrast, only 30% of the control group met criteria for any mood disorder. Rates of alcohol dependence were also elevated among the writers. Similarly, Ludwig [2] examined 59 female writers and an equal number of female controls, applying DSM-III-R criteria alongside the Lifetime Creativity Scale. The writers met diagnostic thresholds for depression or mania far more often than controls and reported suicide attempts at five times the control rate. Other conditions—panic attacks, substance abuse, and eating disorders—were also significantly more common in the creative group.

Jamison [10], studying 47 highly acclaimed poets, playwrights, novelists, and visual artists, found that 38% had been treated for a mood disorder, and over 70% of those treated had received pharmacotherapy with antidepressants or lithium, or had been hospitalized. Poets displayed the highest rates of psychopathology: one-third had received treatment for depression, and 17% had been treated or hospitalized for mania. Interestingly, systematic inquiry into hypomania was difficult, meaning that the prevalence of bipolar disorder may have been underestimated. Her data revealed genre-specific patterns. Novelists and poets most often reported episodes of mood elevation; playwrights and visual artists more frequently reported severe mood fluctuations; biographers reported virtually no mood changes, resembling the general population. This is notable given that biographers often produce substantial written output but are not typically considered as creatively expressive as poets or novelists. An additional dimension of Jamison's work examined "periods of heightened creativity" as reported by the participants. Nearly 90% of the artists described such episodes, often lasting about 2 weeks, characterized by increased energy, self-confidence, rapid associative thinking, and elevated mood—features reminiscent of hypomania. However, behaviors such as excessive spending, sexual activity, or pressured speech were rare, suggesting that these creative highs might represent milder, more focused versions of hypomanic states. Whether these are qualitatively distinct from hypomania or simply lower-intensity manifestations remains an open question. Seasonal variation also emerged as a relevant factor. Over a 36-month observation period, treated artists tended to show mood elevation in summer but with a corresponding decline in productivity, whereas untreated artists' creative output often rose in parallel with mood elevation. Jamison offered two interpretations: artists whose elevated mood is linked to high productivity may be less likely to seek treatment, and conversely, when mood elevation represents true hypomania, it may actually disrupt sustained creative work. Andreasen [11] similarly observed that, in some writers, hypomanic energy was unfocused, dissipating into social or personal activities rather than creative projects.

Studies on Creativity in the General Population and Analyses of National Registry Data

While the above studies center on exceptional creative achievement, creativity is by no means confined to elite artistic circles. Understanding its distribution and determinants in the general population is important for both science and public policy. Larger samples can be recruited, but measurement remains a challenge: creativity is multidimensional, and standard psychometric tools may not capture its full scope.

Two influential studies from the 1980s found that individuals with cyclothymia scored higher on creativity measures than control participants, and that relatives of patients with bipolar disorder also scored above controls [12, 13]. In contrast, individuals with bipolar I disorder did not exhibit higher creativity scores, suggesting that functional preservation may be necessary for any mood-related creative advantage to manifest.

Large-scale registry studies from Sweden, conducted by Kyaga and colleagues [14], have provided population-level evidence. In one analysis of 300,000 individuals diagnosed with schizophrenia, bipolar disorder, or major depressive disorder—along with their relatives—bipolar patients and relatives of patients with schizophrenia or bipolar disorder were more likely to work in creative professions. Schizophrenia patients were not overrepresented in creative occupations overall but were more prevalent in arts-specific roles. No increased likelihood was seen for major depression patients or their relatives. In a subsequent study extending to all psychiatric diagnoses, Kyaga's team examined over 1.17 million patients identified over a 40-year period, plus their families. Only bipolar disorder was associated with a generally higher probability of employment in creative occupations. However, when focusing specifically on the profession of writing, significant associations emerged with bipolar disorder, schizophrenia, major depression, anxiety disorders, substance abuse, and suicide. Moreover, certain familial links were notable: first-degree relatives of patients with schizophrenia, bipolar disorder, or anorexia nervosa, and siblings of individuals with autism spectrum disorder, were more likely to work in creative fields [15].

Hypotheses on the Relationship Between Creativity and Bipolar Disorder

Creativity as a Manifestation of Illness Features

A substantial number of artists and writers recount their most prolific periods as being marked by elevated, expansive, and even euphoric moods—states closely paralleling hypomania. These phases often coincide with accelerated thought processes and increased fluency in expression, both hallmark features of hypomania. The acceleration of thinking is accompanied by a proliferation of associative links, which can also alter the quality of thought. Guilford [16] described creative thinking as involving multiple components, particularly fluency, spontaneous flexibility, and adaptive flexibility. Other investigators have observed that manic states—unlike both schizophrenia and normal mental states—often produce a distinctive form of "combinatory thinking," in which sensory impressions, concepts, and imagery are freely merged. Andreasen and Glick [4] similarly found that individuals in manic states tend to merge disparate elements into single, ambiguous constructs more readily than those with schizophrenia.

In word association experiments, individuals in a manic phase generated roughly triple the number of unusual associations compared with their euthymic periods, while their production of conventional responses dropped to about one-third. Furthermore, the extent of change in their associative patterns was positively related to the severity of manic symptoms [17]. Some reports indicate that hypomania can raise performance scores on the Wechsler Adult Intelligence Scale [18] and may enhance certain creative problem-solving abilities [19]. In many accounts—both autobiographical and empirical—creative surges align with mood elevation, while depressive episodes tend to suppress output. Consequently, the cognitive profile of hypomania—rapid ideation, fluency, and openness to novel connections—

bears considerable resemblance to the mental states associated with creative work. Nonetheless, creativity is not automatically conferred by cognitive acceleration alone; individuals without imaginative capacity will not become creative simply through heightened thought speed, and in those who are creative, severe mania can derail productivity through disorganized or incoherent thinking.

Temperament or Personality Traits Linked to Both Creativity and Bipolar Disorder

A parallel line of inquiry considers temperament or personality traits that might bridge creativity and bipolarity. Persistent themes in studies of accomplished creators include perseverance, self-confidence, willingness to take risks, independence, and a sense of abundance—traits reminiscent of hypomanic or cyclothymic temperament. Some research emphasizes two particularly relevant attributes: fluency of thought and disinhibition, the latter defined as receptivity to a wide array of environmental stimuli. Supporting this, a study of Harvard University students found that those identified as highly creative scored significantly lower on measures of inhibition than their less creative peers [20]. The authors proposed that a combination of high cognitive flexibility and low inhibitory control might, in extreme cases, result either in psychiatric disturbance or in exceptional creative output.

Work from a research team at Stanford University School of Medicine has provided empirical support for this overlap. They reported that both individuals with bipolar disorder and creative controls outperformed non-creative controls on creativity assessments, and that the temperamental profiles of the first two groups were strikingly similar [21]. Analyses based on the Five-Factor Model of personality identified two dimensions—openness to experience and neuroticism—as being elevated in both bipolar patients and creative individuals [22]. The group suggested that openness might contribute cognitive advantages, while emotional intensity and affective variability could offer an emotional depth conducive to creative work [23].

Creativity Emerging from Illness Experience

Beyond illness features of bipolar disorder and temperament traits, some creators attribute their work directly to the lived experience of mood disorder. They argue that severe emotional hardship can yield profound insights, enriching the thematic and emotional resonance of their art. Intense depressive episodes or other psychiatric crises can fundamentally alter one's worldview, perspectives on existence, and even one's sense of the divine. Numerous authors have documented in detail the suffering and transformation brought by prolonged depression, describing both coping strategies and the translation of these experiences into their work.

Notably, poets Anne Sexton and John Berryman—both Pulitzer Prize winners, recurrently hospitalized for bipolar disorder, and ultimately lost to suicide—considered psychological suffering to be integral to their creativity, cautioning against efforts to avoid such pain. Hypomanic phases, in contrast, may propel artists toward heightened social interaction, sometimes fostering relationships that, whether constructive or destructive, shift their creative perspectives. Subsequent milder depressive episodes can provide a period of reflection, enabling critical reassessment of the ideas and experiences generated during mood elevation.

Field-Specific Variations in the Creativity–Bipolar Link

The influence of bipolar disorder on creativity appears to vary markedly across professional and artistic fields. Epidemiological studies indicate that poets are overrepresented among those with bipolar disorder, whereas scientists show comparatively lower prevalence. For poetry, the benefits of heightened emotion, energy, cognitive agility, and enriched experience may outweigh the disadvantages of disrupted work patterns. Conversely, in scientific disciplines, the instability associated with bipolar disorder can be more detrimental than advantageous. Occupational demands likely play a role: poets and composers may achieve recognition without formal qualifications or continuous employment, while careers in law or medicine require sustained performance over many years, a challenge for those with substantial mood variability. Even within the literary arts, genre matters. Novelists, whose craft demands extended structural coherence, may find mood swings disruptive, whereas poets—whose work often depends on imagery, rhythm, and concentrated bursts of inspiration—may be more able to harness mood elevation. The dream-like, non-linear qualities of poetry also align more closely with certain hypomanic cognitive styles.

The potential advantages and drawbacks of bipolar disorder thus depend heavily on the domain of activity. From a mood perspective, elevated affect, confidence, and emotional intensity can benefit both artistic and entrepreneurial pursuits. Energetic drive and reduced need for sleep can also be useful assets. Cognitively, the rapid, unconventional thinking and heightened sensory acuity seen in hypomania may support innovative work in some artistic or scientific contexts, while in domains such as politics or business, the interpersonal dynamism of hypomania may prove more advantageous than its cognitive effects.

Taken together, these hypotheses delineate a multidimensional framework in which creativity and bipolar disorder intersect across temperamental, cognitive, and contextual levels. Rather than implying a direct causal link, they suggest a complex reciprocity between vulnerability and potential, pathology, and productivity. This conceptual synthesis inevitably invites a practical question: if certain features of bipolarity appear to facilitate creative expression, how should such traits be appraised and managed in clinical and cultural contexts? The following section explores this dilemma, addressing the risks of romanticization and the ethical tension between safeguarding creativity and ensuring mental health.

Can Bipolar Disorder Be Positive for Creativity?

If the notion that bipolar disorder has positive aspects becomes widely accepted, it may negatively affect patients' recognition of the illness and their willingness to adhere to treatment. Many high-achieving individuals with mood disorders are reluctant to seek treatment, and some even wish to re-experience the extremes of mood associated with the disorder. Certain individuals view the symptoms of severe mood disorders as an essential part of the human condition. In particular, some artists regard such suffering as an unavoidable price for possessing artistic temperament and heightened sensitivity. As a result, they may reject psychiatric treatment under the belief that it will extinguish their creativity.

What, then, should a clinician do when an aspiring artist voices such concerns during a consultation? In real clinical settings, can the psychopathology of mania be sharply delineated from an artistic lifestyle? Is it therapeutically helpful to explain an artistic lifestyle solely as psychopathology? If patients are simply told that bipolar disorder has no positive aspects and that they must take medication continuously, they may resist and fail to engage with treatment. Even if mood disorders are illnesses, it may be beneficial to acknowledge that mild mood elevation can, in some cases, have positive and productive aspects. Recognition of such aspects can enhance patients' trust in their clinicians and strengthen the therapeutic relationship.

But does psychiatric treatment actually diminish creativity? Many artists and writers express considerable hesitation and concern regarding psychiatric treatment, particularly pharmacotherapy. They worry that medication will negatively affect their creativity, work patterns, and cognitive abilities. While such beliefs are partly shaped by prejudice and preconception, some studies have produced tentative findings that mood stabilizers may adversely influence productivity or creativity. From early studies of lithium onward, it has been well recognized that, while lithium alleviates the elevated mood of hypomania through its therapeutic effects, it can also reduce energy and libido, and may cause cognitive slowing and memory impairment as side effects. Reports from healthy volunteers taking lithium indicate that it can induce mild generalized fatigue and detachment from one's surroundings, leading to passivity. They also describe a reduced drive for intellectual activity, accompanied by a perceived decline in concentration and memory [24]. Of course, many patients do not report such side effects, and when weighed against the risks of remaining untreated, these side effects are unquestionably minor. However, for individuals who place high value on cognitive function—particularly artists—such effects are far from trivial.

According to artists who have been highly productive during hypomanic states, taking lithium feels like applying the brakes to their creative work. They report diminished creativity and drive, making it impossible to continue their projects, and that during depressive episodes they feel so low that they are unable to work at all [25]. Some, therefore, state a preference for maintaining a cyclothymic state—with mood fluctuations that include occasional periods of elevation—over the stable but mildly depressed mood they experience on lithium. Observational studies of artists with bipolar disorder have reported that, among those taking lithium, approximately three-quarters experienced no change or an improvement in their creative work, whereas about one-quarter reported a decline [26, 27]. This variation suggests that individual responses to lithium differ, likely depending on clinical factors such as the duration and severity of symptoms, personal habits in utilizing hypomanic periods, and individual sensitivity to medication. Ultimately, treatment should aim to maximize the benefits of controlling bipolar disorder while minimizing potential adverse effects on cognitive function and creativity, thereby optimizing therapeutic strategies for each individual.

Conclusion

The association between mood disorders and artistic creativity is supported by a growing body of evidence. Biographical accounts and studies of artists suggest that highly creative individuals may be more likely to experience extreme emotional states and are more frequently affected by mood disorders. Systematic research supporting these observations has also been gradually increasing. However, it is important to recognize that psychiatric symptoms are not, on the whole, highly prevalent among artists. That is, the majority of creative individuals do not suffer from significant psychopathology, and conversely, most people with mood disorders are not exceptionally creative. Caution is warranted when discussing the connection between creativity and mood disorders, particularly bipolar disorder, as highlighting a few notable cases of artists with bipolar illness may lead to unintended consequences. These include the risk of diminishing the value of their creative accomplishments or trivializing a serious psychiatric condition that requires appropriate treatment. Any conclusion regarding this association must take such concerns into account.

It is indeed true that mood disorders—especially bipolar disorder—and associated temperamental traits such as cyclothymia or hyperthymic temperament are linked to creativity. Nevertheless, this relationship is not typically of major clinical or social significance. Bipolar disorder and major depression are undoubtedly serious conditions that cause suffering, functional impairment, and even pose risks to life; therefore, they require proper treatment during acute episodes. During the maintenance phase, carefully tailored treatment plans can help preserve creativity without undermining it. Most available evidence suggests that creativity is not significantly impaired by treatment in the majority of cases. Indeed, many individuals have been able to sustain creative output over longer periods with the help of appropriate treatment. That said, potential side effects of psychotropic medications—particularly those affecting cognitive functions—may occasionally interfere with creativity, and minimizing such effects should be an important goal of treatment planning.

With recent advances in neurobiology, foundational studies on human affect and emotion have gained momentum. Future research is, therefore, needed to further clarify the relationship between creativity and mood, including how cognitive functions change across depressive and manic states, how creative capacities are influenced, and what the neurobiological underpinnings of creativity may be.

Declarations

Competing Interests The author(s) has no competing interests to declare that are relevant to the content of this manuscript.

Ethics Approval The author(s) declares that this manuscript does not include primary research with human participants.

The author(s) declares that this manuscript does not include primary studies involving animals.

References

1. Goodwin FK, Jamison KR. Manic-depressive illness: bipolar disorders and recurrent depression. 2nd ed. New York: Oxford University Press; 2007.
2. Ludwig AM. Reflections on creativity and madness. Am J Psychother. 1989;43(4):4–14.
3. Drevdahl J, Cattell R. Personality and creativity in artists and writers. J Clin Psychol. 1958;14:107–12.
4. Andreasen NC, Glick ID. Bipolar affective disorder and creativity: Implications and clinical management. Compr Psychiatry. 1988;29:207–17.
5. Post F. Creativity and psychopathology: A study of 291 world-famous men. Br J Psychiatry. 1994;165:22–34.
6. McKinnon DW. Personality and the realization of creative potential. Am Psychol. 1965;20:273–81.
7. Richards RL, Kinney DK, Benet M, Merzel AP. Assessing everyday creativity: characteristics of the lifetime creativity scales and validation with three large samples. J Pers Soc Psychol. 1988;54:476–85.
8. Lange-Eichbaum W. The problem of genius. Paul E, Paul C, translators. New York: Macmillan; 1932.
9. Juda A. The relationship between highest mental capacity and psychic abnormalities. Am J Psychiatry. 1949;106:296–307.
10. Jamison KR. Mood disorders and seasonal patterns in British writers and artists. Psychiatry. 1989;52:125–34.
11. Andreasen NC, Canter A. The creative writer: Psychiatric symptoms and family history. Compr Psychiatry. 1974;15:123–31.
12. Richards R, Kinney DK, Lunde I, Benet M, Merzel AP. Creativity in manic-depressives, cyclothymes, their normal relatives, and control subjects. J Abnorm Psychol. 1988;97:281–8.
13. Coryell W, Endicott J, Keller M, Andreasen N, Grove W, Hirschfeld RM, et al. Bipolar affective disorder and high achievement: a familial association. Am J Psychiatry. 1989;146:983–8.
14. Kyaga S, Lichtenstein P, Boman M, Langstrom N, Landen M. Creativity and mental disorder: family study of 300,000 people with severe mental disorder. Br J Psychiatry. 2011;199:373–9.
15. Kyaga S, Landen M, Boman M, Hultman CM, Langstrom N, Lichtenstein P. Mental illness, suicide and creativity: 40-year prospective total population study. J Psychiatr Res. 2013;47:83–90.
16. Guilford JP. A revised structure of intellect: Studies of aptitudes of high-level personnel. Report No. 19. Los Angeles: University of Southern California, Psychological Laboratory; 1967.
17. Henry GM, Weingartner H, Murphy DL. Idiosyncratic patterns of learning and word association during mania. Am J Psychiatry. 1971;128:564–74.
18. Donnelly EF, Murphy DL, Goodwin FK, Waldman IN. Intellectual function in primary affective disorder. Br J Psychiatry. 1982;140:633–6.
19. Isen AM, Johnson MS, Mertz E, Robinson GF. The influence of positive affect on the unusualness of word associations. J Pers Soc Psychol. 1985;48:1413–26.
20. Carson SH, Peterson JB, Higgins DM. Decreased latent inhibition is associated with increased creative achievement in high-functioning individuals. J Pers Soc Psychol. 2003;85:499–506.
21. Nowakowska C, Strong CM, Santosa CM, Wang PW, Ketter TA. Temperamental commonalities and differences in euthymic mood disorder patients, creative controls, and healthy controls. J Affect Disord. 2005;85:207–15.
22. Strong CM, Nowakowska C, Santosa CM, Wang PW, Kraemer HC, Ketter TA. Treatment-creativity relationships in mood disorder patients, healthy controls and highly creative individuals. J Affect Disord. 2007;100:41–8.
23. Srivastava S, Childer ME, Baek JH, Strong CM, Hill SJ, Warsett KS, et al. Toward interaction of affective and cognitive contributors to creativity in bipo-

lar disorders: A controlled study. J Affect Disord. 2010;125:27–34.
24. Schou M. Lithium in psychiatric therapy and prophylaxis. J Psychiatr Res. 1968;6:67–95.
25. Polatin P, Fieve RR. Patient rejection of lithium carbonate prophylaxis. JAMA. 1971;218:864–6.
26. Marshall MH, Neumann CP, Robinson M. Lithium, creativity, and manic-depressive illness: review and prospectus. Psychosomatics. 1970;11:406–8.
27. Schou M. Artistic productivity and lithium prophylaxis in manic-depressive illness. Br J Psychiatry. 1979;135:97–103.

GPSR Compliance

The European Union's (EU) General Product Safety Regulation (GPSR) is a set of rules that requires consumer products to be safe and our obligations to ensure this.

If you have any concerns about our products, you can contact us on ProductSafety@springernature.com

In case Publisher is established outside the EU, the EU authorized representative is:

Springer Nature Customer Service Center GmbH
Europaplatz 3
69115 Heidelberg, Germany

Batch number: 10731395

Printed by Printforce, the Netherlands